GENETICS OF AUTOIMMUNITY

The Novartis Foundation is an international scientific and educational charity (UK Registered Charity No. 313574). Known until September 1997 as the Ciba Foundation, it was established in 1947 by the CIBA company of Basle, which merged with Sandoz in 1996, to form Novartis. The Foundation operates independently in London under English trust law. It was formally opened on 22 June 1949.

The Foundation promotes the study and general knowledge of science and in particular encourages international co-operation in scientific research. To this end, it organizes internationally acclaimed meetings (typically eight symposia and allied open meetings and 15–20 discussion meetings each year) and publishes eight books per year featuring the presented papers and discussions from the symposia. Although primarily an operational rather than a grant-making foundation, it awards bursaries to young scientists to attend the symposia and afterwards work with one of the other participants.

The Foundation's headquarters at 41 Portland Place, London W1B 1BN, provide library facilities, open to graduates in science and allied disciplines. Media relations are fostered by regular press conferences and by articles prepared by the Foundation's Science Writer in Residence. The Foundation offers accommodation and meeting facilities to visiting scientists and their societies.

Information on all Foundation activities can be found at http://www.novartisfound.org.uk

Novartis Foundation Symposium 267

GENETICS OF AUTOIMMUNITY

2005

John Wiley & Sons, Ltd

Copyright © Novartis Foundation 2005
Published in 2005 by John Wiley & Sons Ltd,
The Atrium, Southern Gate,
Chichester PO19 8SQ, UK

National   01243 779777
International (+44) 1243 779777
e-mail (for orders and customer service enquiries): cs-books@wiley.co.uk
Visit our Home Page on http://www.wileyeurope.com
or http://www.wiley.com

All Rights Reserved. No part of this book may be reproduced, stored in a retrieval system or transmitted in any form or by any means, electronic, mechanical, photocopying, recording, scanning or otherwise, except under the terms of the Copyright, Designs and Patents Act 1988 or under the terms of a licence issued by the Copyright Licensing Agency Ltd, 90 Tottenham Court Road, London W1T 4LP, UK, without the permission in writing of the Publisher. Requests to the Publisher should be addressed to the Permissions Department, John Wiley & Sons Ltd, The Atrium, Southern Gate, Chichester, West Sussex PO19 8SQ, England, or emailed to permreq@wiley.co.uk, or faxed to (+44) 1243 770620.

This publication is designed to provide accurate and authoritative information in regard to the subject matter covered. It is sold on the understanding that the Publisher is not engaged in rendering professional services. If professional advice or other expert assistance is required, the services of a competent professional should be sought.

Other Wiley Editorial Offices

John Wiley & Sons Inc., 111 River Street, Hoboken, NJ 07030, USA

Jossey-Bass, 989 Market Street, San Francisco, CA 94103-1741, USA

Wiley-VCH Verlag GmbH, Boschstr. 12, D-69469 Weinheim, Germany

John Wiley & Sons Australia Ltd, 33 Park Road, Milton, Queensland 4064, Australia

John Wiley & Sons (Asia) Pte Ltd, 2 Clementi Loop #02-01, Jin Xing Distripark, Singapore 129809

John Wiley & Sons Canada Ltd, 22 Worcester Road, Etobicoke, Ontario, Canada M9W 1L1

Wiley also publishes its books in a variety of electronic formats. Some content that appears in print may not be available in electronic books.

Novartis Foundation Symposium 267
viii+251 pages, 34 figures, 5 tables

British Library Cataloguing in Publication Data

A catalogue record for this book is available from the British Library

ISBN-13 978-0-470-02137-8 (HB)
ISBN-10 0-470-02137-3 (HB)

Typeset in $10\frac{1}{2}$ on $12\frac{1}{2}$ pt Garamond by Dobbie Typesetting Limited, Tavistock, Devon.
Printed and bound in Great Britain by T. J. International Ltd, Padstow, Cornwall.
This book is printed on acid-free paper responsibly manufactured from sustainable forestry, in which at least two trees are planted for each one used for paper production.

Contents

Symposium on Genetics of autoimmunity, held at the Novartis Foundation, London, 22–24 June 2004

Editors: Gregory Bock (Organizer) and Jamie Goode

This symposium is based on a proposal by Abul K. Abbas, David A. Hafler and John D. Rioux

Abul Abbas Chair's introduction 1

Mark J. Daly Patterns of genetic variation in humans and mice 2
Discussion 8

David B. Goldstein Haplotype tagging in pharmacogenetics 14
Discussion 19

Simon J. Foote, Justin P. Rubio, Melanie Bahlo, Trevor J. Kilpatrick, Terence P. Speed, Jim Stankovich, Rachel Burfoot, Helmut Butzkueven, Laura Johnson, Chris Wilkinson, Bruce Taylor, Michele Sale, Ingrid A. F. van der Mei, Joanne L. Dickinson and **Patricia Groom**
Multiple sclerosis: a haplotype association study 31
Discussion 39

Juha Kere Mapping genes for asthma and psoriasis 46
Discussion 52

Linda S. Wicker, Carolyn L. Moule, Heather Fraser, Carlos Penha-Goncalves, Dan Rainbow, Valerie E. S. Garner, Giselle Chamberlain, Kara Hunter, Sarah Howlett, Jan Clark, Andrea Gonzalez-Munoz, Anne-Marie Cumiskey, Paul Tiffen, Joanna Howson, Barry Healy, Luc J. Smink, Amanda Kingsnorth, Paul A. Lyons, Simon Gregory, Jane Rogers, John A. Todd and **Laurence B. Peterson** Natural genetic variants influencing type 1 diabetes in humans and in the NOD mouse 57
Discussion 65

Srividya Subramanian and **Edward K. Wakeland** The importance of epistatic interactions in the development of autoimmunity 76
Discussion 88

Timothy J. Vyse, Angela M. Richardson, Emily Walsh, Lisa Farwell, Mark J. Daly, Cox Terhorst and John D. Rioux Mapping autoimmune disease genes in humans: lessons from IBD and SLE   94
Discussion 107

Martin C. Wapenaar and Cisca Wijmenga A combined genetics and genomics approach to unravelling molecular pathways in coeliac disease   113
Discussion 134

Timothy W. Behrens, Robert R. Graham, Chieko Kyogoku, Emily C. Baechler, Paula S. Ramos, Clarence Gillett, Jason Bauer, Ward A. Ortmann, Keli L. Hippen, Erik Peterson, Carl D. Langefeld, Kathy L. Moser, Patrick M. Gaffney and Peter K. Gregersen Progress towards understanding the genetic pathogenesis of systemic lupus erythematosus   145
Discussion 160

Vigo Heissmeyer, Fernando Macián, Rajat Varma, Sin-Hyeog Im, Francisco García-Cozar, Heidi F. Horton, Michael C. Byrne, Stefan Feske, K. Venuprasad, Hua Gu, Yun-Cai Liu, Michael L. Dustin and Anjana Rao A molecular dissection of lymphocyte unresponsiveness induced by sustained calcium signalling   165
Discussion 174

Adrian Liston and Christopher C. Goodnow Genetic lesions in thymic T cell clonal deletion and thresholds for autoimmunity   180
Discussion 192

Lalitha Vijayakrishnan, Jacqueline M. Slavik, Zsolt Illés, Dan Rainbow, Laurence B. Peterson, Arlene S. Sharpe, Linda S. Wicker and Vijay K. Kuchroo An autoimmune disease-associated CTLA4 splice variant lacking the B7 binding domain signals negatively in T cells   200
Discussion 212

Adrian Ting, Stefan Lichtenthaler, Ramnik Xavier, Soon-Young Na, Shahrooz Rabizadeh, Tara Holmes and Brian Seed Large-scale screens for cDNAs with *in vivo* activity   219
Discussion 229

Jenny Ting Genomic mining of new genes and pathways in innate and adaptive immunity   231
Discussion 239

Index of contributors 242

Subject index 244

Participants

Abul K. Abbas (*Chair*)   Department of Pathology, University of California San Francisco, 505 Parnassus Avenue, Room M-590, San Francisco, CA 94143-0511, USA

Timothy W. Behrens   Center for Immunology, Department of Medicine, University of Minnesota, 6-126 BSBE Building, 312 Church Street, SE, Minneapolis, MN 55455, USA

Anne Bowcock   Department of Genetics, Box 8232, Washington University School of Medicine, 4566 Scott Avenue, St Louis, MO 63110, USA

William Cookson   Wellcome Trust Centre for Human Genetics, University of Oxford, Oxford, OX3 7BN, UK

Mark J. Daly   Whitehead Institute for Biomedical Research, Cambridge, MA 02142, USA

Simon J. Foote   Walter and Eliza Hall Institute of Medical Research, 1G Royal Pale, Parkville 3050, Victoria 3050, Australia

David B. Goldstein   Department of Biology, Darwin Building, Gower Street, London WC1E 6BT, UK

Christopher C. Goodnow   Australian Phenomics Facility, John Curtin School of Medical Research, JCSMR Building, 54, Australian National University, Canberra, ACT 2601, Australia

David A. Hafler   Center for Neurologic Diseases, Harvard Medical School, Brigham and Women's Hospital, 77 Avenue Louis Pasteur, Boston, MA 02115, USA

Juha Kere   Karolinska Institutet, Department of Biosciences, Novum, 7th Floor, SE-141 57 Huddinge, Sweden

Vijay K. Kuchroo Department of Neurology, Center for Neurologic Diseases, Brigham and Women's Hospital, HIM Room 786, 77 Avenue Louis Pasteur, Boston, MA 02115, USA

Cecilia Lindgren (*Novartis Foundation Bursar*) Clinical Research Center, Department of Biosciences at Novum, Karolinska University Hospital, SE-141 86 Stockholm, Sweden

Anjana Rao Center for Blood Research, Harvard Medical School, 200 Longwood Avenue, Warren Alpert Building, Boston, MA 02115, USA

John D. Rioux Inflammatory Disease Research Group, Human Medical and Population Genetics, The Broad Institute of MIT and Harvard, One Kendall Square, Building 300, NE83-G535, Cambridge, MA 02139-1561, USA

Brian Seed Harvard Medical School, Massachusetts General Hospital, 55 Fruit Street, Molecular Biology, Wellman 911, Boston, MA 02114, USA

Jenny Ting Lineberger Comprehensive Cancer Center CB#7295, University of North Carolina, Chapel Hill, NC 27599, USA

Dale Umetsu Division of Immunology and Allergy, Department of Pediatrics, Stanford University, Stanford, CA 94305-5208, USA

Timothy J. Vyse Rheumatology Section, Imperial College, Faculty of Medicine, Hammersmith Hospital, Du Cane Road, London W12 0NN, UK

Edward K. Wakeland Center for Immunology, The University of Texas Southwestern Medical Center at Dallas, 5323 Harry Hines Boulevard, Dallas, TX 75390-9093, USA

Linda S. Wicker Cambridge Institute for Medical Research (CIMR), Wellcome Trust/MRC Building, Addenbrooke's Hospital, Hills Road, Cambridge CB2 2XY, UK

Cisca Wijmenga Complex Genetics Group, Department of Biomedical Genetics, University Medical Center, Utrecht, Universiteitsweg 100, 3584 CG Utrecht, The Netherlands

Jane Worthington Arthritis Research Campaign Epidemiology Unit, Manchester University, Stopford Building, Oxford Road, Manchester M13 9PT, UK

Chair's introduction

Abul Abbas

Department of Pathology, University of California at San Francisco, 505 Parnassus Avenue, Room M-590, San Francisco, CA 94143-0511, USA

We are trying to do something unusual at this meeting. We have two groups of scientists in this room who don't often interact at scientific sessions: geneticists and immunologists. This poses some challenges.

I'd like to introduce this symposium by listing a few general questions that I have generated with help from co-proposers David Hafler and John Rioux. I will warn you these are very general and we may not get to concrete answers. They are also not necessarily specific to autoimmune disease, and may apply to all complex multigenic disorders. Having said this, these are the sorts of questions that we think are important and need to be tackled by the group collectively.

(1) How do we go from large regions (or haplotypes), to individual genes, to functions? This question has major implications for the genetics of disease, and for translating genetics to biology. The issue that none of us has answered in any concrete way is what are the criteria by which we choose candidate genes? This is one big picture question we should try to address.

(2) What is the evidence for causality? This bothers all of us. Is strong association enough?

(3) An issue dear to me: lots of us are MDs in this room where 'MD' stands for 'mouse doctor'! How can we best exploit animal models? What can we learn from them?

(4) Issues specific to autoimmunity. This is something I have left open. All of these things that I have listed in points 1–3 are not specific to autoimmunity but apply to all complex diseases. I am leaving it up to the rest of you to come up with issues that might be a little more specific for autoimmunity.

Patterns of genetic variation in humans and mice

Mark Daly

Whitehead Institute, Cambridge, MA 02142, USA

> *Abstract.* Positional cloning of genes underlying the heritability of autoimmune disease, as in many complex diseases, has largely been a frustrating exercise with few replicated positive findings despite enormous efforts at linkage and association mapping over the past ten years. Similar difficulties have been encountered by researchers attempting to identify such genes in murine models of autoimmunity. One reason is the lack of primary knowledge of genetic variation patterns that would enable the more efficient design and interpretation of comprehensive genetic association studies. We here describe progress towards haplotype maps of both the human and mouse genomes including their current application in the search for genes underlying autoimmune and inflammatory disorders.
>
> *2005 The genetics of autoimmunity. Wiley, Chichester (Novartis Foundation Symposium 267) p 2–13*

The promise and excitement surrounding human genetics lies in the opportunity to discover the fundamental basis of heritable disease and in the potential long-term impact on treatment of disease that lies beyond such discoveries. While this dream of personalized medicine and rational therapeutic development was one of the driving forces behind the recently completed Human Genome Project, such goals have largely been elusive, particularly for autoimmune and other common, complex diseases. One of the main obstacles towards realizing some of these future benefits has been the difficulty in identifying the genetic factors underlying risk, severity and therapeutic response — seen as a critical first step towards the improved biological understanding and diagnostic classification that is required to accelerate progress towards better treatment and prevention.

By contrast, enormous success has been achieved in the identification of genes and mutations underlying monogenic (Mendelian) disorders — with more than 1000 successful efforts to date (Botstein & Risch 2003). In Mendelian disorders, the presumption of monogenicity and complete penetrance of the mutations has enabled the rapid identification of small disease intervals because affected relative pairs must share these necessary and sufficient mutations. In this scenario, single recombination events that break the obligate sharing among affected close relatives are sufficient to delineate a critical region conclusively. With the examination of a substantial family collection, nearby recombination events can efficiently narrow the critical region, within which the causal mutation lies, very effectively — with subsequent gene-based sequencing most often revealing mutations which obviously severely disrupt the coding sequence of the involved gene.

With such a suite of successfully used tools to identify Mendelian genes after initial linkage mapping, why have experiences with complex human disease, as well as gene identification after mouse quantitative trait locus (QTL) mapping, been so painfully intractable? Part of the answer lies in the observation that in complex disease, contributing mutations are invariably neither necessary nor sufficient on their own to cause disease. For nearly every documented genetic factor in complex disease, there are many individuals with disease that do not carry the factor and, with the exception of rare instances of 'Mendelian-like' mutations that predispose to severe, early-onset forms of common disease (e.g. severe *BRCA1* and *2* mutations in breast cancer, maturity onset diabetes of the young [MODY] gene mutations), there are many individuals in the population who carry these risk factors yet do not develop disease. This might be because they require the presence of other interacting genetic factors, certain environmental triggers, or simply because they affect human biology in a subtle quantitative fashion (which may additively combine with other genetic and non-genetic factors to cross a threshold medically defined as disease), it is clear that many genetic risk factors for complex disease act in a probabilistic (i.e. incompletely penetrant alleles which attenuate risk) rather than deterministic (i.e. completely penetrant as in Mendelian disorders) fashion.

Because this is the case, allele sharing among any individual pair of relatives is not required at any given susceptibility locus and thus linkage analysis is significantly weakened. In addition, individual recombination events cannot be used to convincingly delineate a critical region since pairs of affected individuals are not required to share alleles at the causal location. Put another way, there will be many individuals with disease who will not share any specific mutation and the haplotype on which it arose while many unaffected individuals may very well carry that mutation and haplotype. In this probabilistic scenario, it has become clear that statistical association to genetic variation over large population-based samples of cases and controls is the most powerful approach to identifying causal mutations — larger samples being required as penetrance is diminished. In fact Risch & Merikangas (1996) pointed out that in many circumstances, such studies are orders of magnitude more powerful than the standard linkage studies. However, testing genetic variation exhaustively, via complete sequencing, is prohibitively expensive, especially when considering the thousands of samples that may be required for complex disease mapping.

It has been recognized for some time that linkage disequilibrium (LD), the non-random association of alleles at nearby variable sites, may offer us a way of thoroughly testing genetic variation in a region without complete sequencing. While theoretical expectations were such that LD in the general worldwide population would be quite modest and have little useful structure (Kruglyak 1999), many recent studies have described the discovery and empirical characterization of unexpected genetic variation patterns in both humans (Daly et al 2001, Patil et al 2001, Gabriel et al 2002) and classical strains of inbred laboratory mice (Wade et al 2002, Wiltshire et al 2003). These patterns contrast starkly with theoretical expectations, appear to have arisen because of a combination of population demography and recombinational inhomogeneity, and offer unique and promising paths forward for the positional cloning of genes involved in complex phenotypes in both organisms. Confirmation of these early observations has quickly led to efforts to characterize genetic variation throughout these genomes, most notably the International Human Haplotype Map Project (HapMap) which by the end of 2004 should near 1 000 000 single nucleotide polymorphisms (SNPs) examined in 270 worldwide samples.

The goal of HapMap is to accelerate medical genetic research by through the identification and public release of the common patterns of DNA sequence variation throughout the human genome (International HapMap Consortium 2003). Specifically, this resource is a critical step towards the ability to study more thoroughly the influence of genetic variation on complex disease phenotypes. For example, one of the early studies supporting the utility of a haplotype map, the identification of the Crohn's disease locus on 5q31, several years of resequencing and SNP genotyping, followed by the development of analytic methods to dissect the unexpected haplotype and recombination patterns, were required to identify genetic variation replicably associated to disease. With a completed haplotype map in hand (and with technological improvements in SNP genotyping), the effort required to map that locus could be undertaken in weeks. The association to Crohn's disease, while very modest, has since been replicated in five out of five published population samples, underscoring that the approach of indirect association mapping using a haplotype map can in fact identify very modest genetic risk factors for diseases that were previously inaccessible to standard linkage and positional cloning efforts.

The approach of indirect association (i.e. the use of a subset of genetic variation in a region [HapMap]) to serve as surrogates for untested or undiscovered genetic variation in the same genomic region, makes the obvious assumption that the tested subset either contains the causal allele or a marker highly correlated with the causal allele. As the HapMap has been developed, it has become clear that the majority of genome falls into segments with extensive linkage disequilibrium, suggesting that many of the roughly 10 million common SNPs in the genome

TABLE 1 *IBD5* replication attempts

Study reference	Sample	P value	Odds-ratio
Negoro et al 2003	282 trios	P < 0.01	1.43 [1.12, 1.82]
Mirza et al 2003	511 trios	P < 0.01	1.29 [1.06, 1.57]
Mirza et al 2003	684/701 case/con	P < 0.01	1.23 [1.06, 1.43]
Giallourakis et al 2003	368 trios	P < 0.01	1.31 [1.05, 1.62]
Armuzzi et al 2003	330/870 case/con	P < 0.001	1.38 [1.15, 1.66]

P values are one-sided tests of a single SNP identified as associated in Rioux et al (2001). The combined significance of the five replication attempts is 2.3×10^{-10}.

have groups of neighbours that are all nearly perfectly correlated with each other and for which one can serve as a proxy for the others in an association screen. Thus it has been proposed that once the variation patterns are characterized for a given region (Johnson et al 2001, Gabriel et al 2002), a subset of tag SNPs can be selected that would be adequate for subsequent association testing.

The degree to which this is true is an empirical question that the HapMap project has generated supplemental data to address. Ten 500 kb regions have been resequenced in 48 individuals and all SNPs discovered (as well as all in dbSNP) are being typed on the 270 HapMap DNA samples (roughly a density of a SNP every 300 bp). These data (*http://www.hapmap.org/downloads/encode1.html.en*) have provided a first look at haplotype patterns at ultra high density, which in turn has provided the project with the ability to test the performance of methods and inferences on incomplete data by 'hiding' some of the SNPs from consideration and evaluating results based on those hidden SNPs. While the examination of high-density patterns of LD has been informative (indeed inferences regarding the segmental nature of LD are strengthened rather than weakened at high-density and this data, interpreted by methods developed by Peter Donnelly's lab; McVean et al 2004), it has provided much stronger evidence of the widespread nature of recombinational hotspots), it is this latter ability to evaluate the performance and completeness of HapMap that is proving the most critical.

For example, through the examination of subsets of markers from these high-density regions, we observe that with a marker selected at random every 5 kb across the genome, we capture 75% of the common variation (minor allele frequency >0.05) in the genome with an r^2 of 0.8. Thus already, we see that by typing ∼5% of the common variation in a region, we would be confident that at least three-quarters of the full complement of common variants would be adequately tested in an association study. At the eventual HapMap target of 3 000 000 SNPs (expected to be reached in mid 2005), this number should exceed 90%. Importantly, however, the characterization of LD provided by HapMap enables us to take advantage of the considerable redundancy among SNPs at high density. We therefore predict that the typing of between 250 000 and 500 000 tag SNPs selected from this HapMap would be able to assay the common variation with minimal loss of power. In other words, the ability to choose the *best* SNPs from a characterized set of 3 000 000 will enable the description of the vast majority of common genetic variation through the examination of only a few percent—rendering screens for association across large sets of candidate genes, regions of linkage, and very soon the whole genome, feasible in a way that was inconceivable 5 years ago.

As these findings in humans have surfaced, I and others have begun to research what patterns, if any, might exist across the panel of classical inbred mouse strains that pervade nearly every avenue of biomedical research. Positional cloning of genes for complex phenotypes in mouse crosses is recognized as an even more acute bottleneck than in human mapping because, unlike direct human mapping in which linkage has by and large been unsuccessful in detecting regions involved in disease, murine QTL mapping has been enormously successful at defining genomic regions containing genes that contribute to complex and quantitative traits. Because large crosses between inbred strains of mice with divergent phenotypes of interest can be created easily, and because these crosses afford control of the environment, critical in many complex phenotypes, and which cannot be achieved in human studies, even genes that contribute only small fractions of the overall phenotypic variance are easily detected with QTL linkage mapping. However, the positional identification of the genes underlying these effects has been nearly as impenetrable in mice as it has traditionally been in humans.

Through comparison of the emergent C57BL/6 genome sequence with sequences previously generated from other strains, it quickly became clear that there were much more striking patterns of divergence and identity shared between pairs of inbred strains over megabase-sized regions. This research culminated in the description for the first time of the long-suspected mosaic structure of genetic variation among lab mice (Wade et al 2002) and refined a model of the origins of the laboratory mouse. This unified the recent human-driven formation of the inbred strains with the unique evolutionary history of the multiple subspecies of *Mus musculus*. The proposed model of haplotype structure in mice has significant ramifications for accelerating the positional cloning of QTLs through merging cross and strain phenotype information from multiple experiments with the ancestral haplotype patterns to identify small regions where the QTL mapping and ancestral variation patterns are concordant. For example, if a QTL is present between two strains, the genetic difference will (almost by definition) be found in the one-third of the genomic region that is ancestrally diverged between the two strains and contains nearly all of the sequence differences. Dramatic acceleration can thus be attained by comparing the haplotype patterns of many strains that have either been directly used in QTL mapping (positively or negatively) in the region of interest or by correlation of strain phenotype with ancestral haplotype (Wade et al 2002, Wiltshire et al 2003) — the relevant phenotype variation must map to a segment containing genetic variation patterns that are consistent with the QTL map data and strain phenotypes.

As with the high density regions studied by the human HapMap, several recent studies (Yalcin et al 2004, Frazer et al 2004) have extended these results to greater precision and across panels of inbred mice (rather than focusing on pairs of strains). In combination, these studies examined deep sequence data across 10 Mb of genome and while confirming the general findings of the earlier study, offer a much more detailed look at the structure of variation across inbred strains. Specifically, the mouse genome falls into simple segments (on the order of one to several hundred kilobases in length) within which the panel of classical inbred strains generally share two to four distinct ancestral haplotypes. Most importantly, nearly all variable sites (over 98%) are described by these few simple patterns, suggesting that a murine haplotype map requires far fewer markers in order to efficiently characterize the patterns across these mice.

Taken as a whole, meaningful progress is clearly underway in the understanding of the genetics of complex disease. This has been sparked by a better understanding and characterization of genetic variation across the human and mouse genomes and novel approaches to disease genetics using this information. In fact multiple confirmed genetic contributors have been identified in type I and II diabetes, inflammatory bowel disease, Alzheimer's disease and many others. However, realistically we must acknowledge that we are in the infancy of our understanding of the genetics of complex disease. Moreover, this understanding is only the first step in the path towards the development of more effective prevention and treatment for disease. Further experimental and computational developments will be needed to move us ahead in this endeavour. Greater integration of our understanding of genetics with biology and medicine will be needed before we reach this ultimate goal.

References

Armuzzi A, Ahmad T, Ling KL et al 2003 Genotype-phenotype analysis of the Crohn's disease susceptibility haplotype on chromosome 5q31. Gut 52:1133–1139

Botstein D, Risch N 2003 Discovering genotypes underlying human phenotypes: past successes for mendelian disease, future approaches for complex disease. Nat Genet 33:228–237

Daly MJ, Rioux JD, Schaffner SF, Hudson TJ, Lander ES 2001 High-resolution haplotype structure in the human genome. Nat Genet 29:229–232

Frazer KA, Wade CM, Hinds DA et al 2004 Segmental phylogenetic relationships of inbred mouse strains revealed by fine-scale analysis of sequence variation across 4.6 Mb of mouse genome. Genome Res 14:1493–1500

Gabriel SB, Schaffner SF, Nguyen H et al 2002 The structure of haplotype blocks in the human genome. Science 296:2225–2229

Giallourakis C, Stoll M, Miller K et al 2003 IBD5 is a general risk factor for inflammatory bowel disease: replication of association with Crohn disease and identification of a novel association with ulcerative colitis. Am J Hum Genet 73:205–211

International HapMap Consortium 2003 The International HapMap Project. Nature 426: 789–796

Johnson GC, Esposito L, Barratt BJ 2001 Haplotype tagging for the identification of common disease genes. Nat Genet 29:233–237

Kruglyak L 1999 Prospects for whole-genome linkage disequilibrium mapping of common disease genes. Nat Genet 22:139–144

McVean GA, Myers SR, Hunt S et al 2004 The fine-scale structure of recombination rate variation in the human genome. Science 304:581–584

Mirza MM, Fisher SA, King K et al 2003 Genetic evidence for interaction of the 5q31 cytokine locus and the CARD15 gene in Crohn disease. Am J Hum Genet 72:1018–1022

Negoro K, McGovern DP, Kinouchi Y et al 2003 Analysis of the IBD5 locus and potential gene-gene interactions in Crohn's disease. Gut 52:541–546

Patil N, Berno AJ, Hinds DA et al 2001 Blocks of limited haplotype diversity revealed by high-resolution scanning of human chromosome 21. Science 294:1719–1723

Rioux JD, Daly MJ, Silverberg MS et al 2001 Genetic variation in the 5q31 cytokine gene cluster confers susceptibility to Crohn disease. Nat Genet 29:223–228

Risch N, Merikangas K 1996 The future of genetic studies of complex human diseases. Science 273:1516–1516

Wade CM, Kulbokas EJ 3rd, Kirby AW et al 2002 The mosaic structure of variation in the laboratory mouse genome. Nature 420:574–578

Wiltshire T, Pletcher MT, Batalov S 2003 Genome-wide single-nucleotide polymorphism analysis defines haplotype patterns in mouse. Proc Natl Acad Sci USA 100:3380–3385

Yalcin B, Fullerton J, Miller S 2004 Unexpected complexity in the haplotypes of commonly used inbred strains of laboratory mice. Proc Natl Acad Sci USA 101:9734–9739

DISCUSSION

Goldstein: You mentioned a proof of principle, finding variants using some kind of linkage disequilibrium (LD) scaffolding approach. There are now a lot of examples of that. Allan Roses and colleagues did a study like this with *APOE4*, showing association for multiple markers in the gene because they were in LD with the variant that influences disease risk (Martin et al 2000). There has been a study like this with an adverse reaction to abacavir (Hosford et al 2004). This showed that it was possible to pick up an effect on hyperbilirubinaemia. There are quite a few proofs of concept like this. Many of them are in pharmacogenetics, where the association between the genetic variation and response is stronger than in disease predisposition. We can consider the LD approach to be experimentally validated with those kinds of designs.

Abbas: Aren't many of these examples of what Mark Daly described as single, highly penetrant traits?

Goldstein: No, *APOE4* is complex in the sense that there are multiple factors that influence predisposition to Alzheimer's. In terms of the spectrum of variants it's a relatively large effect, but it is certainly complex. Abacavir hypersensitivity is complex.

Wijmenga: They did the same recently for the factor V Leiden mutation (van Hylckama Vlieg et al 2004).

Goldstein: There are a lot of examples like that. One can consider that there has been proof of concept for linkage disequilibrium mapping.

Cookson: With single gene disorders, yes. But I wouldn't bet my shirt on it.

Goldstein: There are two separate issues under discussion here. Firstly, does the indirect association design work? The answer is yes, it can work. There is the entirely separate issue of the nature of the variants that influence common disease. These might be generally relatively intractable in the association framework. This is a separate point, and I have a lot of concern in that direction. But the basic idea of using a marker as a proxy is well established.

Cookson: At least some of the time.

Goodnow: What about when you have three separate mutations in three different haplotypes. Does this come unstuck then?

Goldstein: This makes it harder. The statistical machinery that we all use is actually predicated on the single variants.

Rioux: To a certain extent it will depend on the circumstances. If we take the *CARD15* gene in Crohn's disease as an example, our work demonstrates that the three known causal mutations (Hugot et al 2001, Ogura et al 2001) arose independently (Vermeire et al 2002). It so happens that these three mutations occurred on chromosomes that shared the same ancestral haplotype in the block that contains the *CARD15* gene, and different haplotypes in the flanking blocks. Furthermore, there are SNPs that have alleles that uniquely tag the risk haplotype. Typing any of these tagging SNPs gives a strong association signal and therefore would lead a researcher to the identification of this disease gene. Had the mutations arisen on completely unrelated haplotypes this certainly would have decreased the power of detection.

Goldstein: There are two issues here. One is original detection and the other is fine localization. For fine localization it is going to matter whether the genetic model is right or not. This is going to be quite a challenge. If you have a hit in a region and then you want to try to use all the association data you have to estimate where in the region the variant is likely to be, you can do this in one of two ways. You could assume that it is a single variant and interpret your association data in those terms. What is the evidence that the variants you know about are actually the causal agents? Or you could assume more complicated models of variants that interact to produce the effect. As far as I know, the people taking a statistical approach to fine localization generally assume there is a single variant. This has an effect on how they interpret the association data.

Cookson: There is hardly ever a single variant in a gene for complex disorders. We have looked at a number of loci in some detail. We have comprehensively sequenced SNPs in a number of genes that influence asthma. We find almost invariably that there are several polymorphisms that are influencing what is going on. If you think about this, there is some selective pressure on the gene then it is likely that this selective pressure will find more than one way of modifying the phenotype.

Hafler: There is some degree of evidence that haplotype blocks occur at hotspots of recombination. There may have been biological pressures for this to occur, as certain allelic gene variants may preferentially work together. For this reason, rather than looking at the biological effects of single genes, we might instead want to look at a whole haplotype in terms of how that region is transcribed and translated, and how those different genes work in concert.

Kere: I wanted to make two points. Going back to the monogenic diseases, now that we have this new knowledge about the haplotype structure, it may be that a small subset of mutations that have been described for monogenic disorders are only proxies. The true mutation that is causal for the disease may be something nearby in the same haplotype block. It might be worth going back to some of the monogenic disorders where it has been difficult to understand how the mutation is actually causing the phenotype, and think about the other changes that there are in the sequence, rather than the ones that have been described. The other point is that when we have on average four different alleles for each haplotype, each of these four may have a different quantitative effect on the phenotype that we are looking at. It is not just going to be the risk and the non-risk haplotypes. There might be one a little bit higher risk, one clearly protective and two neutral. This is the picture we should aim at resolving.

Goldstein: The situation is actually much worse that that. There has been too much focus on blocks in complex trait disease genetics. We are almost never in the situation where you can say that the variant that has some effect on phenotype is sitting in this block, and there is no association between variants within this block and nearby blocks, so now I have five common haplotypes in that block and I just need to worry about the effect of these. It is not like that. In fact, there are variable degrees of association extending right across blocks, however you want to define blocks. It doesn't simplify in this way. We need to worry about a large chunk of the genome and exhaustively mine that for variation, not just focusing on a clearly delimited block.

Kere: We should never forget the example provided by cystic fibrosis, where we have a founder mutation in the populations, but on top of that there are hundreds

GENETIC VARIATION IN HUMANS AND MICE 11

of more or less private mutations, some of them also with the characteristics of founder mutations in different populations. Whenever we find that there is a low penetrance haplotype perhaps affecting the risk for some disease, it will be worthwhile to go back and look for rare mutations in the same gene in all the different haplotype backgrounds. It will be especially worth looking for mutations in those haplotypes that don't appear to be the common risk haplotype, because there you will have a good chance of finding private mutations. This goes back to the point in Abul Abbas' introduction about evidence for causality. Whenever we have discovered that there is a common risk haplotype for a disease, we should go back, look at this gene and see whether on top of that at-risk haplotype we also find the individual private mutations in the gene. If we do, this adds a lot of strength to the point that this is the gene, or one of the genes.

Daly: David Goldstein is absolutely right. There is no particular role for blocks or any structural analysis in the scanning for association. What I described for the haplotype map is focused entirely on the initial detection of association. How can we screen regions of the genome to detect association in the most efficient way? It will not succeed in all cases, but we are rapidly coming to the point where we expect a very large number of genes to be involved in each of these complex diseases. If an initial screen can find some of these genes, this will be a very successful first step. The subsequent work to collect a detailed set of genetic variants across those associated regions is not such an intractable computational problem. We have espoused the techniques that Clayton, Cordell and others have described (Cordell & Clayton 2002). If one collects a high density of polymorphism data across a region, one can evaluate whether there is statistical evidence for association and then whether that association can be entirely attributable to a single variant, or whether multiple variants are required. This doesn't necessarily require multi-marker evaluations of epistasis or anything of this nature. One can actually do very well with single marker association effects in an iterative and recursive fashion.

Bowcock: We need to be cautious when describing variants for complex traits on the basis of association. For example, even association with a single haplotype may reflect the presence of more than one predisposing variant on that haplotype in different individuals. This has been seen for the rare autosomal recessive disorder, Bardet-Biedl, where three different mutations were found on a rare haplotype in individuals from Puerto Rico (a founder population). This suggests a bias for mutational events on some haplotypes or a change in the structure of this founder population over time (Sheffield 2004).

I would like to get back to NOD2, because I didn't understand your explanation. My understanding was that there were three different haplotypes, with three different mutations that were reported by the French group. Therefore it was not going to be easy to see association although they did have a very good LOD score. Are you telling me that there is a much larger haplotype on which all the mutations arose or was the ability to detect association a matter of luck?

Rioux: Given that the haplotype on which these causal alleles arose is at approximately 35% in control chromosomes, it is not an unlikely event that the mutations occurred on this one haplotype (Vermeire et al 2002).

Daly: It probably was. When we looked in detail at the gene we found that there were in DB SNP that were in strong linkage disequilibrium with the set of causal mutations as a whole.

Bowcock: On the other hand, the ancestral haplotype may have been more likely than others to undergo mutation within the *NOD2* gene.

Daly: Yes. I don't think we'd assert this on the basis of one mutation, but they could be.

Cookson: Mark Daly, these are terrific data. As the map gets denser there has to be some decision made about what is typed in patient populations and so on. LD and some systematic method of spacing markers is important. But what about the importance of genes themselves? 2% of the genome is genes and their controlling regions: should this be enriched for in any way?

Daly: We would like it to be. The project as a whole is exploring a variety of different ways in which we might synergize our effort with gene-based SNP discovery efforts underway. Failing that, in the future we will engage in more detailed work of that nature.

Behrens: Do you have any current estimates as to how much variation we are dealing with? We think of 1% being a reasonable threshold for a common SNP, so how many of these are there in the human genome?

Daly: The back of the envelope estimate is that there are some 10 million sites of common variation. What we find is that by looking at a haplotype map we can get a good assay for 80–90% of those by looking at fewer than 10%.

Foote: I would like to make a point about mutations occurring on a common haplotype. We have been looking at susceptibility to malaria in Papua New Guinea. We see an original haplotype that occurs in the population and subsequent mutation in the same genes occurring on the same haplotype. It is a bit like affinity maturation in immunoglobulins. A mutation occurs which causes an increase in survival, and then further maturation occurs through additional mutations in the same gene.

Worthington: Illumina are part of the HapMap project, and they talk about releasing in a short time a 100K chip, which is a combination of haplotype tagging and those residing in genes. Do you feel, on the basis of your knowledge of the map, that this will be a useful tool for us to use in association studies?

Daly: It depends on your definition of 'useful'. It is not a right or wrong answer; simply a question of completeness. What is happening is that as you choose more markers, and choose them more efficiently, you get more out of it. You get a description of 30%, then 50%, then 80% of the genetic variation in the genome. The current Affymetrix product offers 120 000 SNPs. These were chosen at random and they cluster in an awkward fashion. His is still a useful product in some senses, even though the curves from the haplotype map data indicate that this gives a reasonable assay perhaps of only 20% of the common genetic variation in the genome. But if you are studying a gene for which there are perhaps 50 different factors in the genome, perhaps you'll catch a few.

References

Cordell HJ, Clayton DG 2002 A unified stepwise regression procedure for evaluating the relative effects of polymorphisms within a gene using case/control or family data: application to HLA in type 1 diabetes. Am J Hum Genet 70:124–141

Hosford DA, Lai EH, Riley JH, Xu CF, Danoff TM, Roses AD 2004 Pharmacogenetics to predict drug-related adverse events. Toxicol Pathol 32(suppl 1):9–12

Hugot JP, Chamaillard M, Zouali H et al 2001 Association of NOD2 leucine-rich repeat variants with susceptibility to Crohn's disease. Nature 411:599–603

Martin ER, Lai EH, Gilbert JR et al 2000 SNPing away at complex diseases: analysis of single-nucleotide polymorphisms around APOE in Alzheimer disease. Am J Hum Genet 67:383–394

Ogura Y, Bonen DK, Inohara N et al 2001 A frameshift mutation in NOD2 associated with susceptibility to Crohn's disease. Nature 411:603–606

Sheffield VC 2004 Use of isolated populations in the study of a human obesity syndrome, the Bardet-Biedl syndrome. Pediatr Res 55:908–911

Van Hylckama Vlieg A, Sandkuijl LA, Rosendaal FR, Bertina RM, Vos HL 2004 Candidate gene approach in association studies: would the factor V Leiden mutation have been found by this approach? Eur J Hum Genet 12:478–482

Vermeire S, Wild G, Kocher K et al 2002 CARD15 genetic variation in a Quebec population: prevalence, genotype-phenotype relationship, and haplotype structure. Am J Hum Genet 71:74–83

Haplotype tagging in pharmacogenetics

David B. Goldstein

Department of Biology, Darwin Building, University College London, Gower Street, London WC1E 6BT, UK

Abstract. Analyses of variation in human populations have become central to understanding how gene variants predispose to disease and influence treatment response. Here I first describe an emerging framework for linkage disequilbrium–(haplotype) based gene mapping focusing on the analysis of patterns of genetic variation in 56 genes that metabolize or transport prescription medicines. Detailed analyses of 754 single nucleotide polymorphisms (SNPs) genotyped in two population samples (European and Japanese) provide a set of haplotype tagging SNPs that economically represent variation in most of the major enzymes that act on prescription drugs. I use these analyses to address a number of outstanding questions relating to haplotype mapping. Following this, I provide a number of applications of haplotype mapping emphasizing the work that needs to be done to translate genotype–phenotype correlations into clinically useful diagnostics, and clinically useful leads concerning new therapeutic targets.

2005 The genetics of autoimmunity. Wiley, Chichester (Novartis Foundation Symposium 267) p 14–30

Here I will give an overview of the current research status of variable drug-response studies and some suggestions as to where they are likely to lead us in the coming years.

The study of variable drug-response represents a simpler means of analyzing complex traits than the direct study of disease predisposition. It is simpler in the sense that there are often obvious candidate genes that may harbour variants which influence drug response, and it is also simpler in that there is often the possibility of more clinical application, for example, with diagnostics that might tell you which drug works best for an individual patient or diagnostics that tell you something about appropriate dosing for an individual patient.

To investigate that claim in more detail, we recently carried out a survey of gene variants that have been associated with drug response in at least two studies (Goldstein et al 2003). We found that 21 of the 42 total variants resided in either the drug target or in the biological pathway in which the drug target resides. Of these 13 were found in genes that directly metabolized the drug or one of its metabolites, while one was found in a transporter for the drug, and seven more in some other category. This review suggested that polymorphisms that are known to influence drug response are often in obvious genes. These figures cannot be taken as an estimate of the proportion of variants that influence drug response in each of the categories, because there is an obvious bias in that the research community have chosen sites where polymorphisms are expected to be found. However, this does show that these obvious candidate genes are home to important pharmacogenetic variants. This suggests that pharmacogenetics is probably simplified by having obvious candidate genes that really do carry gene variants that influence drug responses.

I will now comment on methods for searching for variants that are implicated in drug responses or in common diseases.

Tagging single nucleotide polymorphisms (SNPs)

The basic idea of 'tagging' is to choose a subset of polymorphisms that in some sense represent all the polymorphisms that you don't propose to genotype in clinical material. Figure 1 shows a set of haplotypes in a population in which several polymorphisms are associated with one another, and in this cartoon version a subset of the polymorphisms are sufficient to represent all the existant variation. A commonly-used paradigm for indirect association studies involves genotyping control individuals, which then establishes a linkage disequilibrium data set (LD data set). The patterns of linkage disequilibrium in the LD data set are used to select tagging SNPs, which are typed in phenotyped individuals. However, there are a number of outstanding questions about exactly how to implement such a paradigm for indirect association studies. These questions include:

1. How do we select and test performance of tagging SNPs?
2. How many individuals are required to select adequate tagging SNPs?
3. How does performance depend on allele frequency of 'tagged' SNPs?
4. How does performance depend on the density of the SNPs you have typed in the control or LD data set?
5. Is functional variation is represented as well as non-functional variation?
6. How many more tagging SNPs are required so that the tags perform well in multiple populations?

We have recently published a paper in *Nature Genetics* (Ahmadi et al 2005), which addressed some of these questions. The data set involved genes that encoded many important drug metabolizing enzymes. We genotyped approximately 800 SNPs in these genes in 64 individuals of North European ancestry and 64 of Japanese

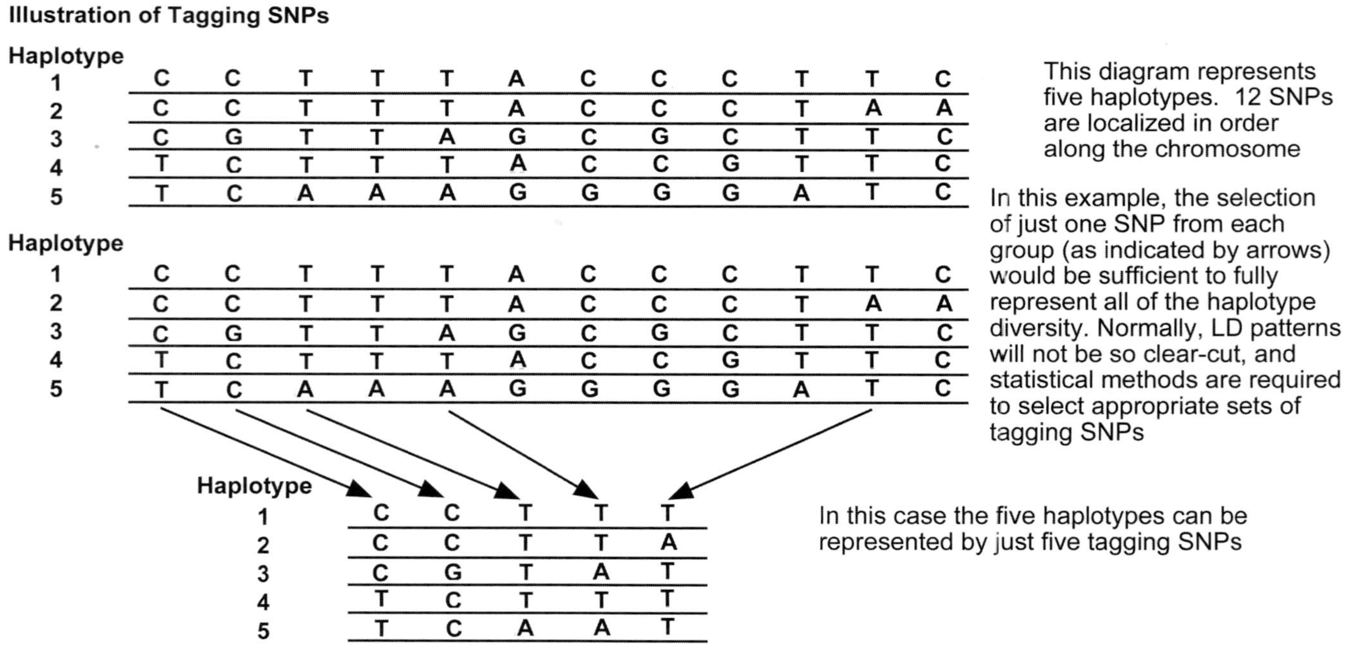

Illustration of Tagging SNPs

Haplotype												
1	C	C	T	T	A	C	C	C	T	T	T	C
2	C	C	T	T	A	C	C	C	T	T	A	A
3	C	G	T	T	G	C	G	C	T	T	T	C
4	T	C	T	T	A	C	C	G	G	T	T	C
5	T	C	A	A	G	G	G	G	A	T	T	C

Haplotype												
1	C	C	T	T	A	C	C	C	T	T	T	C
2	C	C	T	T	A	C	C	C	T	T	A	A
3	C	G	T	T	G	C	G	C	T	T	T	C
4	T	C	T	T	A	C	C	G	G	T	T	C
5	T	C	A	A	G	G	G	G	A	T	T	C

This diagram represents five haplotypes. 12 SNPs are localized in order along the chromosome

In this example, the selection of just one SNP from each group (as indicated by arrows) would be sufficient to fully represent all of the haplotype diversity. Normally, LD patterns will not be so clear-cut, and statistical methods are required to select appropriate sets of tagging SNPs

Haplotype					
1	C	C	T	C	T
2	C	C	T	C	A
3	C	G	A	G	T
4	T	C	T	C	T
5	T	C	A	G	T

In this case the five haplotypes can be represented by just five tagging SNPs

FIG. 1. Illustration of tagging SNPs. (Adapted from Tate & Goldstein 2004.)

ancestry and we developed a framework for asking how well these SNPs represent unknown variation that involves selecting the SNPs in an LD sample in which you have dropped out one of the SNPs from the analysis. Following this the ability of the tSNP set to predict the allelic state of the 'dropped' SNP is assessed in an independent sample. An advantage of using this framework is that it tests how well you can predict the SNPs that you haven't typed in the way the tagging SNPs would actually be used. When we carried out this analysis we found that the unknown SNPs can be very well predicted by the tagging SNPs in all cases where the minor allele frequency of the SNP that you are trying to tag is sufficiently high. The work also suggested that SNPs with low minor allele frequencies are not reliably tagged.

We also found that an approximate density of 1 SNP for every 3 kilobases resulted in a robust set of tagging SNPs. We also addressed the question of how many more SNPs you need to work in multiple human populations. We found that you need 196 SNPs to satisfactorily tag the European population sample, 179 SNPs to satisfactorily tag the Japanese population sample but when you required that the tags performed well in both the European and the Japanese population samples you only required 226 SNPs — roughly 20% more than are needed in the European population sample. This suggests that the patterns of LD between the European and the Japanese population groups are sufficiently similar that you only need a modest increase in the number of tagging SNPs to find a set that works well in both populations. However, I would emphasize that this does not mean that a tagging SNP selected in one of the populations will itself work in the other population. Our results simply show that in order to identify a cosmopolitan tSNP set you don't need that many more SNPs.

We also addressed the question of whether tagging SNPs can adequately represent functional as well as non-functional variation. We made a systematic comparison between the two classes of variation by selecting variants from the literature that had been shown to influence the activity or expression of enzymes and compared these to variants that are not known to be functional. We found that both categories of variation are equally well represented by tagging SNPs. So this analysis does not suggest that there is any particular concern with how well functional variation can be represented by tagging SNPs. To emphasize the power of this tool for mapping further what we find is that around 200 tagging SNPs are sufficient to represent the common variation in all the genes under study, and diversity estimates would suggest that there are on the order of 4000 common polymorphisms within the genes and therefore this tool can provide a remarkable saving in terms of typing effort to comprehensively represent common variation. However, a direct test of the performance of these tagging SNPs in an independent population sample showed that they do a very poor job of representing rare variation so the good news is that common variation is well represented and the bad news that rare variation is very poorly represented.

Finally, I would like to turn to an example of a pharmacogenetics project which we carried out (Tate & Goldstein 2004, Tate et al 2005). Carbamazepine and phenytoin are commonly used anti-epileptic drugs. They are effective and inexpensive, and for these reasons carbamazepine in particular is probably the most widely used anti-epileptic drug and phenytoin is a bit less widely used because it has a slightly worse safety profile than carbamazepine. However, the one difficulty with both these drugs, common in epilepsy and other conditions, is that patients need very different doses to control their seizures. We found that the maximum tolerated doses for phenytoin and carbamazepine ranged, respectively, from 100–900 mg per day and 300–2700 mg per day. We carried out a retrospective study to find gene variants associated with these dose requirements. We considered the obvious candidate genes both for phenytoin and carbamazepine — genes that metabolize the drugs in question and genes that encode the target of the drugs — and we found a polymorphism in the principal agent (that metabolizes phenytoin) associated with dosing of phenytoin. We also found a polymorphism in a gene encoding the target of both phenytoin and carbamazepine — the alpha subunit of a sodium channel — to be associated with their maximum tolerated doses. These results again illustrate the experience that pharmacogenetics provides a simpler means of analyzing complex traits than the direct analysis of common disease predisposition.

It is fair to conclude that association studies will contribute to our understanding of how patients respond to medicines but that this contribution will be subject to an improvement in their design both in terms of basic genetic methodologies and also in terms of the description of the phenotype. In addition, associations should be properly followed up and validated by replication in order to understand their biological basis. It is also fair to conclude that there will soon be a clinical return from the study of variable drug-response. However, it is also fair to say that while the study of disease predisposition is more challenging we may still gain transformational insights generating new possibilities for therapeutic intervention. While pharmacogenetics is an easier strategy the returns might help to optimize the use of medicines as opposed to opening up whole new avenues for therapeutic intervention.

References

Ahmadi K, Weale M, Zhengyu X et al 2005 A single nucleotide polymorphism tagging set for human drug metabolism and transport. Nat Genet, in press
Goldstein DB, Tate SK, Sisodiya SM 2003 Pharmacogenetics goes genomic. Nat Rev Genet 4:937–947

Tate SK, Goldstein DB 2004 Pharmacogenetics and the treatment of cardiovascular disease. Handbook of Experimental Pharmacology: Cardiovascular Pharmacogenetics 160:25–37

Tate SK, Depondt C, Sisodiya SM et al 2005 Genetic predictors of clinical use of the antiepileptic drugs phenytoin and carbamazepine. Proc Natl Acad Sci USA, in press

DISCUSSION

Daly: I agree completely that block analysis can impair the choice of tags. This is why we don't espouse their use in that way. But this sort of analysis is quite helpful in exploring the landscape of variation in NOD. I don't quite agree with your subtle point about association studies and not wanting to have redundant polymorphism. If one has an appropriate statistical method for estimating significance, typing a redundant SNP in your association study should cost you nothing. As a throwaway example of why we might study complex diseases, I think it is quite obvious that gene variants involved in pharmacogenetics are much closer to clinical relevance and utility. I think it is valuable to work on this. By chance, the two confirmed modest associations in type 2 diabetes both occur in already-targeted genes. This may point to a unification of all our interests.

Goldstein: I agree completely. One could take account of the correlation among markers by permutation, but in fact this is very often not done. So use of tags would result in a less conservative test when corrections such as Bonferroni are applied.

Daly: Absolutely. That is a problem that transcends the use of blocks or non-blocks. Even if one chooses tags optimally, there is still correlation there. Simply counting the SNPs and correcting by Bonferroni is conservative under any circumstances and should not be the state of the art.

Goldstein: Agreed, even tSNPs have some correlation, and it is more powerful to assess association with permutation than standard correction for multiple comparisons.

Rioux: You showed that there are variants that are more informative in one population than another. So there are clearly population differences. It may therefore be interesting that for Crohn's disease two genes have been identified in Caucasian populations: *CARD15* and *IBD5*. The associated alleles for these two genes are of either very low frequency or absent in Asian- and African-derived populations. Do you think that it is a coincidence that these variants for the same disease are only found in Caucasians and affect disease susceptibility in those populations and not in others? If not, what would you draw from this?

Goldstein: I have no idea whether it is a coincidence or not. But let's say that it is not a coincidence. What would I infer from that? If it isn't a coincidence the explanation is that functional variation has been influenced by selection and selection pressures haven't been the same across human populations. This is an extremely interesting general question. Is it the case or not that for the variation which I define as associated with common diseases and drug responses, the pattern of geographical variation has been influenced by selection? This is an important question and I suspect that we don't have the data to answer this at the moment. It would be extremely interesting to know the answer. It may be that one of the reasons we have the common disease that we do have is that we have variants that have been selected to do different things in different populations. Then when those variants come into new genetic backgrounds or environments, they can become deleterious. It also could be practically useful to answer this question. If it is true that the variants that influence disease are systematically more likely to have frequency differences among populations, we could use that information in some kind of a weighting scheme when we do our association work.

Rioux: Immunologists can really understand selection!

Hafler: This relates to the potential benefits of admixture studies. For example, multiple sclerosis (MS) is very rare in subjects of African descent, and is a disease predominantly of Caucasian descent. If one looks at African-Americans they appear to have about one-third the incidence of Caucasians. It can be hypothesized that the higher incidence of MS in the African–Americans as compared to Africans is related to the introduction of European ancestry into the African–American population. This raises the issue that there may be MS risk genes that are monomorphic in the Caucasian population and define risk for that whole population; that is, genes that were selected in the bottle-neck out of Africa. In these instances, association studies will not allow us to detect them and the use of a transmission disequilibrium test (TDT) analysis examining Caucasian populations will not show any variation. However, it doesn't mean this variant isn't an important disease risk factor, and the only way we might be able to get to this is to compare the Caucasian populations with African populations by doing these admixture studies.

Seed: In terms of understanding where the biological basis of selection comes from, it is important to recognize that there are probably very different forces at play. I am going to advance a bias of mine about pharmacogenetic influences: that polymorphic and selected variations mostly arise from differences in diet. For example, you can find animals that are capable of eating one kind of food. For example, rabbits can eat tomatoes. The leaves are poisonous to most other species but rabbits can eat them. When you think about the genes that are involved in drug transformation, they are mostly xenobiotic transformations. For the most part we would never have been exposed evolutionarily to the drugs that have recently appeared in our systems. This suggests to me that there ought to be a strong contribution of geographic variation specifically in those genes that are most likely to be affected by pharmacogenetic transformations. You might find isolated populations forced by circumstances to choose a particular food source, and then only those that had a particular resistance to a toxin or ability to use a substrate survived.

Goldstein: For drug metabolism, that is my guess as well. There is even some evidence that differences in diet have influenced patterns of variation in drug-metabolizing enzymes. There is a hypothesis that Magnus Ingelman-Sundberg (Karolinska Institute) put forward that the cline in *CYP2D6* nulls through Europe is influenced by alkaloids. You get a high frequency of nulls in northern Europe, but almost none in the Arabian peninsula. The idea is that there are more alkaloids there, however this hasn't yet been addressed systematically. It would be interesting to take a large set of functional variants of drug-metabolizing enzymes and ask whether their overall pattern of geographic variation is statistically distinguishable from a set of functional variants in another class of genes. This would be interesting to do.

Bowcock: Getting back to Dr Hafler's question, I would like to propose that we will be able to identify autoimmunity genes in a single population, because both predisposing and protective (or non-predisposing) alleles still exist in most populations. For example, we believe that many genes involved in autoimmune disease will be immune system genes. Some of these have arisen due to selection against pathogens. However, different individuals respond differently to pathogens, presumably because of the presence of different immune system alleles. These alleles presumably exist together in the population due to balancing selection. This then leads on to the questions, are individuals with autoimmune disease at one-end of a continuum of allelic distributions and can we find genes for autoimmunity by looking for immune system genes that are under balancing selection? There is already a precedence that some immune system genes are under balancing selection. These include CD4 (Prahalad et al 2003), CCR5 (Bamshad et al 2002) and many genes within the MHC (Hughes et al 1998). In the case of a psoriasis susceptibility locus that we found on chromosome 17, we see two complementary haplotypes that are common in the population (Helms et al 2003). I wonder whether this region, that negatively regulates T cell activation, is subject to balancing selection? I know that Mark Daly has frequently observed the existence of two common complementary haplotypes in the genome and although coalescence theory has been used to explain the presence of many of them, some could exist today due to balancing selection.

Rioux: Could you briefly define for the audience the terms balancing selection and coalescence?

Bowcock: Balancing selection is where two alleles exist stably in a population. The theory is that normally if you have two alleles at a particular location, one is on its way to extinction and one is on its way to fixation. The classical example of balancing selection is the sickle cell mutation in malarial areas, where both the wild-type and mutant forms of the β globin gene are maintained. Both alleles are maintained because the heterozygote is 'fitter' than either homozygote. As soon as you leave the malarial areas the sickle cell mutation is lost. So my question was, have we selected for two alleles within some immune system genes as a result of balancing selection (perhaps due to protection from local pathogens), and are some of these alleles now predisposing us to autoimmunity?

Kere: I'd like to moderate the emphasis on selection. From the little I have learned in the past, when you look at neutral markers which many blood group antigens are supposed to be, there is a lot of variation in their frequencies between populations that is purely drift.

Foote: I strongly disagree.

Cookson: I think that's unlikely, isn't it?

Kere: The point is that we could perhaps pick a set of loci where there are no genes nearby, and see how much variation there is for those. Would we see a difference between drug-metabolizing genes and random genes?

Goldstein: That is a workable approach in principle.

Kere: Classically these blood group genes have been used as markers for assessing drift.

Foote: A lot of blood group markers are still under strong selection.

Kere: Let's take other markers then.

Foote: Are there any neutral markers? The entire genome has to be under some sort of selection. Just because we don't know what the selection is doesn't mean that it isn't present.

Kere: I agree that a lot of the genome must be under selection. What I am saying, however, is that the drift that has occurred across human populations may be an even stronger player than selection.

Goldstein: There are almost certainly parts of the genome that can be thought of as neutral, in the sense that any selected variant has a zone of influence, depending on the strength of selection and the recombination rate. It will influence some set of neighbouring sites. It will be hard to be absolutely certain that you have a set of variants that are not under selection. You could, however, have a set of variants that are much less likely to be under selection than coding variants, for example. You could take a large set of such variants and try to use them to get a background picture of the amount of differentiation among populations. This could be used as a comparator for asking questions about specific variants. A tiny bit of work has been done in this direction, and what we know is that it is hard to do.

Kere: Perhaps one measure would be how many different allelic structures there are in the gene. If you only have two, or if you have 12, this might be signifying something about their function or selection.

Wakeland: In terms of the relationship between autoimmune susceptibility alleles and balancing selection, HLA is an outstanding example. Many HLA class

I and class II allelic lineages have extremely long coalescence times, to the extent that lineages of alleles can be traced back through multiple primate species. Many of these same allelic lineages are associated strongly with autoimmune disease in human populations, indicating that autoimmune susceptibility alleles can have extremely ancient origins. Some type of balancing selection must be responsible for maintaining these alleles in natural populations. In mice there is a good opportunity to show that coalescence times are long, because there are a variety of well-documented subspecies. By comparing alleles in various sub-species, it is possible to trace allelic lineages on an evolutionary timescale. We have actually done this for *TIM1*, *CTLA4* and the *CD150* family and this analysis indicates that the allelic lineages associated with autoimmunity for these genes are often very common and can have origins that predate sub-speciation events in mice. This suggests that many autoimmune disease alleles are common in natural populations, possibly being maintained by pathogen-driven selection.

Goodnow: What is coalescence?

Wakeland: It refers to the most recent evolutionary timepoint at which you can say that two alleles had a common ancestor.

Abbas: Isn't selection for genes that maintain various control mechanisms fairly obvious? Are you implying that there is a selection for polymorphisms associated with autoimmunity?

Wakeland: Selection for polymorphism, termed balancing selection, is not very common. This type of selection is distinct from purifying selection, in which a specific single function is being maintained during evolutionary divergence. Balancing selection refers to a situation in which two different versions of a gene's function are maintained in a natural population.

Seed: The natural extension of that would be gene duplication and the natural representation of both alleles. Do you see any examples of that?

Wakeland: In the case of gene families such as the HLA complex, there are clearly duplications occurring, as well as balancing selection. A limited number of HLA molecules do the bulk of antigen presentation to T cells, which may indicate that too much duplication in this function is deleterious for the development of an efficient immune system. However, limitations in the number of presenting molecules leads to gaps in the presentation of all possible peptides in the immune system of any individual, which is thought to lead to selective pressures to maintain polymorphic forms of HLA molecules that exhibit changes in peptide presentation properties. Whatever the evolutionary mechanism may be, the HLA gene complex exhibits both genetic duplications affecting many functional loci, as well as extensive genetic polymorphisms affecting the structures of the peptide binding grooves.

Rao: You raised the specific example of phenytoin. Allele number three had variant copies. If you combined those polymorphisms there was a 130 mg variation in dose. But the actual variation that you mentioned across the entire patient population was 800 mg. Clearly there are other genes affecting this, and it would seem mostly not to be drug metabolism but actually targeted genes for the drug itself.

Goldstein: There are other things affecting dose sensitivity. I don't know whether there are other gene variants. I was struck that we saw association despite not controlling for various non genetic factors. Patients are on a whole bunch of other drugs and phenytoin is just added in, some are on monotherapy, all sorts of epilepsies are represented, and so on. All these factors are not actually being taken into account. It is a broad range of doses: there may be other genetic factors but there may not be. The rest of the variation might be largely environmental.

Hafler: Did you look at drug levels?

Goldstein: Typically, that is not done for phenytoin in the UK. We don't have pharmacogenetic data.

Cookson: What was the r^2 for the variation?

Goldstein: Together the *SCN1A* and *CYP2C9* variants explain only about 4% of the total variation in tolerated dose in this unselected retrospective study.

Ting: I wanted to follow up the issues of the environment and the *CARD15* association with IBD in Caucasians but not in Japanese. IBD is likely affected by diet changes and perhaps also local bacterial populations. A very important line of studies in colon cancer has examined different ethnic groups raised in different places. In those cases colon cancer and high blood pressure can be shown to have a major dietary component. Has this been studied with IBD and *CARD15* association?

Rioux: The first question that has to be addressed is the epidemiology of the disease across different populations. Those studies for IBD are quite limited. Another related question is that since these variants have been identified, we can now look at how these variants are associated with intermediate phenotypes and the interactions with environmental influences. This is currently revealing some interesting findings. Comprehensive studies of environmental influences are hindered, as is the case with many diseases, by the fact that most epidemiological studies have not coupled to genetic studies and vice versa.

Wakeland: I have a question on a topic raised in Mark Daly's talk. We have been fine-mapping various regions of the genome and find that recombinational 'hotspots' are a common feature of recombination within a given area. However, they are not necessarily in the same place in all crosses, thus their locations appear to be strain dependent. What is the current thinking about recombinational hotspots in the human genome? Are they very stable, or is this a vague concept that may be dependent on the two chromosomes that are undergoing recombination?

Daly: A little bit of each. Within humans they are relatively stable from one population to another, with the LD patterns largely conserved. In the African populations there is a much greater history of mutation and recombination so there are additional sites of recombination. Interestingly, this does not seem to translate much further back in history. The observations in mice in a variety of settings have indicated variable intensities of hotspots. When we look at chimpanzee LD, the human hotspots are clearly not hotspots of recombination. The hotspots in humans and chimps are positionally unrelated to each other. This is very interesting and suggests that attempts to find common sequence motifs that account for this are destined to failure. What we know from yeast suggests that this probably wasn't going to work out anyway. What this all might propose is that to some degree there might be a great deal of haplotype specificity, or in some other way a connection between recombination and mutation. The hotspots are flaming themselves out over relatively short periods evolutionarily.

Wakeland: How do you distinguish between the end of LD due to historical events and a recombinational hotspot? Because you see an LD block end doesn't mean that there must be a recombinational hotspot.

Daly: In some cases there can be one specific recombinational event occurring early in history that happened to rise to great prominence to break down the LD. There are several sophisticated methods (most developed in Peter Donnelly's lab) that enable us to estimate the recombination rate from population genetic LD data. For example, in the most simplistic terms, if one can see four or five haplotypes in gene A and then four or five in an adjacent gene, but can see 20 or 25 different combinations, many independent events have occurred. On the basis of these sorts of observations, one can actually develop models where the actual underlying recombination rate is estimated. In cases where sperm typing has been done, for example, these methods appear to be quite accurate.

Vyse: I wanted to follow up on the question about susceptibility to infection. The genetics of susceptibility to infection and the genetics of the susceptibility to autoimmune disease are strongly related. These are common issues. We have some data that reflects this. The influence of Fcγ receptor polymorphism is related, for example, to lupus. There is evidence to suggest that this may influence the resistance or otherwise of mice within wild-type populations to infection. This suggests that the data emerging on genetic polymorphisms—in particular populations—affecting the resistance to disease are something we could take advantage of in relation to our analyses of autoimmune diseases.

Abbas: One general question that has been plaguing me is that you could have predicted the polymorphisms in drug sensitivities on the basis of known pathways. So why is this so unsuccessful when we look at autoimmune disease? Is this because of our ignorance of pathways? I don't think we are that ignorant.

Cookson: I think we are completely ignorant about large parts of what the immune system is doing. The traditional view of immunity focused on the adaptive immune system, and it is only recently that we have grudgingly accepted the importance of the innate immune system. The amount of energy spent on immunity in the genome hasn't even been imagined. The only way we will get to this is through genetics. There are likely to be huge numbers of pathways of which we are all unaware.

Abbas: I think we will revisit this question. There are several people in this room who are taking an approach to identifying pathways that is not based on open-ended genomics. In my view, given the challenges of creating genomewide haplotype maps, we have the potential to learn an awful lot without them. Let's just look at 200 genes instead of all of them.

Hafler: As someone who has studied pathways in immunology and autoimmunity, dealing with the cell or pathway *de jour* has been frustrating. There are so many pathways potentially out there and it is so difficult to study them in human diseases, that we need to move to genetics.

Abbas: Linda Wicker knows this better than I do, but identifying a *CTLA4* polymorphism that turns out to be a splice variant was entirely based on knowing a particular pathway and its significance. There was no other rationale for going after this.

Kere: Let's look at what has been discovered. We have four examples of positionally cloned asthma genes, and none of these was ever near a candidate gene for anything we knew from before. For psoriasis we now have 8–10 loci, and for one of these there was an obvious candidate gene, the HLA region. Even then, it is not certain that this is the functional gene.

Abbas: Of course, we don't know if any of them are functional genes. You could always argue that these associations don't count. They are not the right ones because we don't know whether they are functional. If you want to take the devil's advocate extreme approach, you can say that the only functional ones you will find are those related to known pathways, and those you have found by linkage or association analysis are irrelevant.

Cookson: The MHC was only found by genetics. It was a genetic discovery.

Abbas: It was a genetic discovery resulting from a precise question. That illustrates exactly the point I was making. People were looking for genes that controlled graft rejection. That's why it is called what it is.

Wakeland: Actually, Peter Gorer and George Snell were not studying graft rejection, but rather cancer resistance.

Abbas: It turned out to be transplantation the minute they were inbred. It really was graft rejection. If you go looking for a specific gene for a specific pathway will you find it, as in this case?

Bowcock: There are 30–40 000 genes and we only know the function of 5000 or so.

Hafler: How many pathways are left to be discovered?

Goodnow: That is why we are doing genomewide mutagenesis in mice. We don't know how many new pathways there are. My sense is that if you look at the few spontaneous mutants that are popping up which cause autoimmune disease, we are clearly well away from saturation. Take *Foxp3*: we don't understand that pathway. What is upstream or downstream of it? My sense is that we are at the beginnings of this process for autoimmune disease, as opposed to TCR signalling which has been intensely taken apart.

Abbas: Obviously, it is not an all or nothing issue, but if you were to do the next set of analyses, would you go upstream and downstream of *Foxp3*? Is this what we should be doing rather than this open-ended search?

Rao: The best of both worlds is the targeted elimination of every gene, looking for their effects of autoimmunity of any kind.

Abbas: But you will only be detecting the high penetrance single-gene mutations.

Goodnow: You are assuming that one gene makes one protein makes one trait. Yet what we are looking at is much more complex. For example, with *Zap70*, depending upon where you inherit a missense mutation you get immunodeficiency or the paradoxical opposite in Sakaguchi's autoimmunity. Even for the best-studied proteins, in pathways we understand, depending upon the nature of the genetic variant all bets are off as to what is going to happen.

Hafler: The variation in autoimmune diseases is unlikely to be a result of complete ablation but could be affected by common variations with subtle differences in function.

Rao: I agree, we have to go beyond the knockouts.

Kere: We could change every amino acid, one at a time, in each protein!

Seed: I heard an interesting talk by Bruce Beutler, who is doing a forward genetic screen with ENU mutagenesis of innate immunity in mice. He started looking at mice with overt visual phenotypes and found out that about 20% of them had immune deficits of one sort or another. He saw a number of examples among this genre of not fully penetrant alleles which had powerful immune deficiency phenotypes. The immune system is probably a sensitive antenna for collecting all sorts of perturbations to different pathways.

Kere: Some of them are going to be antigenic properties that we are looking at and not functional properties.

Wakeland: Is there a way to detect functional polymorphisms within populations? At a genomewide level can you find genes that are polymorphic in a manner that makes them look as though they are being maintained by balancing selection? Identifying such genes would allow investigations to focus on polymorphisms with functional consequences.

Abbas: How would you do this?

Wakeland: Coalescence times would be one way, or possibly looking at the ratio of synonymous and non-synonymous mutations. If you could demonstrate that certain genes have more amino acid substitutions or that their alleles have much longer lineage coalescence times than would be predicted by neutrality, then this would indicate that their polymorphisms have functional consequences, which would make them excellent candidates for common disease involvement.

Foote: There are examples of that in the mouse. If you do a mouse cross there are certain things you don't see because presumably they are lethal. There are obviously loci that work synergistically, where you have to have two given alleles or you can't have either. When we have good descriptions of the HapMap, will we be able to look at genomewide LD, rather than just blocks of LD, to see whether we can detect LD between loci, presumably starting off with a candidate approach and seeing whether there is LD between distant regions.

Goldstein: There will be examples where a variant that is functional has been under selection. The evidence for this can be seen through some kind of test of neutrality based on variation in one population. There are some examples of this that look convincing, such as *CCR5*. There are lots of population genetic reasons for not being confident that this approach will be powerful enough to show that a variant does something. If you say, let's take a genomewide approach to that, I would not be remotely confident that the seemingly normal variants do anything. One example of this is stabilizing selection. It is very hard to see the effect of something that makes frequencies more similar across populations, because we are very different from one another. Given that we are not very different in the first place a force that makes the frequencies more similar is very hard to detect. Yes, there are some extreme examples where you see it and you ought to be interested in that polymorphism, but it is not a powerful approach overall to organizing the 10 million polymorphisms into those that are likely to do something and those that aren't.

Hafler: Extended haplotype homozygosity (EHH) assesses the age of each haplotype at a gene by measuring the decay of the extended (SNPs far away from the gene) ancestral haplotype, which occurs over time with recombination. Can use of EHH analysis provide information here?

Daly: I agree with David Goldstein: I am not at all confident that we will be able to effectively partition the genome on the basis of evidence of selection, into functional and non-functional categories. Most of the small number of variants that have been confirmed as involved in complex disease do not show any meaningful signature of selection of any specific flavour. On a genomewide basis I don't think that we will be able to identify many regions as outlying to an extent beyond what might arise by drift.

Wakeland: You are referring to humans. In an experimental model system such as the mouse it may be more tractable.

Goodnow: What if you are doing this on a couple of candidate genes, so you have more power? Then would it be possible?

Wicker: We have two regions where we believe that this is true. Although we have yet to prove the identity of the candidate genes by developing knock-in mice having the suspected causal sequence variation, we have two disease-causing intervals containing a relatively small number of genes where of all of the genes within that interval the prime candidate shows the most evidence of selection. This was surprising to us. In addition, although both of these candidates have changes in their protein sequence, it appears as if an alteration in regulation is the functional change causing the disease phenotype.

Goldstein: It doesn't help if they are candidates already.

Wicker: One of them was a completely unknown gene.

Goldstein: The point is, if you want to use this as a guide to parts of the genome that you want to focus more attention on, then you have to implement it on a genomewide scale.

Wicker: This was picking out what should we try first among 10 genes in a 1 Mb interval.

Goldstein: If it is a small number of genes, you do have more power to detect selection, but if you are already focused on this small number then the diversity perspective doesn't add very much. This is the problem.

Kere: If we accept that the human population has expanded over the last 50 000 years or so, with tremendous diasporas across the planet, I would tend to think that drift has been a much more powerful force over this period of history than selection.

Cookson: 100 years ago 50% of children died.

Goldstein: I think both are true. It is quite clear that there has been a lot of selection. I don't mean to say that we won't see anything from selection: we will. For example, in one of the regions, the *CYP3A* locus, there is almost no variation at all in Europe across four or five genes. It looks like there has been a massive selective sweep in this region. In Africa it is diverse. There will be examples like that, but overall it will not allow us to partition the genome into a set of polymorphisms that we do and don't need to worry about.

Rioux: I'd like to make a comment to bring this together for people who aren't thinking about genetics all the time. The likely reality is that there will be a spectrum of different disease-causing alleles in terms of frequency, genetic effect, and influence of selection. Consequently, the various genetic approaches will prove to be complementary, no single approach being perfect and therefore we will need them all.

References

Bamshad MJ, Mummidi S, Gonzalez E et al 2002 A strong signature of balancing selection in the 5' cis-regulatory region of CCR5. Proc Natl Acad Sci USA 99:10539–10544

Hughes AL, Yeager M 1998 Natural selection at major histocompatibility complex loci of vertebrates. Annu Rev Genet 32:415–435

Helms C, Cao L, Krueger JG et al 2003 A putative RUNX1 binding site variant between SLC9A3R1 and NAT9 is associated with susceptibility to psoriasis. Nat Genet 35:349–356

Prahalad S, Wooding S, Dunn D, Weiss R, Jorde LB, Bamshad M 2003 A signature of balancing selection in the human CD4 gene. Am J Hum Genet, Annual Meeting 2003, A27

Multiple sclerosis: a haplotype association study

Simon J. Foote*[†], Justin P. Rubio*[†], Melanie Bahlo*[†], Trevor J. Kilpatrick*[†], Terence P. Speed*[†], Jim Stankovich*[†], Rachel Burfoot*[†], Helmut Butzkueven*[†], Laura Johnson*[†], Chris Wilkinson*[†], Bruce Taylor[‡], Michele Sale[†§], Ingrid A. F. van der Mei[†§], Joanne L. Dickinson[†§] and Patricia Groom[†§]

*The Walter and Eliza Hall Institute of Medical Research, 1G Royal Parade, Parkville, Melbourne, Victoria 3050, †The CRC for the Discovery of Genes for Complex Diseases, ‡The Royal Hobart Hospital, and §The Menzies Centre, Hobart, Tasmania, Australia

> Abstract. Results are presented from a genomewide haplotype association study on multiple sclerosis (MS) cases from Tasmania, an island state of Australia. Cases were ascertained on strict clinical and radiological grounds and on the fact that they had at least one grandparent born in the state. This enriched for early settler chromosomes among present day Tasmanians with MS and increased the chances of finding common haplotype sharing at disease predisposition loci in distant relatives sharing common ancestral haplotypes. Four-to-five close relatives were also collected for each of 170 cases and 105 population-based controls. All were genotyped at a 5 cM resolution, haplotypes reconstructed and sharing estimated using an empirical approach based on sorting haplotypes to find the most common at each locus and then generating a test statistic for excess sharing in the cases based on permutation testing. Five initial loci were found where there was an excess sharing in the cases. These were fine-mapped with 10–12 additional markers. Only loci on chromosomes 6 and 10 remained after fine mapping. These loci demonstrate an increase in sharing of multi-marker haplotypes in MS cases compared to both population control transmitted haplotypes and case non-transmitted haplotypes.
>
> *2005 The genetics of autoimmunity. Wiley, Chichester (Novartis Foundation Symposium 267) p 31–45*

Multiple sclerosis (MS) is a neurodegenerative disease of the CNS characterized by anatomical and temporarily discreet lesions. The disease can lead to severe neurological impairment and the current immunomodulatory therapy is far from effective and is very expensive. It is widely believed that the disease has significant genetic and environmental components. Evidence for a significant genetic influence comes from twin studies where the concordance in monozygotic (MZ) twins is 25%, falling to 3% in dizygotic (DZ) twins (Ebers et al 1986, Sadovnick et al 1993, Robertson et al 1996). Attempts at identification of both the environmental and genetic factors have been pursued with vigour over the last decade (and beyond).

Several affected sib pair (ASP) and other family-based studies have been performed on MS patients from Finland, Europe and America (Sawcer et al 1996, Haines et al 1996, Ebers et al 1996, The Transatlantic Multiple Sclerosis Genetics Cooperative 2001, Akesson et al 2002). The outcome of these studies was disappointing. There was insufficient power to detect susceptibility loci, and even the major histocompatibility complex (MHC) needed seeding for detection in a couple of the studies. However these studies were useful in detecting several 'suggestive' regions and they also answered the question about the anticipated relative risk attributable to susceptibility loci. It will be small. Obviously extremely large numbers of ASPs will be needed in order to find linkage to regions carrying susceptibility genes. Given the incidence of disease and the frequency of affected sibs, this may not be possible. Recognizing this, a large allelic association study has been attempted using cases and controls, pooled and genotyped with simple sequence length polymorphism (SSLP) markers (Sawcer et al 2002, Goedde et al 2002). This study has not been successful, due probably to the insufficient density of markers required to cover the genome and difficulties inherent in the technical approach. This lack of success has not been limited to MS; many other studies of the genetics of complex diseases have foundered on similar difficulties. It may therefore be time to investigate alternative strategies in locus identification in genetically complex diseases.

One way around the difficult problem inherent in complex genetic diseases is to decrease the complexity by working with 'special populations'; this approach has been used to solve several diseases. In appropriate circumstances it can provide a powerful tool to identify regions containing disease genes by linkage disequilibrium. With a founder effect in an isolated population, a given disease haplotype may be enriched, making it easy to identify by either allelic or haplotypic association (Hastbacka et al 1992, Lee et al 2001). Traditionally, the populations used have been old populations where there has been a tight bottleneck and where time has resulted in significant erosion of the disease haplotype. The small size of the residual region in linkage disequilibrium (LD) means that the region containing the disease haplotype must be identified through some other means than association, e.g. linkage. The tight bottleneck means that most affected individuals in the population will share the same disease haplotype. This is fine for diseases where enrichment of a rare disease allele can occur but difficulties arise when the disease is caused by a common allelic variant with a decreased penetrance, as many would claim is the genetic basis for the common, complex diseases.

We have taken an intermediate approach. We have used a population with a recent, fairly wide bottleneck and generated haplotypes in control and case individuals to perform a case-control haplotype association study at a genomewide level. Patients and controls were recruited from Tasmania.

Tasmania is an island state off the south-eastern coast of Australia. Tasmania has a population of about 500 000 and around 60% of this population are descended from the early settlers. These arrived from England and Ireland in the mid 19th century (King 1986). There was little immigration into the state from that time and there was a massive efflux of males in the 1860s when gold was discovered in the neighbouring state of Victoria. Present descendants from a common settler are separated by 10–16 meioses. Modelling and previous studies in Tasmania would suggest the average haplotypic size shared between today's descendants of an early settler would average 25 cM. Obviously this has a large variance. The underlying assumption in this study is that there are present day Tasmanians with MS who share a common ancestor and therefore a common disease haplotype. This haplotype will be present on a large common chromosomal segment and will be detectable by genotyping at a 5 cM resolution. The haplotype common to related MS patients will be found by an increase of haplotypic sharing around the disease gene. There is no assumption that there will be only one haplotype in this population and indeed, it is conceivable that there will be more than one haplotype showing an increase in sharing over that seen in the controls.

Methods

Haplotype reconstruction

Given the paucity of candidate MS susceptibility loci, a genomewide haplotype association study was performed. This requires accurate haplotype reconstruction. We performed simulations with various family structures to determine the best collection of relatives with which to reconstruct haplotypes. Haplotypes were reconstructed with GENEHUNTER. The ideal set of relatives included both parents along with either a couple of sibs or a grandparent. This analysis directed the collection of close relatives of both cases and controls. Four or five relatives were collected for each case and control. These, along with the case and control were genotyped at an average density of 5 cM using the Applied Biosystems HD-5™ marker set. The collection of close relatives not only allowed accurate haplotype reconstruction but was also extremely useful in identifying genotyping errors, which can be very misleading in an association study.

Patient collection

Patients were recruited through the efforts of the local MS Association and through media advertisements. To enrich for patients with immigrant settlers as ancestors, only patients with a grandparent born in Tasmania were recruited. All respondents were interviewed and examined by one of the six participating neurologists. In addition, when available, magnetic resonance images (MRI) were assessed or, at a minimum MRI reports were obtained. The Poser criteria of clinically definite or laboratory-supported definite MS were set as the minimum standard by which patients were included in the study, but in addition, patients were required to have cerebral MRI abnormalities consistent with MS, as defined by the criteria of Paty et al (1988). All patients with a classification of primary progressive MS had to exhibit progressive neurological disability for at least one year, to have no other better explanation for the clinical features and to have not only relevant spinal cord abnormalities but also changes on cerebral MRI consistent with demyelination. 170 cases and 105 closely matched controls were collected. Many of the controls were spouses of the cases. An average of 4.5 individuals were collected per case or control family.

Data analysis

Due to the large number of genotypes called ($\sim 10^6$) we developed a pipeline to manage the data. This was largely written in Perl and the data was first scanned for relationship inconsistencies using PREST (McPeek & Sun 2000). Once pedigree inconsistencies were resolved, the data was scanned for genotyping inconsistencies with PEDCHECK (O'Connell & Weeks 1998). A CGI-PERL script was developed to provide a web interface that generates an easy to review summary of the genotyping errors. This interface assists in data cleaning and file translation. It also makes parsing of large output files from PREST, PEDCHECK and other data summary programs possible. Excess recombination events were detected with the software packages SIBMED (Douglas et al 2000) and MERLIN (Abecasis et al 2002). Allelic inconsistencies were treated by setting the genotype to 'null'.

Genomewide haplotypes were produced from the genotype data. LINAGE-style files were produced using the in-house program LINKPREP. Haplotypes were inferred probabilistically with GENEHUNTER v 2.1 (Kruglyak et al 1996) using the Viterbi algorithm with population allele frequencies estimated from 343 unaffected founders. The accuracy of the haplotype calls was validated by simulation studies using MERLIN. A given pair of haplotypes was strongly preferred over all others for each case and control.

It was anticipated that at a disease locus cases would share an extended haplotype above that seen in the controls. In order to measure sharing, at each individual locus, alleles are sorted on frequency. At the most common allele, sorting is next based on haplotype frequencies using flanking markers. At each new haplotype a test statistic is calculated using a standard permutation procedure. An empirical distribution is generated by randomly assigning haplotypes from the data into 'case' and 'control'. The test statistic is based on a series of two-by-two contingency tables whose significance is evaluated using a standard χ^2 one degree of freedom (d.f.) test statistic. The entries in the contingency table are based on the remaining number of case and control haplotypes sharing the most frequent haplotype as determined by an initial sort of the case haplotypes. The assumption is that the disease haplotypes will be represented by the most frequent allele in case haplotypes at marker i, where sorting commenced. The addition of further χ^2 statistics occurs as long as more than five haplotypes remain in an ancestral cluster. This is analogous to 'growing the haplotype'. This test statistic is valid only for the test performed and is not able to be extrapolated to a genomewide significance level. Computationally, this algorithm is manifest in a Perl program 'HAPLOCLUSTERS' which sorts haplotypes, imputes missing data and produces a test statistic for each marker with a P-value and standard error.

This sharing statistic was computed using the two controls inherent in the study design. Control haplotypes were deduced from the population controls but there were also the non-transmitted haplotypes as deduced from the cases. The use of two sets of controls was important in confirmation of the regions where there was excessive sharing in the cases. It was also possible to calculate the amount of background LD by comparing the two control populations.

Haplotypes demonstrating excess sharing were ranked based on a number of criteria: a sharing statistic more than two orders of magnitude greater than that seen for background LD; sharing stretching over more than one marker; regions showing previous evidence of association or linkage and; regions showing a rejection of the null hypothesis using a Q–Q (quantile–quantile) plot.

Fine mapping

Regions showing excess sharing were genotyped with additional markers in all cases, controls and family members. An additional 10–12 SSLP markers were selected from the region surrounding the peak of association. The analysis of these further haplotypes was as described above.

Results

Candidate MS loci

Five regions were initially chosen as potential MS susceptibility loci. These regions had a P-value more than two orders of magnitude greater than the background LD, the sharing extended over 2 or more markers and they were outliers on the Q–Q plots. These regions can be seen on Fig. 1.

These regions were fine mapped and only two of these regions showed haplotypic sharing with the fine markers. The other three exhibited no sharing at all when the extra markers were added. This indicates that the genomewide haplotypes were identical by state (IBS) and not identical by descent (IBD). It is

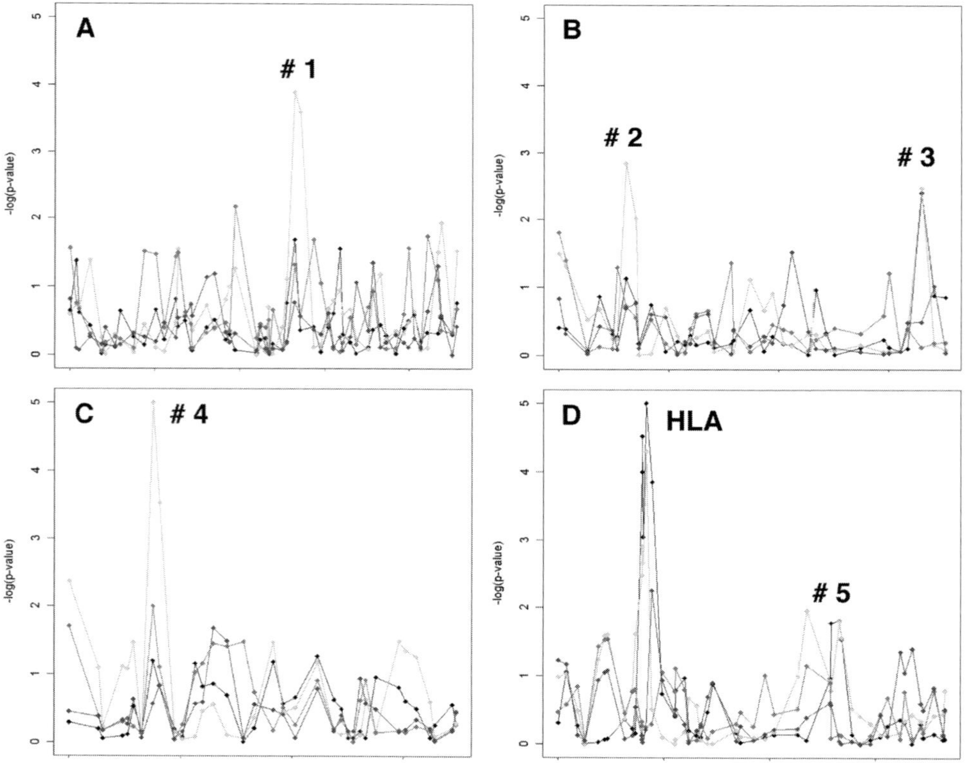

FIG. 1. Genomewide scan data on the five most promising loci. Haplotype sharing was estimated using HAPLOCLUSTER which calculates a P-value based on permutation testing. (A) Chromosome 3; (B) chromosome 10; (C) chromosome 12; and (D) chromosome 6. The following comparisons are presented: transmitted case haplotypes vs. transmitted control haplotypes (black line), transmitted case haplotypes vs. untransmitted case haplotypes (very light grey line), transmitted control haplotypes vs. untransmitted case haplotypes (dark grey line) and untransmitted case haplotypes vs. transmitted control haplotypes (medium grey line)

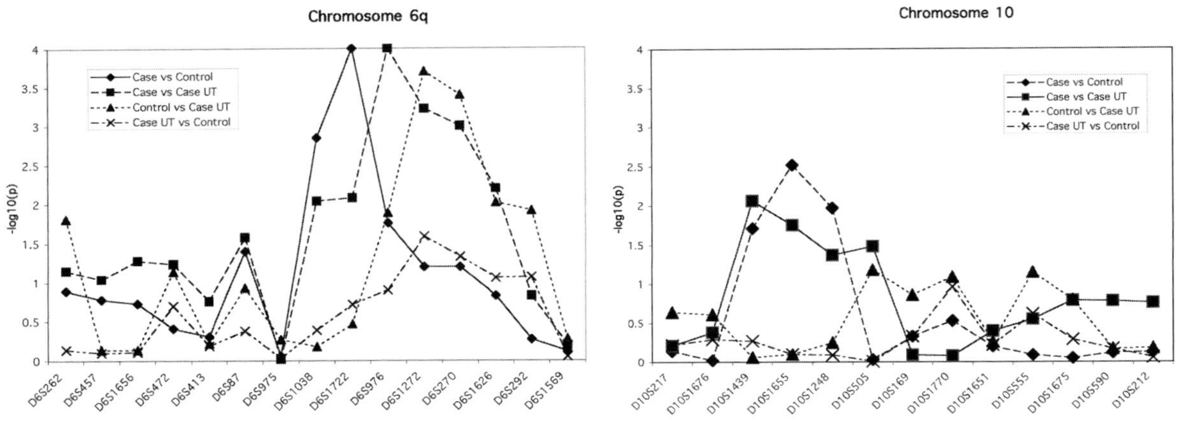

FIG. 2. Fine mapping data on the chromosomes 6 and 10 loci. Haplotype sharing was calculated using HAPLOCLUSTER which calculates a *P*-value based on permutation testing.

likely therefore that the two remaining loci do exhibit IBD, i.e. that these haplotypes do originate from the original Tasmanian settlers. These loci are on chromosomes 6 and 10 (Fig. 2). Chromosome 6 shows some residual background LD, however this is due to one of the original genomewide markers and this disappears if the marker is removed (data not shown). There is no decrease in *P*-value if the sharing statistic is calculated in the absence of the original genomewide scan markers for these two chromosomes indicating that the entire haplotype is shared and therefore it is likely to be IBD.

Interestingly, the MHC region did not appear on the genomewide scan data but was only seen when markers known to be associated with MS were added (Fig. 1).

Discussion

We have used a novel method of finding association of chromosomal segments to disease susceptibility in MS using a Tasmanian population. This method uses a haplotype association approach in a population enabling a course mapping strategy to reconstruct large haplotypes over which sharing can be calculated. The strategy was designed around knowledge of the population structure, the estimated extent of sharing given an inheritance of common, settler chromosomal segments and the family structures needed to reconstruct accurate haplotypes.

Five regions of sharing were identified. Out of these only two remained post-fine mapping. The two that remained (chromosomes 6 and 10) shared one characteristic not present in the other three. Both of these demonstrated *P*-value peaks when the case transmitted chromosome was compared to both control transmitted and case untransmitted. None of the other three loci demonstrated peaks against both controls, despite having greater *P*-values for one of the control comparisons. This confirms the utility of including population-based controls and of not relying on the non-transmitted controls.

There are another four loci where this circumstance is repeated. These loci do not have high *P*-values but there is a peak for both control sets. These are being fine mapped at present.

References

Abecasis GR, Cherny SS, Cookson WO, Cardon LR 2002 Merlin — rapid analysis of dense genetic maps using sparse gene flow trees. Nat Genet 30:97–101

Akesson E, Oturai A, Berg J et al 2002 A genome-wide screen for linkage in Nordic sib-pairs with multiple sclerosis. Genes Immun 3:279–285

Douglas JA, Boehnke M, Lange K 2000 A multipoint method for detecting genotyping errors and mutations in sibling-pair linkage data. Am J Hum Genet 66:1287–1297

Ebers GC, Bulman DE, Sadovnick AD et al 1986 A population-based study of multiple sclerosis in twins. N Engl J Med 315:1638–1642

Ebers GC, Kukay K, Bulman DE et al 1996 A full genome search in multiple sclerosis. Nat Genet 13:472–476

Goedde R, Sawcer S, Boehringer S et al 2002 A genome screen for linkage disequilibrium in HLA-DRB1*15-positive Germans with multiple sclerosis based on 4666 microsatellite markers. Hum Genet 111:270–277

Haines JL, Ter-Minassian M, Bazyk A et al 1996 A complete genomic screen for multiple sclerosis underscores a role for the major histocompatability complex. Nat Genet 13:469–471

Hastbacka J, de la Chapelle A, Kaitila I et al 1992 Linkage disequilibrium mapping in isolated founder populations: diastrophic dysplasia in Finland. Nat Genet 2:204–211 (Erratum in Nat Genet 2:343)

King H 1986 (ed) Epidemiology in Tasmania: historical demography and genetic structure of Tasmania. Brolga press, Canberra

Kruglyak L, Daly MJ, Reeve Daly MP, Lander ES 1996 Parametric and nonparametric linkage analysis: a unified multipoint approach. Am J Hum Genet 58:1347–1363

Lee N, Daly MJ, Delmonte et al 2001 A genomewide linkage-distribution scan localizes the Saguenay-Lac-Satint-Jean cytochrome oxidase deficiency to 2p16. Am J Hum Genet 68:397–409

McPeek MS, Sun L 2000 Statistical tests for detection of misspecified relationships by use of genome-screen data. Am J Hum Genet 66:1076–1094

O'Connell JR, Weeks DE 1998 PedCheck: a program for identification of genotype incompatibilities in linkage analysis. Am J Hum Genet 63:259–266

Paty DW, Oger JJ, Kastrukoff LF et al 1988 MRI in the diagnosis of MS: a prospective study with comparison of clinical evaluation, evoked potentials, oligoclonal banding, and CT. Neurology 38:180–185

Robertson NP, Clayton D, Fraser M, Deans J, Compston DA 1996 Clinical concordance in sibling pairs with multiple sclerosis. Neurology 47:347–352

Sadovnick AD, Armstrong H, Rice GP et al 1993 A population-based study of multiple sclerosis in twins: update. Ann Neurol 33:281–285

Sawcer S, Jones HB, Feakes R et al 1996 A genome screen in multiple sclerosis reveals susceptibility loci on chromosome 6p21 and 17q22 [see comments]. Nat Genet 13:464–468

Sawcer S, Maranian M, Setakis E et al 2002 A whole genome screen for linkage disequilibrium in multiple sclerosis confirms disease associations with regions previously linked to susceptibility. Brain 125:1337–1347

The Transatlantic Multiple Sclerosis Genetics Cooperative 2001 A meta-analysis of genomic screens in multiple sclerosis. Mult Scler 7:3–11

DISCUSSION

Goldstein: The first scan was one marker every 5 cM. So why all this effort for haplotypes when the vast majority of pairs of markers won't have any association?

Foote: They will.

Goldstein: Surely even in Tasmania, most of the markers 5 cM apart don't have high levels of association.

Foote: The idea is that MS cases who are alive today, which actually share an ancestral haplotype, will on average share 25 cM of DNA. We did this by simulation but we have also done this in reality. This study was based on tracing back to a single at-risk haplotype in our founders.

Goldstein: The problem with that is that in a population of 10 000 there is very little effect on diversity. This is a pretty big population unless it stays at 10 000 for a long period. I don't think you are going to have such a big drift effect in that population, or do you have evidence that there is such an effect?

Foote: The idea is that individuals who share a haplotype will share this because they are related. We are looking at large pedigrees.

Goldstein: An at-risk haplotype is unlikely to have been present in a single copy in your original founding population of 10 000. It will have been present in multiple copies. So the time since finding the Tasmanian population is not relevant.

Foote: I disagree: it is completely relevant.

Goldstein: To the extent that there are multiple at-risk haplotypes in the founding population, then the genealogical relationship among those haplotypes at the time of finding is relevant, not the time since.

Foote: I disagree. It is the opposite. There will be multiple disease haplotypes in the founding population.

Goldstein: Let's back up and get some agreement. I could send a population to Mars right now, and they will have some pattern of genealogical variation. The relationships among at-risk haplotypes in that population on Mars have to do with the relationships among the haplotypes that they carried with them when they went to Mars. I guess the point I am making is that the Tasmanian examples exist somewhere in between these.

Foote: In 200 years from now these newly arrived Martians will have expanded their population from 10 000 to say 500 000. Over that time some of the risk haplotypes will have died away and others will have expanded. There will be two dozen copies of them, say.

Hafler: Do we know that? Why wouldn't they just reflect the population that was there at the beginning?

Goldstein: The point I am making is that this is not much drift. A population size of 10 000 for a few generations is very little genetic drift. If you want a lot of genetic drift over a short period you need a very small population size.

Foote: The idea is that if you have 24 individuals who carry the disease haplotype and you can ascertain everyone in that population who has the disease, if that particular haplotype is more common in your MS cases than in controls you will pick it up.

Daly: One of you is talking about haplotypes in different parts in the genome and one of you is talking about haplotypes at the same location.

Kere: You are basically saying that when you are selecting your cases you are selecting for the risk-causing haplotypes. Then you compare whether your net for risk-causing haplotypes has an excess of certain haplotypes when compared with the population background.

Goldstein: That is reasonable. But what I am saying is that the expectation that they will be tracing back to a founder chromosome that has been amped up in frequency to a very different frequency than the source population over a short period is not reasonable.

Foote: That is not what the test is.

Goldstein: What I am saying is that if I am right, then you should not get different results if you went and did this on the Australian mainland than in Tasmania. Your claim is that this is not true.

Foote: It is not possible for us to do this on urbanised populations on the Australian mainland.

Daly: You are looking for something that is rare and penetrant that would look different on Tasmania than on the mainland.

Foote: If you look at the MS population in Melbourne, it isn't even possible to identify association with the HLA. The ethnic background of Melbournians is so eclectic.

Goldstein: That is a different point. Rare variants are expected to be changed by the kind of drift that you might have in the population in Tasmania, but not common ones.

Foote: I don't disagree with that; but this was not the basis on which the study was performed.

Abbas: Have these loci been picked up in other attempts to do haplotype mapping in MS populations?

Foote: To my knowledge there have not been any other studies. The only other study that looks like this is one done on depression in South America, where they used similar haplotype association studies.

Goodnow: If it was like the NOD gene in IBD, where it is a relatively infrequent variant that occurs on two or three haplotypes, then this is like a trait in an F6 intercross in mice. Am I missing something?

Hafler: It is not an F6 cross because you are starting with a broad population. The critical point to understand what David Goldstein is saying is that you start with a large population and make an analysis after a few generations. What you start with and end with is not terribly different. There is not enough of a bottleneck to see a significant effect.

Goldstein: That is exactly right.

Hafler: It is not an F6 cross where you are starting with a bottleneck of two mice. You are starting with a vast number of mice.

Goodnow: But if you were starting with 10 strains intercrossed to make 10 000 mice, and only a few of them actually carried a Mendelian locus, then it would be different.

Hafler: It is not a Mendelian locus: they are common traits.

Goodnow: That's an assumption.

Hafler: One important fundamental issue begs the question: are the autoimmune diseases due to rare mutations, which come together, or are they common variants? We don't know the answer.

Abbas: I want to take Chris Goodnow's reasoning one step further. The prediction is that there won't be many changes from the starting population to the current population. What is the implication of this?

Goldstein: You might expect rare variants to be changed to a degree, but not common variants. The point is that this strategy applied in Tasmania wouldn't be expected to identify long-range at-risk haplotypes because they have been amplified in frequency by the drift process. This is what I understood the expectation to be here. On the basis of the population genetics we would not expect to do better in this population at identifying common variants using this kind of approach than you would in another population that doesn't have stratification issues associated with it. On the other hand, it is true that even populations of that size can have an important effect on very rare variants, and your mapping strategy can be affected by that level of drift. I don't know how that would play out in this strategy because one marker per 5 cM is not a good way of picking up rare variants. The point I am making is that for the common things you don't expect much drift.

Kere: I guess the whole point here is that Simon Foote wanted to go to that population because the relatively short population history after the bottleneck, irrespective of the size of the bottleneck, allows him to see fairly long haplotypes, many of which happen to be true haplotypes. If you go with the same resolution of markers to the more general population, your things wouldn't be haplotypes.

Goldstein: I would like to see some data on this, showing how the long-range LD patterns differ in Tasmania. It is difficult to do this in a statistical way. My expectation from population genetics theory is that the effect would be modest for anything that is common.

Foote: It depends which markers you look at and which population.

Goldstein: Starting with 10 000, I expect that effect to be modest.

Foote: I still think you are missing the point of this study. There are a number of chromosomes present in the early 1800s in Tasmania. Those are going to be transmitted to what are actually large pedigrees. If those are responsible for MS, you will get a haplotype shared among 25 cM in today's population. If you ascertain on a disease then you will enrich for individuals who actually carry your haplotype that was present 200 years prior.

Goldstein: Not if the haplotyes are present in the same frequencies as they where in the base population. What you are saying is predicated on the drift process changing the haplotype diversity for chromosomes that carry at-risk alleles for

MS. If the current Tasmanian population has exactly the diversity for those chromosomes as the founding population then what you are saying does not apply. My point is that this amount of drift does not change common variation much, though certainly it could change rare variation. So it depends on whether you are looking for rare or common variation.

Foote: The haplotype that we are actually looking for is very rare. It is present in perhaps one person in that 10 000 population. This is a reasonable assumption.

Seed: The danger of thinking about pedigrees is that you don't think about the reconstitution or recreation event. This can happen naturally by intercrossing. When you take a look at the whole population, you have an affected haplotype that could propagate but you are also creating that haplotype anew by intercrossing and it may be from a completely different population. At steady state, because there is no selection, you are creating and destroying those haplotypes with equal frequency.

Foote: We know that the average sharing of a particular haplotypic region is about 25 cM. There isn't enough depth in the population to completely destroy those original founding haplotypes.

Seed: It all depends on how many different genetic contributions go into making up the disease.

Foote: It does and it doesn't. When we looked at these pedigrees before we started this MS work, at that stage we had pedigrees that were related. We were trying to do a pedigree approach for mapping genes for glaucoma. We failed completely. There was a gene that was published at that time so we went in to that population and looked at those individuals who actually shared that particular mutation in these pedigrees. They shared a couple of different haplotypes. There were obviously a couple of different founding mutations coming into Tasmania at the time. The average length of shared haplotype was about 25 cM. On the basis of these data we thought if we could ascertain for disease, it would enrich for those haplotypes present in Tasmania in the 1800s.

Abbas: I am trying to understand the implication of this. If we go with the assumption that autoimmunity is caused by a combination of common variants, does this therefore imply that we should not be focusing our haplotype mapping on homogeneous populations?

Goldstein: It doesn't hurt you to do so, it just doesn't help you.

Abbas: If it is a collection of common variants that differ from one person to another, then looking at these homogeneous populations is not going to be informative.

Daly: The advantages they might have are factors such as common environment and diet, not of common genetic history.

Kere: But you are not worse off.

Abbas: If you have to choose a patient population, you have to start with the assumption that it is a collection of common variants, but would you choose a more heterogeneous population?

Seed: It is a winning strategy to use a small interbred population.

Kere: It is easier to screen for longer and therefore fewer than lots of haplotypes.

Rioux: This is based on another assumption. Look at the French Canadian population in the Saguenay Lac St Jean region where we and others have shown for rare Mendelian traits that LD surrounding the causal allele extends 10–20 cM. These are rare alleles that have come into this population through a single founder, who is responsible for the present day population of carriers of that allele. What I think David is saying for the populations that you are discussing is that unless there was a very large difference in the diversity of what came in versus what is there now, you are not going to see that effect. This allele may be very old and have occurred in multiple individuals that have undergone recombination events, such that when they come into that population they will be the same alleles but they will be on different long-range backgrounds. The challenge is to identify the allele — very different than the case of causal alleles for a rare disease in a founder population.

Foote: I have to agree with David in that if the hypothesis that these are very common alleles was true then we wouldn't pick up anything. It is not obvious that this is the correct hypothesis. We don't have enough power to pick up loci where there are 10 000 different haplotypes in Tasmania at the present time.

Goldstein: I don't think that there is much disagreement here. The point is well established that rare variants can be affected by the kind of bottleneck that you are talking about. What one is doing is zeroing in on precisely those examples by looking at diseases that are more common than expected in a given population, and then finding the chromosomes that are responsible. What has happened is that a very rare chromosome has been increased in frequency and resulted in quite a big change for that rare variant between the present and founding populations. The point I am making is that the expectation is that the kind of drift that you are talking about will not have much effect on common variation. Will this help you to identify common variation because you can use a coarser LD map? I think the answer is no.

Daly: In almost all of the isolated founder populations that people study it is often possible to look retrospectively and see that these mutations were unique, as you have done. It is somewhat challenging to go in a forward direction, using a greater density of markers in order to distinguish those haplotypes from others that have arisen through recombination.

Hafler: Do we think we are dealing with common variations or rare ones? Let's make sure that we get back to this.

Abbas: Many people, like me, who look at high-penetrance rare alleles in mice tend to focus on that end, and we clearly demonstrate that they are capable of causing autoimmunity. But what is the cause of common autoimmune diseases? We need to get to this question: are there collections of common variants?

Rioux: It is biology. It is a spectrum; it is not one extreme or the other.

Goodnow: Is the common variant hypothesis an unfalsifiable hypothesis in a Popperian sense?

Wakeland: Many autoimmune disease alleles are very common. The best example at the moment would be disease-associated HLA alleles. All these alleles are relatively common, globally distributed and are very powerful as disease predisposing elements. The insulin promoter polymorphism in diabetes is another example, in that the susceptibility allele is present in about 60% of the population.

Goodnow: But there is an equal number that are quite rare.

Wakeland: Disease alleles that are quite rare within the population usually only contribute to disease susceptibility in a small fraction of the global disease population. Consider C1q deficiency as a cause of lupus in humans. Homozygosity for a defective C1q gene leads to the development of lupus in a highly penetrant fashion, virtually as a single-gene disease. However, only about 40 such individuals have been identified world-wide, and, although virtually all such people have lupus, this accounts for a minuscule portion of the millions of people with lupus in the global population.

Goldstein: The common ones are easier to find.

Wakeland: They are more prevalent and are potentially involved in disease susceptibility in many more individuals, however their effects are generally much less penetrant. Nonetheless, they contribute to the susceptibility in a larger fraction of individuals with a common disease.

Goldstein: How can you know, because it is so hard to find the rare ones? You don't know how many rare ones are out there.

Cookson: It's easy to find rare ones. It is like falling off a log.

Mapping genes for asthma and psoriasis

Juha Kere

Department of Biosciences at Novum, Karolinska Institutet, 14157 Huddinge, Sweden, and Department of Medical Genetics, University of Helsinki, 00014 Helsinki, Finland

Abstract. A property of susceptibility genes for complex diseases is their reduced penetrance, due to the influences of other genes, the environment, or stochastic events. With this in mind, it is possible to devise population genetic strategies and statistical methods to allow their positional cloning. The identification of the relevant effector gene in an implicated locus may provide further challenges and require functional studies. The challenges of positional cloning are demonstrated by two examples: the cloning of *GPRA* and *AAA1* on chromosome 7p14 at a susceptibility locus for asthma and atopy, and the study of *HCR* on chromosome 6p21 at *PSORS1*, the major susceptibility locus for psoriasis. To implicate *GPRA* in asthma and atopy, we studied its isoform-specific expression in bronchial biopsies and other sites for allergic reactions. We also studied its expression in a mouse model of ovalbumin-induced hypersensitivity. To study the role of *HCR* in psoriasis, we engineered transgenic mice with either a *HCR* non-risk allele or the *HCR*WWCC* risk allele controlled by the cytokeratin 14 promoter. The results suggested that while the overexpression of *HCR* in mouse skin is insufficient to induce a psoriasiform phenotype, it appears to induce allele-specific gene expression changes similar to those in psoriatic skin.

2005 The genetics of autoimmunity. Wiley, Chichester (Novartis Foundation Symposium 267) p 46–56

The credibility of genetic and functional studies of complex diseases has suffered in the recent years, because often their results have appeared to contradict each other. Consequently, a consistent picture has not often emerged. The field of asthma susceptibility gene research provides multiple examples of this. A gene may have been implicated by functional studies, but subsequent genetic linkage and association studies have failed to support its important role, leaving a casual observer confused. An example is *IL4*, which undoubtedly plays a key functional role in the pathway of T cell maturation and lineage specification, but has apparently no major genetic polymorphism of relevance to asthma or atopy (Lonjou et al 2000). On the other hand, genes implicated by positional cloning may have been uncharacterized, or may not have fitted in previously known pathways. The recently suggested asthma candidate gene *ADAM33* may provide an example of this situation, as its functional role in asthma remains both unknown and non-intuitive (Van Eerdewegh et al 2002). However, these results that appear inconsistent may be such only superficially and a deeper understanding will be necessary to compile a consistent picture; thus, one should not jump to premature conclusions on the utility of both genetics and functional studies for shedding light on complex disease mechanisms. For example, the results on *IL4* make complete sense when one considers that the control of *IL4* expression may not be in *cis* in the gene itself but instead operate in *trans* from another important locus that may remain uncharacterized.

In this presentation, I shall describe case studies on two common complex diseases involving immune mechanisms in their pathogenesis, namely asthma and psoriasis. For asthma, I shall focus on our recent positional cloning effort that led to the identification of *GPRA* as a candidate gene for asthma susceptibility, supported even by initial functional evidence for its role in asthma. The second example is on psoriasis and the *PSORS1* locus near HLA-C, where strong association of a long DNA segment to psoriasis has been frustrating for detailed genetic analyses aiming at single-gene resolution of association. We have studied functionally one of the *PSORS1* region genes, *HCR*, with initial functional evidence for its role in psoriasis, even though the roles of the *PSORS1* locus genes remain controversial and in part unsolved. Neither of these cases can be considered closed or completely understood for the time being, and therefore this presentation should be considered merely a record of the current status of affairs.

Positional cloning of asthma susceptibility genes on chromosome 7p

In the hope of reducing both diagnostic and allelic heterogeneity, we chose to study asthma and high serum IgE levels in families from the Finnish Kainuu province with a population size of 100 000. The choice of the subpopulation for study was made based on our previous experiences of working with rare recessive diseases in the region; results of those studies had suggested enrichment of rare disease alleles to 1–2% carrier frequencies (de la Chapelle & Wright 1998, Kere 2001). Even though the strategy could not be defended at the time with more than theoretical arguments (Lander & Schork 1994), it was intuitively safer than the opposite strategy adopted by the Collaborative Study of the Genetics of Asthma (CSGA 1997), choosing to ensure genetic heterogeneity in their sample. A genome scan with 86 pedigrees, totalling 443 subjects, implicated with statistical significance a locus on chromosome 7p14-p15, which could then also be replicated in a French Canadian and a second Finnish sample set (Laitinen et al 2001). This locus was among those that had been suggested by the first genome scan for asthma among Australian and British families (Daniels et al 1996), but not found in a number of other genome scans (CSGA 1997, Illig & Wjst 2002). Because significant, replicated linkage suggested that at least in some populations a gene on 7p would play a role in asthma, we adopted a sequential fine-mapping strategy to test the hypothesis of chromosome segments shared identical-by-descent more often in patients than in controls (Laitinen et al 2004). This strategy led us to focus on a 130 kb conserved haplotype, including a haplotype block with only 7 alternative allelic SNP structures with frequencies >2% in any of the three populations (Finnish Kainuu and North Karelian, French Canadian). The four most closely related haplotypes associated with risk for high IgE values or asthma in all three populations, whereas the three remaining haplotypes most different from those four were non-risk. Genetic association in distinct populations sharing only a common ancient European origin, the risk haplotype frequencies (Laitinen et al 2004), and linkage in Australian and British samples (Daniels et al 1996), together suggest that the gene might be of interest in many populations other than just Finns and Canadians.

Detailed study of gene content across the implicated segment identified an untranslated, alternatively spliced gene named *AAA1* and an unannotated orphan G protein-coupled receptor gene named *GPRA* (synonymous to *GPR154*). *GPRA* showed other properties compatible with a role in the pathogenesis of asthma. One of its two alternatively spliced mRNAs produced *GPRA* protein isoform B that was differentially expressed in bronchial epithelial cells and smooth muscle cells from asthmatic subjects as compared to healthy subjects. The result was distinctly consistent between 8 biopsies from asthmatic and 10 biopsies from healthy subjects, suggesting that the dysregulation of *GPRA* isoform B may be a common feature in the majority of asthma patients. An up-regulation of *Gpra* (mouse orthologue of *GPRA*) mRNA levels in lungs was also observed in a mouse model of ovalbumin-induced hypersensitivity. Taken together, these genetic and molecular findings suggest the specific involvement of *GPRA* in the pathogenesis of asthma and atopic disorders. Because *GPRA* is a virtually unannotated gene, it may provide a tag to a previously uncharacterized pathway with a role in the development of asthma.

What next in asthma genetics?

The number of positionally cloned 'second generation' candidate genes for asthma and related disorders is now at least four, counting *ADAM33*, *DPP10*, *PHF11* and *GPRA* (Van Eerdewegh 2002, Allen et al 2003, Zhang et al 2003, Laitinen et al 2004, Weiss & Raby 2004). These findings allow the direct testing of well-motivated polygenic models for asthma. Is the risk for asthma additive or multiplicative if one carries not only one, but two or more risk alleles for the different genes? Are some combinations of genes particularly high-risk? One can also go back to the previously identified but much weaker or uncertain risk genes. For example, is the weak effect seen for the chromosome 5q interleukin gene cluster stronger in the presence of one or another of these positionally cloned susceptibility genes? Another interesting gene is *IL9R*, located in the pseudoautosomal region of Xq and Yq, that has consistently yielded significant associations to asthma-related phenotypes (Melén et al 2004). Even though one will be testing more than one hypothesis in these studies, the problems of multiple hypothesis testing should be much less pronounced than in two-locus models without *a priori* evidence for the role of some loci. One can also start to look for common cellular links between these candidate genes and mechanisms, and those of already known regulatory pathways, such as those affecting T cell maturation. Hopefully, these studies will also shed light on the immediate mechanisms of action for some of these new genes. Undoubtedly, there will also be several more new candidate genes coming, because other loci that have been implicated in genome scans are still being pursued by positional cloning methods at the laboratory bench. However, it may not be too early to predict that the end-game for identifying key regulatory networks in asthma pathogenesis has begun.

Psoriasis and the *PSORS1* locus

In another project aiming at characterizing the major susceptibility gene for psoriasis that resides in the *PSORS1* locus on chromosome 6p21, we have used both genetics and transgenic mice to assess a positional candidate gene. Genetic analysis of *PSORS1* with samples from 419 families from six populations suggested that a specific allele of the *HCR* gene, residing 113 kb from the HLA-C susceptibility candidate gene, may have comparable risk ratios (Asumalahti et al 2002). The study size was however clearly insufficient to distinguish with significance the risk effects of these two genes. Other studies using comparable sample sizes yielded more-or-less the same result, that definitive distinction between the risk effects of several genes across the *PSORS1* region was not easily obtained because of strong linkage disequilibrium (Nair et al 2000, Veal et al 2002). Some results suggested that the strongest genetic effects may be closest to the HLA-C gene, but even if that was the case, the functional role of HLA-C in psoriasis has remained unsolved despite two decades of research. On the other hand, *cis*-acting regulatory elements may act over tens of kilobases, and thus the effector role of any gene within *PSORS1* cannot safely be ignored.

In an approach to assess the role of *HCR* as an effector gene in the *PSORS1* locus, we engineered transgenic mice with either the *HCR* common allele or the *HCR*WWCC* risk allele controlled by the cytokeratin 14 (K14) promoter

(Elomaa et al 2004). The choice of promoter and transgenic (rather than knockout) models were motivated by the physiological expression of *HCR* in basal keratinocytes of human skin and the seemingly dominant effect of *PSORS1* on psoriasis susceptibility. Several independent lines of mice were obtained with both transgene constructs, and all lines with verified expression of the transgene mRNA and protein showed normal development, phenotype, and fertility. Specifically, no histological features of the skin of transgenic mice allowed one to distinguish them from wild-type mice. Animals followed up to more than one year of age remained equally unaffected, but initially, no attempts were made to challenge their skin with irritants to simulate known external risk factors in human. To monitor subtle effects of transgenes on cellular biochemistry, we measured mRNA changes by Affymetrix arrays from skin samples from 4, 4 and 3 animals representing risk, non-risk and wild-type genotypes, respectively. The results revealed that *HCR* transgenes had allele-specific effects on the expression of especially cytoskeletal genes. A complete listing of genes with altered expression levels in transgenes compared to wild-type mice, and risk transgenes compared to non-risk transgenes included numerous overlaps with genes shown previously to have altered expression levels in human psoriatic skin (Elomaa et al 2004). These results suggest that while the overexpression of *HCR* in mouse skin is insufficient to induce a psoriasiform phenotype, it appears to induce gene expression changes reminiscent of psoriatic skin. Thus, *HCR* should be considered a candidate effector gene within the *PSORS1* locus.

These results undoubtedly complicate the field of research further, because they challenge us to try to understand the detailed cellular roles of other genes in the *PSORS1* locus as well, before the genetic mechanism for psoriasis susceptibility can be considered solved. Functional analyses, however, are much hampered by the lack of fully representative animal models; indeed, no other species than human is known to have a corresponding skin disorder. Because of the complexities of unique recognition and subtle differences inherent in the immune systems between human and mouse or other model species, testing of hypotheses for the role of *HLA-Cw6* is riddled with ambiguities. Indirect evidence of the roles of several other genes in the *PSORS1* region suggest that they are not obvious candidates for susceptibility genes, with the possible exception of *CDSN*. Again, the suggested roles of these genes do not invite researchers to look at their roles in similar models as our transgenic mice, and thus the results may remain asymmetrically available for functional assays of these genes. In the best case, the problem will be solved by results that overwhelmingly implicate a mechanism that explains in a sweep the genetic association, the suggested functional effects of the relevant gene, and environmental influences into a unifying model.

Lessons learned

These examples may give many ideas or concerns for future work, but I would like to emphasize three points. First, persistent application of positional cloning with appropriate genetic models to guide detailed strategies has started to yield results in the form of interesting and credible susceptibility genes in complex diseases. The widespread pessimism that followed early genome scans with inconsistent results was clearly unwarranted. The recent successes suggest instead that genetic association studies with current high-density maps and genotyping methods might yield interesting results on suggestively linked loci that may have been ignored. Second, these results reveal the advantages and limits of genetic analyses. Haplotype blocks are immensely helpful in studying genetic associations, but at the same time, they set the limit for resolution in implicating individual genes. When the thousands of past generations in human populations cannot any more provide recombinations to resolve the effects of neighbouring genes, one is left only with the guidance provided by functional studies, and their design and interpretation may not always be obvious. Third, results of these and other recent studies serve to highlight our lack of understanding of molecular pathways and regulatory networks within cells and tissues. Genetic studies of complex diseases will continue to link together unexpected genes, poorly characterized pathways, and common diseases.

Acknowledgements

I wish to thank especially Drs Tarja Laitinen, Lauri A. Laitinen and Tom Hudson for long-term collaboration on asthma genetics. Drs Kati Asumalahti, Outi Elomaa and Ulpu Saarialho-Kere are key members of our psoriasis team. Most significant support for our work is provided by Academy of Finland, Sigrid Jus³lius Foundation and Medical Research Council of Sweden.

References

Allen M, Heinzmann A, Noguchi E et al 2003 Positional cloning of a novel gene influencing asthma from chromosome 2q14. Nat Genet 35:258–263
Asumalahti K, Veal C, Laitinen T et al 2002 Coding haplotype analysis supports HCR as the putative susceptibility gene for psoriasis at the MHC PSORS1 locus. Hum Mol Genet 11:589–597
Collaborative Study on the Genetics of Asthma (CSGA) 1997 A genome-wide search for asthma susceptibility loci in ethnically diverse populations. Nat Genet 15:389–392
Daniels SE, Bhattacharrya S, James A et al 1996 A genome-wide search for quantitative trait loci underlying asthma. Nature 383:247–250
de la Chapelle A, Wright FA 1998 Linkage disequilibrium mapping in isolated populations: the example of Finland revisited. Proc Natl Acad Sci USA 95:12416–12423
Elomaa O, Majuri I, Suomela S et al 2004 Transgenic mouse models support HCR as an effector gene in the PSORS1 locus. Hum Mol Genet 13:1551–1561
Illig T, Wjst M 2002 Genetics of asthma and related phenotypes. Paediatr Respir Rev 3:47–51

Kere J 2001 Human population genetics: lessons from Finland. Annu Rev Genomics Hum Genet 2:103–128
Laitinen T, Daly MJ, Rioux JD et al 2001 A susceptibility locus for asthma-related traits on chromosome 7 revealed by genome-wide scan in a founder population. Nat Genet 28:87–91
Laitinen T, Polvi A, Rydman P et al 2004 Characterization of a common susceptibility locus for asthma-related traits. Science 304:300–304
Lander ES, Schork NJ 1994 Genetic dissection of complex traits. Science 265:2037–2048
Lonjou C, Barnes K, Chen H et al 2000 A first trial of retrospective collaboration for positional cloning in complex inheritance: assay of the cytokine region on chromosome 5 by the consortium on asthma genetics (COAG). Proc Natl Acad Sci USA 97:10942–10947
Melén E, Kere J, Pershagen G et al 2004 Influence of male sex and parental allergic disease on childhood wheezing: role of interactions. Clin Exp Allergy 34:839–844
Nair RP, Stuart P, Henseler T et al 2000 Localization of psoriasis-susceptibility locus PSORS1 to a 60-kb interval telomeric to HLA-C. Am J Hum Genet 66:1833–1844 (Erratum in Am J Hum Genet 70:1074)
Van Eerdewegh P, Little RD, Dupuis J et al 2002 Association of the ADAM33 gene with asthma and bronchial hyperresponsiveness. Nature 418:426–430
Veal CD, Capon F, Allen MH et al 2002 Family-based analysis using a dense single-nucleotide polymorphism-based map defines genetic variation at PSORS1, the major psoriasis-susceptibility locus. Am J Hum Genet 71:554–564
Weiss ST, Raby BA 2004 Asthma genetics 2003. Hum Mol Genet 13(Spec No)1:R83–89
Zhang Y, Leaves NI, Anderson GG et al 2003 Positional cloning of a quantitative trait locus on chromosome 13q14 that influences immunoglobulin E levels and asthma. Nat Genet 34:181–186

DISCUSSION

Abbas: HCR doesn't look like a transcriptional regulator, does it?

Kere: We see it in both the nucleus and cytoplasm in skin sections. It is an unannotated gene.

Ting: We have been using Affymetrix chips to look at gene expression in disease models. The specific model we are using has a toxin-induced demyelination phase, and when the toxin is taken away it goes through a remyelination phase. We are looking for genes associated with these two phases. We found some that went up 20–50-fold. Some of these are well known genes such as class I, and others are unknown genes with very few functional data. To examine the effects of these genes, we have used mice lacking MHC-I expression or mice lacking some of these unknown genes. In neither case can we see any effect of gene deletion on the disease outcome and pathology. To us, this was a little disappointing. How many people have had this experience where there is a dramatic change in gene expression with very little measurable outcome? It makes me worry a bit about extrapolating how important it is that a gene changes significantly in these chip assays.

Abbas: I think we will come back to this precise issue later. There are at least four or five people here who have used expression arrays to identify candidate genes in disease.

Goodnow: We have put new ENU mutants on arrays to see whether it explains the phenotypes. We find lots of big changes. We do mixed bone marrow chimeras, because most of them go with haemopoeitic cells. Then we repeat the experiments with sorted cells shown in the mixed chimeras to be a primary cellular site of action for the inherited abnormality profiling side-by-side mutant and wild-type cells as closely matched as possible. Almost all the changes go away as secondary effects of the mutation. My sense is that if you are lucky you might pick the right gene, but there are a lot of secondary effects.

The question would be, in the human setting can you find the equivalent culture system where you can subtract out all those secondary changes and make them common, so you can actually see the primary causal effects. A beautiful example of this is Brian Kotzin's work (Rozzo et al 2001) in mouse lupus, narrowing the inherited differences to a single congenic interval and then profiling expression changes that tracked with that interval.

Kere: There are different ways of using Affymetrix chips. Looking for expression differences is not the only strategy. A typical approach is to take cases and controls and look for differences: lots of things are different. Another way of using chips is when you have a candidate gene and you engineer it in your mice, and then you see what downstream effects it has.

Cookson: I wanted to ask about asthma. Looking for shared haplotypes is a highly innovative approach. You didn't give any P values. If you just do simple TDT-type statistics, what sort of P values do you get?

Kere: When the haplotype pattern mining procedure was under development by the computer scientists the scoring was based on associations and Chi-square tests, evaluated for significance by randomizations. That algorithm doesn't use TDT.

Cookson: What P value do you get with TDT in the Finnish families with those SNPs?

Kere: I don't remember. Something like 0.05. The nominal Chi-square association was 0.00001.

Cookson: How rigorous was the correction for the comparisons that you must have made? You put a sliding window across that region, so how does this work out?

Kere: Basically, what the haplotype pattern mining does is that we use as input chromosomes or haplotypes that come from cases and then control haplotypes that are the untransmitted parental chromosomes. Then we see what differences exist between these two groups. To assess how significant these different levels of Chi-square are, we put all these chromosomes back into a bag and then compare how often we get a certain level of Chi-square.

Cookson: The sort of figures about the extent of linkage disequilibrium we have heard so far at this meeting are around 100 kilobases to 250 kilobases. How far does LD extend across disease chromosomes in the Finnish and Canadian populations?

Kere: At the beginning we hoped that we would find very large stretches of LD in accordance with the finding in Tasmania and with the experience with monogenic diseases in Finland in that particular geographical region. What we discovered was that the LD does not extend any further. It is the same distance in the Finnish and the French Canadian population; it is short. I would expect to see exactly the same association in the British population and other European populations. The point is, the bottleneck in that kind of region was not that tight that it would have allowed us to see only a single haplotype background, with a long LD pair. This is a very frequent risk allele and so what we are seeing for the LD pattern is the pan-European association.

Kuchroo: I am interested in the GPRA isoform B. Besides being expressed on the target tissue, is it also expressed differentially in the immune system?

Kere: We are currently looking at this in the immune system cells. I can't give you details about the different cell types, because I am not yet confident about all the results. But it does seem to be expressed in the immune system as well.

Cooskon: Epithelial cells are part of the immune system!

Umetsu: I had a related question about *GPRA*. There are many different forms of asthma. Do you think that *GPRA* might be an atopy gene that affects other related atopic diseases such as allergic rhinitis and eczema, or is it an organ-specific gene that might only affect asthma?

Kere: This appears to be associated with high IgE levels as well. I would expect it to be an atopy gene. In fact, we are now looking at associations in eczema and other atopic disorders.

Kuchroo: The fact that there is an association with IgE levels suggests multiple different atopic diseases.

Kere: It is expressed in the gut as well, which is interesting, in relation to food allergies.

Umetsu: Have you looked in the mucosa of the nose? Is it expressed there and does it affect allergic rhinitis?

Kere: No, we haven't looked.

Seed: I didn't know about the Cw6 association and how penetrant it is. This reminds me a lot of the HLA–B27 story. This is a dominant allele that is not too prevalent in the population. Not everyone who has B27 gets ankylosing spondylitis. When they tried to put this into mice, nothing happened, but when they put it into rats they got the disease. It might it be productive to outcross your trait deliberately to see whether you can find some rare episodic coincidence of genes.

Kere: To my knowledge, nobody had tried to put the HLA-C into mice.

Abbas: There are lots of interesting issues. Many people here know about B27, but it is only in infected animals that you get the disease. If the animals are made germ free, the disease goes away.

Goldstein: How does the statistical test work? You said that the user can set different window sizes within which the comparison is made. Do you scan possible maximum window sizes to look for the strongest association?

Kere: No. We decide the window size on the basis of the population history and marker density.

Goldstein: So you don't look at the data and then pick a window size on the basis of the data, which would then mess up the statistics you do. Has anyone looked at *GPRA* and its association with response to asthma medications?

Kere: Not to my knowledge.

Foote: Psoriasis and MS are similar in that one sees foci of disease surrounded by normal tissue. We have no idea why this happens: it is a major question in MS.

Hafler: If you do spectroscopy on the 'normal' white matter, it is not that normal.

Goodnow: This is true for all immune disease if you have the right resolution. Pemphigus is a classical example, where the antibody and its epidermal target antigen are ubiquitously distributed, yet antibody/antigen reactions and bullous lesions are focal, typically at areas of flexure.

Foote: There is definitely a focus of disease which gives a neurological sign that associates with the anatomical focus.

Hafler: Every autoimmune, organ-specific disease has a 'geometry' to the inflammatory lesions.

Bowcock: When we did our gene expression study on psoriasis we saw over 1300 differentially expressed genes in involved skin (Zhou et al 2003). But we also saw 54 differences between normal and uninvolved skin, although these were small-fold changes. Some of these differences in gene expression may have been triggered by circulating cytokines, but it is also possible that they were triggered by genetic susceptibility factors. If this was the case you could identify individuals at risk of developing psoriasis on the basis of expression differences in their skin, prior to disease manifestation.

Rao: I have a question about the alternative reading frame on the opposite strand that encoded this non-coding RNA. Knowing what we do today, it is not inconceivable that this might also be implicated. But when you did your heterozygous/homozygous analysis and showed that the *GPRA* isoform homozygosity correlated with an increased risk for asthma, was there any likelihood that you were missing the non-coding RNA?

Kere: Genetics cannot differentiate between these two genes. When we talk about disease genes we should be more specific and talk about effector genes, those coding for a protein that interacts with other proteins to affect the phenotype.

Rao: The RNA can affect the phenotype.

Kere: These RNA genes are regulatory genes whose only effect is to regulate some other gene. I like to make the distinction between a regulatory gene and an effector gene, and regulatory polymorphism and effector polymorphism. Within the locus this may be going on. The RNA may well be regulating the *GPRA* gene, but it may be that protein that is having a final effect in the cell. To answer the question, we would need to understand whether the different forms of RNA can modulate the expression of the other genes.

Rao: I am not talking about that. Let's suppose you had some micro RNA that affected, for example, the haemopoietic differentiation into IgE-producing cells or one of the stages of B cell differentiation.

Abbas: That is an interesting question. In the past most of us have not paid attention to possible regulatory functions of micro RNAs. Most of us who do this kind of work look for open reading frames and proteins. It is not going to make life any easier, that's for sure.

Foote: The problem with that has been that there have been relatively few simple Mendelians that have mapped onto small RNA genes.

Kere: There is one well characterized example, which is cartilage hair hypoplasia, where the gene has been shown to be an RNA gene.

References

Rozzo SJ, Allard JD, Choubey D et al 2001 Evidence for an interferon-inducible gene, Ifi202, in the susceptibility to systemic lupus. Immunity 15:435–443

Zhou X, Krueger JG, Kao M-C et al 2003 Novel mechanisms of T-cell and dendritic cell activation revealed by profiling of psoriasis on the 63,100-element oligonucleotide array. Physiol Genomics 13:69–78

Natural genetic variants influencing type 1 diabetes in humans and in the NOD mouse

Linda S. Wicker, Carolyn L. Moule, Heather Fraser, Carlos Penha-Goncalves, Dan Rainbow, Valerie E. S. Garner, Giselle Chamberlain, Kara Hunter, Sarah Howlett, Jan Clark, Andrea Gonzalez-Munoz, Anne Marie Cumiskey*, Paul Tiffen, Joanna Howson, Barry Healy, Luc J. Smink, Amanda Kingsnorth, Paul A. Lyons, Simon Gregory†, Jane Rogers†, John A. Todd and Laurence B. Peterson*

*Juvenile Diabetes Research Foundation/Wellcome Trust Diabetes & Inflammation Laboratory, Cambridge Institute for Medical Research, Wellcome Trust/ MRC Building, Addenbrooke's Hospital, University of Cambridge, Cambridge CB2 2XY, UK *Department of Pharmacology, Merck Research Laboratories, Rahway, New Jersey 07065, USA, and †The Wellcome Trust Sanger Institute, Wellcome Trust Genome Campus, Hinxton, Cambridge CB10 1SA, UK*

> *Abstract.* The understanding of the genetic basis of type 1 diabetes and other autoimmune diseases and the application of that knowledge to their treatment, cure and eventual prevention has been a difficult goal to reach. Cumulative progress in both mouse and human are finally giving way to some successes and significant insights have been made in the last few years. Investigators have identified key immune tolerance-associated phenotypes in convincingly reliable ways that are regulated by specific diabetes-associated chromosomal intervals. The combination of positional genetics and functional studies is a powerful approach to the identification of downstream molecular events that are causal in disease aetiology. In the case of type 1 diabetes, the availability of several animal models, especially the NOD mouse, has complemented the efforts to localize human genes causing diabetes and has shown that some of the same genes and pathways are associated with autoimmunity in both species. There is also growing evidence that the initiation or progression of many autoimmune diseases is likely to be influenced by some of the same genes.

2005 The genetics of autoimmunity. Wiley, Chichester (Novartis Foundation Symposium 267) p 57–75

Genes causing human type 1 diabetes

Three loci are now well established in human type 1 diabetes: the HLA class II genes, the promoter region of the insulin gene (*INS*) and the *CTLA4* gene. These gene associations underpin the presumed T lymphocyte-associated immune-mediated mechanism of type 1 diabetes that results in a chronic and complex inflammatory response against the insulin-producing β cells of the pancreatic islets. HLA class II molecules present peptides derived from self proteins, including insulin and its precursors, in the thymus. Depending on the class II alleles and self proteins present, the T cell repertoire is established. Most high affinity self-reactive T cells are deleted in the thymus, a process known as central tolerance. The expression of insulin in the thymus is under the control of the disease susceptibility locus (Barratt et al 2004) at the promoter region of *INS*. This genetically-controlled differential expression of insulin in the thymus most likely influences the efficiency of deleting insulin-specific T cells (Chentoufi & Polychronakos 2002, Chentoufi et al 2004, Anderson & Kuchroo 2003). CTLA4, a negative-signalling member of the CD28 co-stimulatory family (Rudd & Schneider 2003) regulates T cell activation and expansion. In particular, the *CTLA4* gene encodes a soluble version of the molecule, and it is the levels of the mRNA of this isoform that correlate with susceptibility to both type 1 diabetes and autoimmune thyroid disease (Ueda et al 2003). Ongoing research in our laboratory is directed towards understanding the biological consequences of the variation of soluble CTLA4 in human peripheral blood cells. This is of special interest since an artificial soluble form of CTLA4 (an Ig fusion protein) has therapeutic effects in clinical trials of autoimmune disease (Kremer et al 2003).

Recently, Bottini et al (2004) described the association with type 1 diabetes of a non-synonymous single nucleotide polymorphism (SNP) in the gene encoding a tyrosine phosphatase that is a negative regulator of T cell activation, *PTPN22/LYP* (Cloutier & Veillette 1999, Hasegawa et al 2004). This result has now been confirmed (Smyth et al 2004). *PTPN22/LYP* has also been shown to be associated with rheumatoid arthritis (Begovich et al 2004), lupus (Kyogoku et al 2004), and Graves' disease (Smyth et al 2004). The fact that both *CTLA4* and *PTPN22* are strongly implicated in type 1 diabetes as well as other autoimmune diseases suggests that the regulation of T cell reactivity is vital for controlling susceptibility to multiple autoimmune diseases. Moreover, these two proteins and Cbl-b, which when mutated in a rat model of type 1 diabetes predisposes to the disease (Yokoi et al 2002), are all negative regulators of lymphocyte activation and expansion, indicating the central importance of T cell development and homeostasis in protection against autoimmunity.

Todd and co-workers have convincing evidence for a fifth locus in type 1 diabetes in the interleukin 2 (IL2) receptor α chain gene (*IL2RA/CD25*) region on chromosome 10p15-p14 (Vella et al 2005). Since IL2 has a non-redundant role in the generation of regulatory T cells (Malek et al 2002), a reduction in the expression or function of the α chain gene, which is critical to form the high affinity trimeric IL2 receptor, could contribute to autoimmune disease susceptibility.

Limitations in identifying disease susceptibility genes in mouse models

In a model of disease such as the NOD mouse, key tools in defining genes include the development of congenic strains that are protected from autoimmune diabetes because of a genetic region derived from a disease resistant strain (Wicker et al 1995). Ultimately, because of biological (recombination hot and cold spots) and practical (the number of potentially recombinant mice that can be screened) issues, the best that can be obtained from such strains is the narrowing of a region containing the disease gene to 0.5 to 3 Mb, depending on the frequency of recombination in the region under study. At this point, a systematic gene identification strategy is to obtain a complete sequence of the defined region, determine the gene content, and from comparative sequencing of the same region in other inbred strains, identify all potentially relevant SNPs. Unfortunately, these steps remain time-consuming and expensive and only represent the beginning of the search for the causative SNP(s) in a multigenic disease. It will be rare for a susceptibility gene to be identified from sequence information alone. One case would be if the susceptible and resistant strains are identical-by-descent in the defined genetic interval and there is a single functional *de novo* mutation that has occurred in one of the two strains being compared. Unfortunately, as is the case for all of the loci currently under analysis in our laboratory, *Idd5.1* and *Idd5.2* on chromosome 1 (Wicker et al 2004), *Idd3* (Lyons et al 2000a), *Idd10* (Penha-Goncalves et al 2003), and *Idd18* (Podolin et al 1998, Lyons et al 2001) on chromosome 3, and *Idd9.1*, *Idd9.2* and *Idd9.3* (Lyons et al 2000b) on chromosome 4, the susceptible and resistant parental strains have distinct ancestral haplotypes (Wade et al 2002, Wiltshire et al 2003, Yalcin et al 2004) in the narrowly defined *Idd* intervals and, therefore, many DNA variants are present (>20 SNPs per 10 kb) in essentially all of the interval's genes. This makes the identification of potentially causal SNPs much more difficult and definitive proof of a causative variation even more challenging.

Proving causality for an SNP (or SNPs)

To prove that a variant gene within a disease-modifying genetic interval is *the* disease-causing gene requires that the SNP change the *course of the disease*. This is true even for a gene with alleles having a compelling functional difference. Ultimately, in most cases, definitive proof for an *Idd* gene can only be obtained from a carefully designed gene replacement strategy, and that genetic alteration will have to be analysed on the NOD background (Brook et al 2003) in the context of other disease susceptibility genes. Simple addition of wild-type alleles by transgenesis would often lead to uninterpretable results because precise expression levels are not achieved or a particular splice variant is not produced. An additional complexity comes when there is more than one compelling candidate gene within an interval each having potentially causative SNPs. In this case the replacement strategy must proceed initially focusing on the 'best guess' between the two or more loci. Because 'proving' causality requires a large commitment of resources, even though such experiments are clearly scientifically valuable and desirable to perform, we have chosen not to make this our experimental priority. Rather, our current priority is to define each putative NOD *Idd* gene to a level where the candidacy is compelling because of sequence polymorphisms and functional distinctions. An example of building a case for a candidate SNP is our recent work on the *Idd5.1* locus where we hypothesized the disease gene was *Ctla4* and the diabetes-predisposing sequence variation determined the ability to produce one of the three CTLA4 splice variants (Ueda et al 2003, Wicker et al 2004, Vijayakrishnan et al 2004, Greve et al 2004).

CTLA4 and ICOS are encoded within the *Idd5.1* interval

Fine-mapping narrowed the *Idd5.1* region significantly (Hill et al 2000, Wicker et al 1994), reducing the number of candidate genes to four, including *Ctla4* and *Icos*. In addition to the previously described full-length and soluble forms of CTLA4 (Fig. 1), we discovered a new isoform of mouse CTLA4 lacking the B7-binding domain which we named ligand independent CTLA4 (liCTLA4) (Ueda et al 2003).

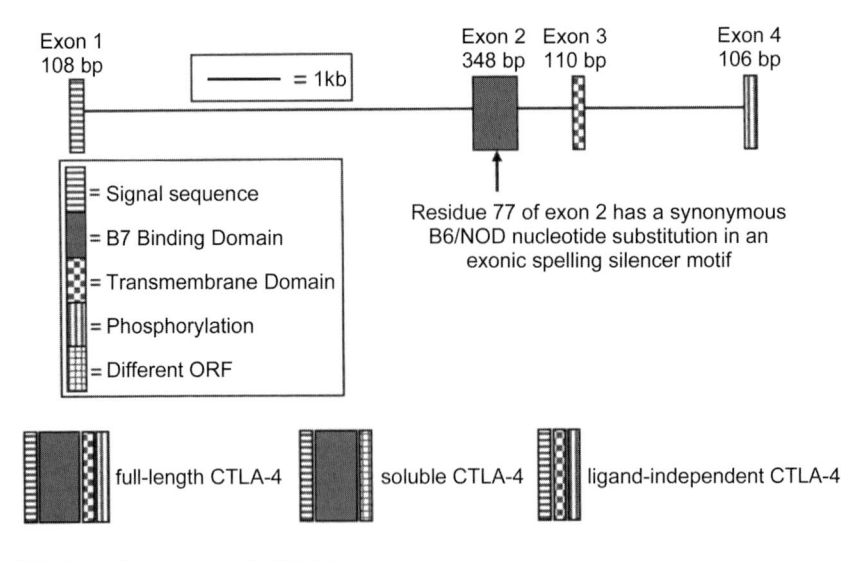

FIG. 1. The structure of CTLA4.

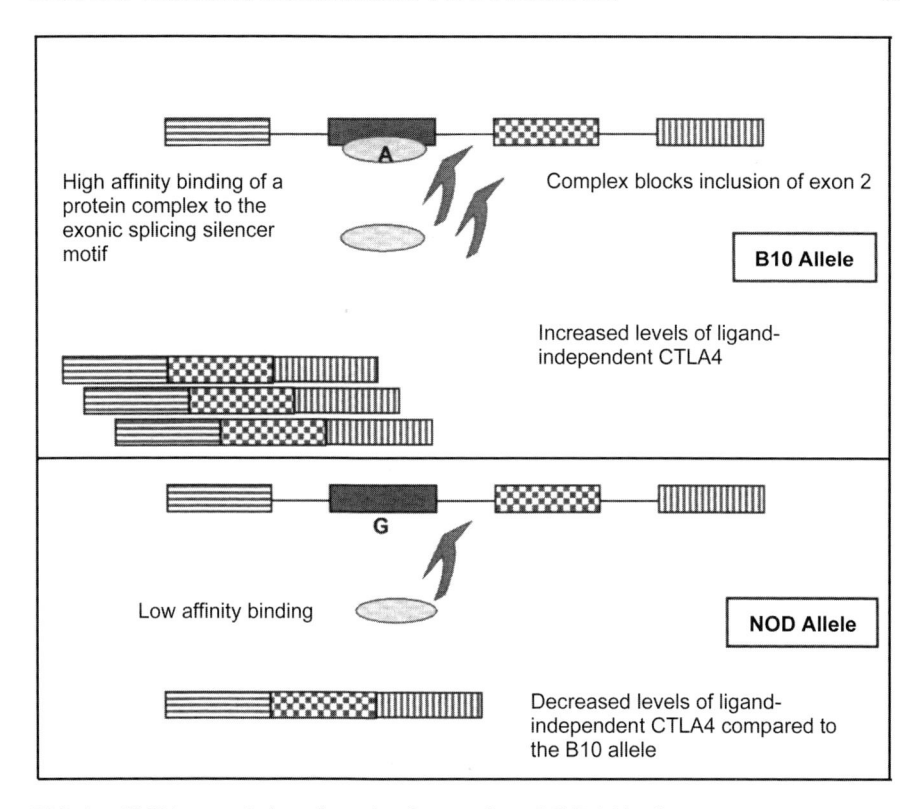

GENETIC VARIANTS INFLUENCING TYPE 1 DIABETES 61

FIG. 2. SNP in exon 2 alters the ratio of expression of CTLA4 isoforms.

The expression of liCTLA4 mRNA is dependent on the *Idd5.1* genotype with the resistant *Idd5.1* B6 allele producing fourfold higher levels (Ueda et al 2003, Wicker et al 2004) than the NOD allele (Fig. 2). The differential expression is determined by a NOD/B6 synonymous SNP at residue 77 in exon 2 of *Ctla4* within an exonic splicing silencer (ESS) motif (Ueda et al 2003) that is remarkably similar (Fig. 3) to the motif described previously for *CD45* (Lynch & Weiss 2001). The motif is disrupted in the cases of human and rat CTLA4 genes and we have failed to detect mRNA for the liCTLA4 isoform in these two species (Ueda et al 2003). In collaboration with Vijay Kuchroo, vectors encoding liCTLA4 were developed and liCTLA4 was shown to mediate negative signalling in T cells (Vijayakrishnan et al 2004). In unpublished data, Kuchroo's laboratory has recently shown that the liCTLA4 transgene can rescue CTLA4 knockout mice from the spontaneous and rapid lethal autoimmune syndrome that characterizes this strain.

Further collaborative studies with the Kuchroo laboratory demonstrated that in addition to encoding functionally variant CTLA-4 alleles, the *Idd5.1* region also

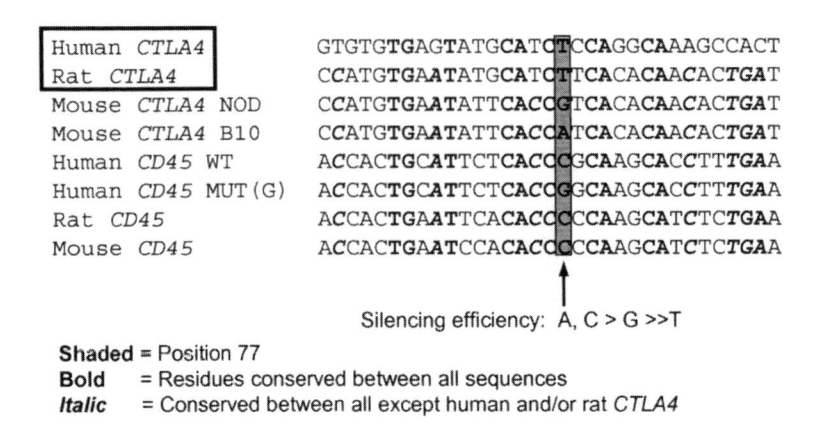

```
Human  CTLA4          GTGTGTGAGTATGCATCTCCAGGCAAAGCCACT
Rat    CTLA4          CCATGTGAATATGCATCTTCACACAACACTGAT
Mouse  CTLA4 NOD      CCATGTGAATATTCACCGTCACACAACACTGAT
Mouse  CTLA4 B10      CCATGTGAATATTCACCATCACACAACACTGAT
Human  CD45 WT        ACCACTGCATTCTCACCCGCAAGCACCTTTGAA
Human  CD45 MUT(G)    ACCACTGCATTCTCACCGGCAAGCACCTTTGAA
Rat    CD45           ACCACTGAATTCACACCCCCAAGCATCTCTGAA
Mouse  CD45           ACCACTGAATCCACACCCCCAAGCATCTCTGAA
```

Silencing efficiency: A, C > G >> T

Shaded = Position 77
Bold = Residues conserved between all sequences
Italic = Conserved between all except human and/or rat *CTLA4*

FIG. 3. ESS Motif in *CTLA4* and *CD45* genes.

causes differential expression of ICOS (Greve et al 2004). Using T cells from NOD and NOD.B10 *Idd5* congenic strains, we found that strains with the resistant B10 *Idd5.1* allele up-regulated less ICOS on the cell surface than strains with the susceptible NOD *Idd5.1* allele. Higher ICOS expression also correlated with more IL10 production by NOD T cells compared with T cells from B10 *Idd5.1* mice (Greve et al 2004).

Since expression differences for both CTLA4 and ICOS were observed when comparing the NOD and B10 *Idd5.1* alleles, the question arose as to whether the ICOS expression difference was a downstream consequence of the differential expression of liCTLA4 or a variation that was directly dependent on ICOS SNPs. And in the grander scheme of autoimmunity, are one or both genes responsible for the diabetes phenotype controlled by *Idd5.1*? Experiments are in progress to address these questions by developing congenic strains of mice that have ancient recombination events between the CTLA4 and ICOS alleles defined in the NOD and B10 strains. If these experiments support the hypothesis that the CTLA4 polymorphism controls the disease phenotype, a knock-in strategy replacing residue 77 in exon 2 of the NOD CTLA4 gene with the B10 residue could be employed to provide final proof for the identity of the *Idd5.1* locus.

Human *CTLA4*

In the publication by Ueda et al (2003), we demonstrated a correlation between the differential expression of the soluble isoform of CTLA4 with the *CTLA4* genotype in normal human volunteers. We noted that more mRNA encoding the soluble form of CTLA4 was produced by human CD4$^+$ T cells having the

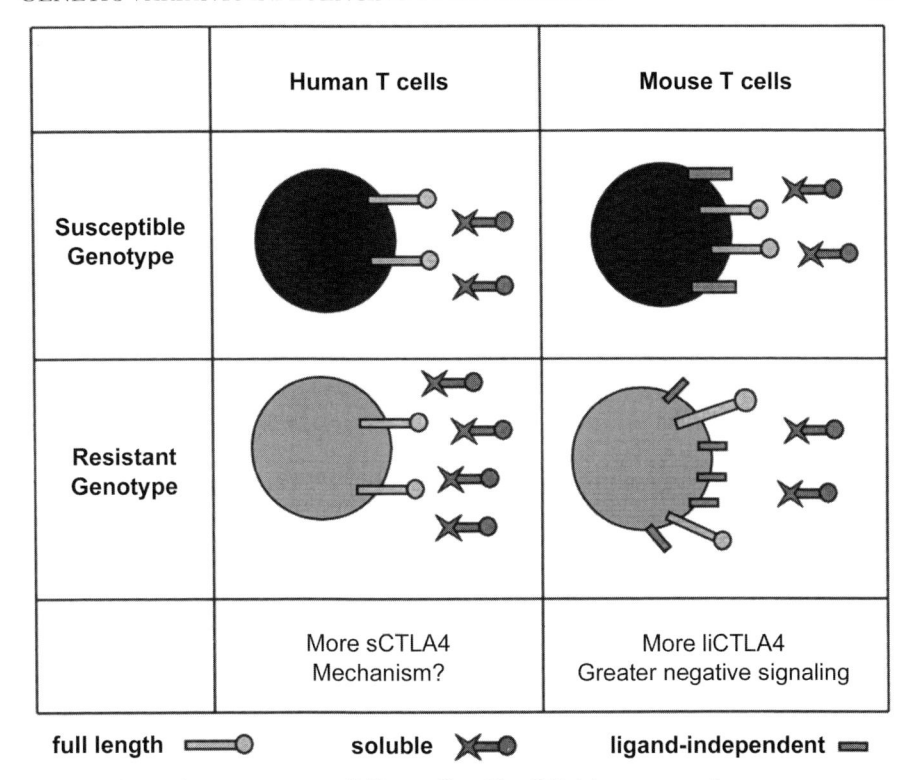

	Human T cells	Mouse T cells
Susceptible Genotype		
Resistant Genotype		
	More sCTLA4 Mechanism?	More liCTLA4 Greater negative signaling

full length   soluble   ligand-independent

FIG. 4. Protection versus susceptibility mediated by CTLA4: two strategies.

protective genotype compared with CD4$^+$ T cells isolated from humans with the disease-susceptible haplotype (Fig. 4). Thus, in the mouse the liCTLA4 isoform varies as determined by genotype while in humans where there is no liCTLA4, it is the amount of the soluble isoform that correlates with the disease-associated genotype. Because the same gene is being affected in both species, we are increasingly confident that the pathways involving key molecules leading to diabetes in humans and in NOD mice are shared between species. This additional example of a shared genetic control in human autoimmune diabetes and the NOD mouse was an important discovery since we rely heavily on the NOD mouse to provide genetic insights into the pathogenesis of human type 1 diabetes.

An ongoing focus in our laboratory is the mechanism of action of the soluble isoform of CTLA4. Although termed the 'soluble form', it is actually not known whether the sCTLA4 isoform functions within the cell or as a secreted product, or both. While some functional studies with an Ig fusion protein of CTLA4 have been performed (Kremer et al 2003), the mechanism of action of the natural 'soluble' CTLA4 protein, which may function as a monomer as compared to the

CTLA4–Ig dimer, has not been well-characterized. Soluble CTLA4 may have unique or only partially overlapping properties with the engineered CTLA4 fusion protein. In a parallel fashion to the discovery of the liCTLA4 isoform in the mouse, investigation of the functionality of natural soluble CTLA4 may provide insights into new therapeutic opportunities in the future.

Acknowledgements

Linda S. Wicker, Paul A. Lyons, and John A. Todd are supported by grants from the Juvenile Diabetes Research Foundation (JDRF) and the Wellcome Trust. The availability of NOD congenic mice through the Taconic Farms Emerging Models Program has been supported by grants from the Merck Genome Research Institute, NIAID and the JDRF.

References

Anderson AC, Kuchroo VK 2003 Expression of self-antigen in the thymus: a little goes a long way. J Exp Med 198:1627–1629
Barratt BJ, Payne F, Lowe CE et al 2004 Remapping the insulin gene/*IDDM2* locus in type 1 diabetes. Diabetes 53:1884–1889
Begovich AB, Carlton VE, Honigberg LA et al 2004 A missense single-nucleotide polymorphism in a gene encoding a protein tyrosine phosphatase (PTPN22) is associated with rheumatoid arthritis. Am J Hum Genet 75:504–507
Bottini N, Musumeci L, Alonso A et al 2004 A functional variant of lymphoid tyrosine phosphatase is associated with type I diabetes. Nat Genet 36:337–338
Brook FA, Evans EP, Lord CJ et al 2003 The derivation of highly germline-competent embryonic stem cells containing NOD-derived genome. Diabetes 52:205–208
Chentoufi AA, Polychronakos C 2002 Insulin expression levels in the thymus modulate insulin-specific autoreactive T-cell tolerance: the mechanism by which the *IDDM2* locus may predispose to diabetes. Diabetes 51:1383–1390
Chentoufi AA, Palumbo M, Polychronakos C 2004 Proinsulin expression by Hassall's corpuscles in the mouse thymus. Diabetes 53:354–359
Cloutier JF, Veillette A 1999 Cooperative inhibition of T-cell antigen receptor signaling by a complex between a kinase and a phosphatase. J Exp Med 189:111–121
Greve B, Vijayakrishnan L, Kubal A et al 2004 The diabetes susceptibility locus Idd5.1 on mouse chromosome 1 regulates ICOS expression and modulates murine experimental autoimmune encephalomyelitis. J Immunol 173:157–163
Hasegawa K, Martin F, Huang G et al 2004 PEST domain-enriched tyrosine phosphatase (PEP) regulation of effector/memory T cells. Science 303:685–689
Hill NJ, Lyons PA, Armitage N et al 2000 NOD *Idd5* locus controls insulitis and diabetes and overlaps the orthologous *CTLA4/IDDM12* and *NRAMP1* loci in humans. Diabetes 49:1744–1747
Kremer JM, Westhovens R, Leon M et al 2003 Treatment of rheumatoid arthritis by selective inhibition of T-cell activation with fusion protein CTLA4Ig. N Engl J Med 349:1907–1915
Kyogoku C, Langefeld CD, Ortmann WA et al 2004 Genetic association of the R620W polymorphism of protein tyrosine phosphatase PTPN22 with human SLE. Am J Hum Genet 75:504–507
Lynch KW, Weiss A 2001 A CD45 polymorphism associated with multiple sclerosis disrupts an exonic splicing silencer. J Biol Chem 276:24341–24347

Lyons PA, Armitage N, Argentina F et al 2000a Congenic mapping of the type 1 diabetes locus, *Idd3*, to a 780-kb region of mouse chromosome 3: identification of a candidate segment of ancestral DNA by haplotype mapping. Genome Res 10:446–453

Lyons PA, Hancock WW, Denny P et al 2000b The NOD *Idd9* genetic interval influences the pathogenicity of insulitis and contains molecular variants of *Cd30*, *Tnfr2*, and *Cd137*. Immunity 13:107–115

Lyons PA, Armitage N, Lord CJ et al 2001 Mapping by genetic interaction: high-resolution congenic mapping of the type 1 diabetes loci *Idd10* and *Idd18* in the NOD mouse. Diabetes 50:2633–2637

Malek TR, Yu A, Vincek V, Scibelli P, Kong L 2002 CD4 regulatory T cells prevent lethal autoimmunity in IL-2Rbeta-deficient mice. Implications for the nonredundant function of IL-2. Immunity 17:167–178

Penha-Goncalves C, Moule C, Smink LJ et al 2003 Identification of a structurally distinct CD101 molecule encoded in the 950-kb *Idd10* region of NOD mice. Diabetes 52:1551–1556

Podolin PL, Denny P, Armitage N et al 1998 Localization of two insulin-dependent diabetes (Idd) genes to the *Idd10* region on mouse chromosome 3. Mamm Genome 9:283–286

Rudd CE, Schneider H 2003 Unifying concepts in CD28, ICOS and CTLA4 co-receptor signalling. Nat Rev Immunol 3:544–556

Smyth DJ, Cooper JD, Collins JE et al 2004 Replication of an association between the lymphoid tyrosine phosphatase locus (*LYP/PTPN22*) with type 1 diabetes, and evidence for its role as a general autoimmunity locus. Diabetes 53:3020–3023

Ueda H, Howson JM, Esposito L et al 2003 Association of the T-cell regulatory gene CTLA4 with susceptibility to autoimmune disease. Nature 423:506–511

Vella A, Cooper JD, Lowe CE et al 2005 Localization of a type 1 diabetes locus in the *IL2RA/CD25* region using tag single nucleotide polymorphisms. Am J Hum Genet, in press

Vijayakrishnan L, Slavik JM, Illes Z et al 2004 An autoimmune disease-associated CTLA-4 splice variant lacking the B7 binding domain signals negatively in T cells. Immunity 20:563–575

Wade CM, Kulbokas EJ, 3rd, Kirby AW et al 2002 The mosaic structure of variation in the laboratory mouse genome. Nature 420:574–578

Wicker LS, Todd JA, Prins JB et al 1994 Resistance alleles at two non-major histocompatibility complex-linked insulin-dependent diabetes loci on chromosome 3, *Idd3* and *Idd10*, protect nonobese diabetic mice from diabetes. J Exp Med 180:1705–1713

Wicker LS, Todd JA, Peterson LB 1995 Genetic control of autoimmune diabetes in the NOD mouse. Annu Rev Immunol 13:179–200

Wicker LS, Chamberlain G, Hunter K et al 2004 Fine mapping, gene content, comparative sequencing, and expression analyses support *Ctla4* and *Nramp1* as candidates for *Idd5.1* and *Idd5.2* in the nonobese diabetic mouse. J Immunol 173:164–173

Wiltshire T, Pletcher MT, Batalov S et al 2003 Genome-wide single-nucleotide polymorphism analysis defines haplotype patterns in mouse. Proc Natl Acad Sci USA 100:3380–3385

Yalcin B, Fullerton J, Miller S et al 2004 Unexpected complexity in the haplotypes of commonly used inbred strains of laboratory mice. Proc Natl Acad Sci USA 101:9734–9739

Yokoi N, Komeda K, Wang HY et al 2002 *Cblb* is a major susceptibility gene for rat type 1 diabetes mellitus. Nat Genet 31:391–394

DISCUSSION

Foote: I have a very general point. The only way to make absolutely sure that your candidate gene is the gene that is involved is to do a knock-in. I have been guilty of sitting back and looking at the biology of my favourite candidate gene in an animal with a relatively small congenic interval, building up a story that convinces me that this is the right gene, only to have the whole thing disappear with one recombination event. To a certain degree, biological examination of candidate genes is essentially data dredging. While it is very important in helping us understand how things work, it doesn't necessarily mean that your gene is actually involved.

Wicker: That is why I was pointing out which are the more tractable knock-ins in this system so far, such as 4-1BB. If your natural variant is a natural knockout, like *Nramp1*, you could approach genes such as this with knockouts. This is like the *Il2* knockout: if your hypothesis is that a 50% reduction can make a difference, then if you can show that when all the other genes in the interval are kept constant and you only change the candidate gene by 50%, which then changes the phenotype, you can make fairly strong statements. It really depends on how convinced you are by the biology you have found when studying the natural variants. For the ICOS/CTLA4 problem, if you have a natural recombinant, you test it, and if it is carrying along the phenotype of the *Ctla4* SNP rather than the *Icos* SNP, do you want to spend US$150 000 making your own point mutation via a knock-in strategy? It depends on where you want to leave your story.

Foote: If you do the knock-in and get a change of phenotype, then that is the end of the story, there is no more discussion.

Wicker: I disagree. The real hard part is what is downstream, and how the gene works. When you have limited resources, this is the most important part because this is the only place where you will find out whether it is therapeutically feasible to do anything. What cell type is it hitting? This is why I am so excited by the transgenic systems we are studying in collaboration with Pere Santamaria. We have a 50% knockout of IL2 changing the disease phenotype similar to that of the natural variant which reduces IL2, but only in some cell types. If people still don't believe that the *Idd3* gene is the *Il2* gene, let them make the knock-in of this full segment. We believe we have compelling *Il2* expression data that are explained by 5′ UTR sequence variation and that we can now start building the functional story working back from the downstream cellular consequences. We have progressed in our understanding so much further than we ever did without the genetic clue that *Il2* expression differences are determined by the 5′ UTR variation between *Il2* alleles.

Foote: But this is still data dredging. There is no hypothesis that you are trying to disprove. The only way you can have a disprovable hypothesis is by regenerating your mutation somehow.

Wicker: If we had put the 50% *Il2* knockout onto the NOD background and hadn't changed the disease frequency it would have been inconsistent with the hypothesis that a twofold reduction in IL2 makes a difference.

Hafler: At the end of the day, the reason we are studying this is for its relevance to human disease. Until you go into a clinical trial and show an amelioration of disease associated with specifically targeting something identified in a mouse study, do you really know it is of importance? This is a key question in allocating resources to provide more and more evidence in the mouse models.

Foote: If you are actually working on the wrong gene in the mouse, you will definitely not identify the right pathway in humans.

Abbas: Let's take this one step further. Following David Hafler's reasoning, does this mean that if we really want to identify genes in order to do something about human disease, we should only be studying those in which there is a homologous polymorphism in patients? Let's take an extreme view. You could say that if there is no 5′ UTR abnormality in patients with type 1 diabetes, forget it — it is interesting biology but nothing to do with diabetes.

Hafler: Let me argue the opposite. If it still regulates the immune response, whether it's involved in diabetes or not, it still may be relevant.

Wicker: It doesn't have to be polymorphic in humans for it to be usable as a therapeutic.

Abbas: If you take that argument, we don't need any of this sophisticated mouse genetics! I could have told you 10 years ago that in the absence of IL2 there is serious disease. Or if you want to take the regulatory T cell reasoning, you can say forget all the genomics: it is completely irrelevant. We know that T_{reg} cells control autoimmunity, so treat them.

Wicker: Would you have thought that less than a twofold difference in the amount of IL2 would have made a difference on the basis of those previous experiments? It is genetics that has led us to the quantitative observation.

Abbas: It may or may not make a difference.

Rioux: I think that the mouse studies can lead to the identification of pathways that can lead to a given disease. In your example, IL2 may have no therapeutic effect on humans and no relevance to why some people get disease and others don't, and why some respond and others don't.

Seed: I'd like to raise this to another level. Even if we understand fundamentally how a disease is caused, say schizophrenia, there is no guarantee that our understanding of the molecular mechanism will lead us to a better cure. Just as these other implications in related systems may help us to derive a treatment which is effective, for this reason alone it is justifiable to pursue this. If you look at chronic granulomatous disease, it is a plasma membrane cytochrome oxidase that is responsible. The treatment for this is γ interferon, which causes generalized activation of the immune system and has nothing to do with the mechanism of disease *per se*, but nonetheless is an important viable therapeutic option.

Abbas: In some ways this leads back to one of the questions I raised in my introduction. The reason why many labs study animal models is because they are valuable for understanding pathways. We don't worry too much about whether they are a model for a human disease. I think transgenic models are awful models for studying type 1 diabetes, but they are spectacular models for understanding the choice between tolerance and autoimmunity. A lot of people get hung up on this issue of whether or not certain transgenic models are good models of the human disease. I don't think that's terribly important.

Wakeland: There is a common notion that you must produce a knock-in animal with the disease allele to prove that a gene causes a disease. What is needed specifically is an approach that allows genetic phenotypes that are only detectable *in vivo* to be genetically manipulated and assayed *in vivo*. This could be via the production of allelic knock-ins, a genetic knockout, or the production of a BAC transgenic. For example, if an autoimmune phenotype is recessive or is at least partially rescued in a heterozygote with the wild-type allele, and you have the wild-type allele in a BAC clone, then you can make a BAC transgenic and attempt to rescue the normal phenotype in a mouse homozygous for the disease allele. If transgenic mice carrying a specific BAC cause a diminution in the phenotype, then the causative allele must be present on that BAC. This approach was used first by Takahashi to identify the gene carrying the clock mutation and can be used to localize a disease gene within a congenic interval onto a single BAC clone. Presently, this is much simpler to do than a knockout or knock-in.

Wicker: I guess I am concerned that in the case of *Idd3*, you could overexpress IL21 or IL2 and perhaps both would affect the phenotype.

Foote: We have an example where we have overexpressed a gene through multiple copy-BAC transgenesis and got a phenotype similar to the one that we were studying which ended up being relevant.

Wakeland: When trying to identify a disease gene within a congenic interval, you can produce transgenic mice with each of the BACs in the tiling path. Theoretically, only the BAC containing the disease gene should impact the phenotype. It is really a matter of picking your poison, with respect to which technique to use—they all have difficulties. However, at least there are direct approaches available in the mouse. Whatever strategy you use to demonstrate *in vivo* that a specific gene causes a disease is fine. In the end, knowing the genes is the most important point, while understanding the specific mutation is probably less important than understanding the functional consequences.

Foote: We have been in a similar position where we had a seductive candidate in our congenic interval where we were absolutely certain the gene mediated the phenotype and then we get one recombination event that separates it from the phenotype. It is frustrating.

Kere: One of the reasons it makes a lot of sense to figure out the polymorphic gene effects in humans is that if they are druggable targets, you could mimic the normal physiology in your therapeutic approach. If you have a variation that is the cause of the disease, if you could modify that back by targeting the molecule, you could create a very physiological therapeutic system.

Goodnow: Rate limiting phenomena are interesting. The IL2 knockout tells you that if you take IL2 away all hell breaks loose in regulation. IL2 is a rate limiting component for negative regulation, but it doesn't seem to be rate limiting for activation of the immune response. Is this more likely to be a QTL in a polygenic trait than something that is less rate-limiting?

Seed: What does the IL2 heterozygote knockout look like in this respect?

Wicker: In terms of disease it is actually more diabetic than the NOD mouse.

Abbas: For those of you who don't know the IL2 story, it is now turning out that it is required for the generation and maintenance of regulatory T cells. Take IL2 away these mice get very sick with bad autoimmune disease.

Kuchroo: What is the importance of IL2 in deletion of effector T cells versus generation of regulatory T cells?

Abbas: Deletion is the other pathway in which IL2 is active. Most of us now think that although IL2 clearly has an effect on potentiating cell death in some populations, this is probably its minor role.

Rao: I was confused about one of your points. You referred to a structural polymorphism that involved a glycosylation change. At this point it is irrelevant to the disease because you can have the same structural polymorphism but not have the disease. Is that correct?.

Wicker: Yes, and what is striking to me is that there are at least nine alleles of IL2 known to have an altered exon 1 sequence involving the glycosylation site. This region of the IL2 molecule doesn't seem to be used for binding to the IL2 receptor. There is a microsatellite embedded in exon 1 which appears to account for the many alleles of *Il2* in mice.

Rao: So what are you now attributing to the 5′ regulatory region?

Wicker: We would have to say that the causative variation could be 5′, 3′ or intronic. It is all one giant haplotype.

Kere: Are the different alleles expressed at different levels?

Wicker: Yes. You can either have high or low expression.

Abbas: If it is correct that the expression difference is only seen in CD8 cells, then we have to say that normally CD8 cells make the IL2 that drives the generation of CD4 regulatory T cells. This becomes very complex and unclear. It goes through a lot of hoops and it is a very complicated way of looking at this. Judgement needs to be reserved, for the moment, about whether this is going to be a relevant pathway.

Vyse: Since the phenotype you got in one of your congenics was very specific to a certain kind of immunological scenario, when you are trying either to construct or dismantle your phenotype by breeding congenics together, might you not expect that by mixing particular congenics together you would get much more of a suppressive effect, or no effect. This would depend on whether the congenic that you were bringing in happened to interact specifically with that specific pathway in your original congenics. I think in your model you tried to suppress the phenotype.

Wicker: Empirically, when we try to mix and match them, sometimes two protective congenic strains that are both 50% protected separately, when combined show no increase in protection above the 50%, but with other combinations of partially protected strains, we observe epistasis.

Vyse: Might you not have expected that given this very specific set of circumstances that you had to produce to generate this phenotype? Once you get an angle on something quite specific in relation to the way that something is acting, it is then going to open the way for you to explore other congenics that you showed positively interact with that.

Wicker: Yes. Actually, many other *Idd* loci are showing effects in the TCR systems I discussed that we haven't been able to dissect out yet in the spontaneous disease. It will help.

Cookson: Do the NOD mice develop diabetes if they are raised in sterile circumstances?

Wicker: Yes, even in gnotobiotic conditions.

Abbas: You have to remember that they are the exception to the rule: we all look for infections being triggers for autoimmunity. All you have to do is infect a NOD mouse and you will cure it. You don't even have to infect it: a little bit of complete Freund's adjuvant will cure it.

Kuchroo: I don't know whether it is the exception, because in the SJL mouse, where you have the endogenous repertoire for myelin proteolipid protein (PLP), if you put them in germ-free conditions the autoreactive repertoire expands.

Cookson: So there are all these strong environment factors acting in these diseases. How does this tie in with the genetic findings?

Wicker: The environment can influence the immune system. I don't see any problem with this. The infections change the myeloid cell system.

Cookson: Can you say anything more specific?

Goodnow: We can speculate. T cells might be making more IL2 and correcting the qualitative deficit.

Cookson: It has to be more specific than that.

Bowcock: Do NOD mice have to be a certain age for infection to cure them?

Wicker: They are most pliable when they are young.

Bowcock: Can they still be cured when their thymus have degenerated?

Abbas: In mice the thymus persists for much longer than in people with the same problem. There is also a strong gender bias in the NOD disease that is not anywhere as well documented in human type 1 diabetes. There are some peculiar things about the disease which no one understands.

Foote: Can you make a C57BL/6 diabetic by putting NOD loci into it?

Wicker: No, this has been tried without success. There are a lot of genes that we haven't found yet.

Abbas: It is a heck of a long way away. This comes back to an issue I raised earlier: every one of those genes you would have predicted based on what we know. You didn't need to do positional cloning. If you listed the 100 genes that are involved in regulating T cells you would have found all of them.

Wicker: These are potent natural variations that must be able to be fine-tuned differently than other immune genes. I think it is incredible that there are so many genes that are being defined that can vary in both species in a functional way. A lot of knockouts aren't conducive to life.

Abbas: My question was if you had sat down with a list of all the genes that regulate T cell function, you would probably end up with 50 or so involved ones.

Wicker: We now know that we can modulate these particular genes a small amount and get an effect.

Abbas: My point was that you would have ended up in the same place. If you had sequenced those 50 in the NOD mouse you would have found all those you found by positional cloning. But you would not have found NOD2 in IBD if you had taken that approach, and probably many others.

Bowcock: Most of us don't believe that there are as many as 50 genes for each of the complex autoimmune diseases. We believe there are perhaps 10 for each. A lot of those others regions that have been reported to potentially harbour autoimmunity loci are spurious linkages where neither associations nor genes will be found.

Abbas: Why do you believe that?

Bowcock: In psoriasis there have been 10 genomewide scans, and there have been approximately 20 loci reported. A subset of these have been replicated at least once, or have a LOD score indicating evidence for linkage, but a number of others appear to be spurious. However, the corollary to that is that some loci with weak effects may not have been reported in initial linkage scans. For example, a meta analysis of six genomewide scans has shown that at a locus on chromosome 4 that had a weak signal in many scans is likely to be real. It has also been in a separate linkage scan in Han Chinese. Hence, although the number of loci appears to be far less than 50, we may not yet have the power or the correct approach to identify the major psoriasis loci. *Hafler:* How powerful are linkage scans using microsatellites?

Abbas: There are two points. That is one, but the second is that you are actually looking at a disease with an extremely restricted phenotype, compared to the NOD disease. NOD mice get a large number of endocrine organs involved, so they have much more systemic or widespread autoimmune manifestations. What is a human disease like? It would depend on whether you are looking at lupus and rheumatoid arthritis on one hand versus psoriasis on the other.

Hafler: Let's get back to the point about the linkage. I understand that the previous linkage analyses didn't have the power.

Bowcock: That may be true, although you may be able to determine the approximate number of susceptibility loci by determining the lambda sub S (λ_s) for a particular disease, and then by looking at the individual lambdas contributed by your identified loci. The caveat to this is that you may need to have identified the variants in question to perform this type of analysis.

Behrens: However, you are dealing with families so you are only looking at 5–10% of all the cases of psoriasis. The same is true of lupus and MS: it is always a small proportion of cases with familial disease, and everyone else has 'sporadic' disease. I wonder how much of this is just small families, where there aren't enough sibs to show additional cases in a low-penetrance disease. Linkage peaks are going to have limited value in identifying genes. We have an example now of potent genes that do not lie under linkage peaks. I suspect the number of genes is going to be very high.

Goodnow: We know in NOD that there are all these things that don't show up if you read the whole scan. They are very replicable.

Kere: One of the reasons why the linkage studies have been so difficult to replicate is that it has not really been appreciated that the individual gene effects have such low relative risks. For this reason, practically every genome scan has been underpowered to start with. You're lucky to find anything.

Abbas: So family-based linkage studies will underestimate association.

Cookson: Linkage studies will detect genes with greater effect because they are not very powerful. There is quite a lot of literature underlying the theoretical basis of how many genes you would expect to influence a complex trait. The answer is many. The feeling from the literature is that there are likely to be a few genes of larger effect, and then there are many others of smaller effect (or smaller effect in certain circumstances).

Behrens: Or genes of powerful effect which just do not show up on linkage scans. We see in systemic lupus that HLA shows up on some genome screens but not in others. Yet when you go to the same collection of families that showed no signal by linkage, and test for association, there is a strong signal. This is happening for reasons I don't understand.

Kere: Is anyone able to quote a gene with a relative risk of higher than 2?

Bowcock: HLA, even for psoriasis.

Seed: The fact that you can't pin these things down points to more genes rather than fewer. Pick a model organism: how many times have we been able to generate a human-like disease in a model organism by knocking out genes for which we have no reasonable suspicion in the human case? Look at IBD for example. This has been caused numerous times in mice by various gene deletions or overexpression. It may be difficult to estimate the total number but my suspicion would be that it is large.

Rioux: Knocking out a gene and getting some sort of inflammatory component in a part of the body is not in any way relevant to the human disease.

Seed: I am just saying that in terms of the number of genes that could be contributing to a given phenotype, if you take a model organism approach, this suggests potentially tens or hundreds of ways to get IBD.

Rioux: The reality is that this doesn't give you a clear idea of the true number of genes that are variant in the human population and which predispose to disease.

Seed: If you wait long enough the population will give you all of those.

Abbas: The issue of phenotype is that you can knock out a lot of genes and get features that look like colitis, but it is not obvious that this is the same as Crohn's disease in humans.

Rao: But would you not argue that even though they may not all correspond to Crohn's disease in humans, the genes are likely to be on the same pathway that leads to the set of disease symptoms?

Rioux: Yes, you could make that argument. I think we are addressing a number of different areas here. If the primary question is an estimate of the number of genes in a human population that confer risk to a given phenotype, that approach does not give you the answer. It may give you potential candidate pathways to examine in human disease as you state.

Rao: If there are 20 genes in a biochemical pathway and only two of them are represented in the human population, nevertheless the therapies could be applied to one of the other 18.

Hafler: We should get back to the issue of rare and common genes.

Abbas: I want to ask the geneticists a question. At the moment, would you say that the most reliable way to directly identify disease-associated polymorphisms in people is some version of haplotype mapping?

Cookson: It is some version of association mapping. You want large numbers of samples, cases and controls, lots of intermediate phenotypes, expression array phenotypes perhaps, and lots of SNPs.

Bowcock: Sometimes you also need to perform haplotype analyses to pinpoint a region with a causative variant.

Abbas: We still don't have a reasonably cost-effective method of doing this, or, even worse, going from haplotypes to genes and then to function.

Cookson: You can do a genomewide association for US$600 on one individual. The cost is coming down all the time. We are not quite there yet, but we are nearly there.

Abbas: So we have the technology for doing fast associations, or we are getting there. The first question I posed in my introduction was how are we going to go from regions or associations to genes, to functions? We don't have any reasonably rapid and cost-effective way of doing this.

Wicker: You could knock-in the human variant to the mouse gene.

Abbas: One approach everyone is talking of is doing knock-ins. You need the right embryonic stem (ES) cells and it takes a year or so to do a knock-in.

Wicker: Maybe that is a more important experiment to do than the knock-in of a mouse gene to prove its candidacy. It really depends whether you think that the resulting mouse strain might provide a human-specific screen for an inhibitor or a target for a therapeutic antibody.

Kere: How about comparing the allelic effects of different forms of the human gene? You could compare by phenotype to start with and then if there is no difference in phenotype you could go for biochemical detail.

Rao: I think biochemistry is very different from organismal phenotype. Sometimes you don't see changes of more than twofold or even 1.5-fold, which are very hard to pick up biochemically. Over the length of time an animal or individual matures there are profound physiological effects that make it very difficult to mix biochemistry with phenotype. I think you could get a negative result, and it wouldn't mean anything.

Kere: Negative results don't mean anything with animal models.

Rioux: The challenge is that haplotypes that are associated with a given disease will often extend over a region that contains multiple genes. From a genetic association perspective, all of the genes on this haplotype are equally good candidate genes. If you follow-up with functional work (e.g. mRNA expression profiling) on only one of the genes while ignoring the rest, you are almost certain to see some difference between disease and normal tissue, but that is not a definitive answer. The challenge that we face is how do we take an associated region that contains multiple genes and prove actual causality to human disease?

Rao: These days one would have to think about the non-coding transcripts. This doubles or triples the problem.

Goodnow: The other thing that makes autoimmune disease so much harder than the example Juha Kere gave us, is that if the gene is acting in T cells such as those that Linda Wicker is talking about, then the intermediate phenotype may only be active in autoreactive T cells. These are a tiny fraction of the inflammatory fraction of blood cells that we can pull out of a patient. Even in the mouse it is only when you start looking at the clonal level by crossing onto a TCR transgene that you can start to see intermediate phenotypes for these subtle genes. How can we translate this kind of thing to a human situation?

Hafler: It will be very difficult.

Bowcock: Would you know the triggering antigens, so you could then get those T cells to proliferate?

GENETIC VARIANTS INFLUENCING TYPE 1 DIABETES

Goodnow: In the case of diabetes, this is the holy grail: to be able at least to score the number of insulin-reactive T cells. No one has come up with a peripheral blood assay that works.

Ting: This is a poor man's approach. You could use retrovirus RNAi. You can infect your primary haemopoeitic cells and put them back into animals.

Abbas: Chris Goodnow has used bone marrow chimeras brilliantly over the years. There is a lot you can do with them.

Kuchroo: Many of these cases may occur as haplotypes. What is very telling is that if you break the haplotype you get rid of the phenotype, so they have to come together not as a single gene but as multiple genes. The phenotype may not be the outcome of one gene but they may all be involved in giving the phenotype. To say that there is a single gene in that region and that is giving you the phenotype is probably dreaming.

Abbas: At least with RNAi, in theory you can do multiple knock downs in a haemopoietic cell. My sense, Jenny Ting, is that you are correct: this will be a fairly proximal assay.

Rao: No, the reason it won't is because it is not a knockdown, but a single point mutation.

Ting: That is why I prefaced it by saying it is not a knock-in, but you can use it to get some idea of the function of the gene.

Abbas: As a proximal assay, it is so much quicker than knock-ins.

Hafler: The whole point of looking for one 'holy grail' immune defect doesn't make much sense any more. The genetics suggest that the immune defects that we should look for functionally will be minor variations that may be difficult to detect. We should not expect the immune defect to be specific for one autoimmune disease and found only in patients with that disease. Instead we need to develop ways of rapidly looking at multiple different immunological measures at the same time. In the way that geneticists take those data together of different haplotypes and lead to a disease risk, we may have to do the same thing in conjunction with the genetics in terms of multiple immune measures to see which ones in concert lead to higher risk for disease. The differences in immune function may be subtle.

Kuchroo: There is more than one way to get there. You can make a deletion by one mechanism and get regulation that could compensate for it. This might result in the same phenotype but different genes may be involved in the process. The power is diluted because there is more than one way to get to the end phenotype.

Wijmenga: That is the problem, because not every mutant in itself is sufficient to get the disease phenotype. How are you going to reconsititute this in an animal model or an *in vitro* system?

The importance of epistatic interactions in the development of autoimmunity

Srividya Subramanian and Edward K. Wakeland[1]

Center for Immunology, University of Texas Southwestern Medical Center, Dallas, TX 75390-9093, USA

Abstract. Genetic predisposition is the main element in susceptibility to a variety of autoimmune diseases, including systemic lupus erythematosus (SLE). Epistatic interactions between susceptibility loci play a major role in the progression of autoimmunity, as our recent work, associating a common haplotype of the SLAM/CD2 receptor family with autoimmune susceptibility in specific genomic contexts, has illustrated. Furthermore, these interactions can be abrogated in the presence of appropriate modifier loci. We postulate that susceptibility to autoimmunity may be a consequence of imbalances in immune regulation that are elicited by specific combinations of common alleles at multiple, immunoregulatory loci.

2005 The genetics of autoimmunity. Wiley, Chichester (Novartis Foundation Symposium 267) p 76–93

The genetic complexity underlying susceptibility to the autoimmune disorder systemic lupus erythematosus (SLE) has rendered identification of causal, predisposing alleles a challenging task. This has proven true in both human lupus genetic studies as well as those undertaken in spontaneous, inbred murine lupus models such as NZM2410, BXSB and MRL/*lpr* (reviewed in (Wakeland et al 2001, Tsao 2004, Raman & Mohan 2003). This inherent genetic intricacy is further complicated by the fact that SLE is a multi-faceted, chronic autoimmune disorder with a highly heterogenous clinical presentation. Thus, although the most common autoimmune characteristic of SLE is the presence of high titres of serum anti-nuclear autoantibodies (ANAs), particularly anti-dsDNA, the resulting clinical consequences and end-organ pathogenesis can be quite diverse.

---

[1]This paper was presented at the symposium by Edward K. Wakeland to whom correspondence should be addressed.

We have utilized a congenic dissection strategy to characterize the immunological functions of susceptibility loci identified via linkage analysis of the NZM2410 murine lupus model (Morel et al 1994, 1999a). Mice made congenic for NZM2410-derived susceptibility loci on the C57Bl/6J (B6) genome have unique phenotypes that recapitulate what is seen in the parental NZM2410, yet no locus by itself develops highly penetrant and severe lupus nephritis (Morel et al 1997, Mohan et al 1997, 1998, 1999a). Genetic reconstitution experiments have revealed that of these loci, the chromosome 1 locus *Sle1*, is necessary for the initiation and development of fatal autoimmunity in this model system, despite having in isolation a relatively benign phenotype of high ANA titres (Morel et al 2000).

The *Sle1* locus is in turn comprised of a series of sub-loci, in relative close proximity to each other, designated *Sle1a–Sle1d*. Of these, *Sle1b* is the most potent and mediates a highly penetrant, female-biased loss in tolerance to chromatin that results in high titres of serum ANAs, similar to that seen with the entire interval (Morel et al 2001). Furthermore, when *Sle1b* is combined with lupus accelerating mutations on the B6 background, it leads to systemic, pathogenic autoimmunity, similar to the whole locus (Croker et al 2003). Interestingly, the syntenic human interval to *Sle1b*, 1q23, has also been linked to lupus susceptibility (Moser et al 1998, Cantor et al 2004).

The characterization of the phenotypic properties of each susceptibility locus, in isolation or when genetically reassembled, indicate that lupus susceptibility loci act at different stages of the disease process. This has also been noted in other spontaneous models of autoimmunity and, combined with observations from lupus-prone strains produced by genomic manipulation, suggests a model in which SLE susceptibility genes broadly fall into three pathways (Wakeland et al 2001). Pathway 1 genes, such as *Sle1a*, *Sle1b*, or the recently described *roqin* mutation (Vinuesa et al 2004), play a key role in disease initiation and lead to defects in the immune system's ability to maintain tolerance to nuclear antigens. Introduction of other genes like *Sle2*, *Sle3* and *Yaa* can lead to pathogenic autoimmunity when they interact epistatically with Pathway 1 genes, due to their ability to alter or dysregulate the immune system. The third category of genes plays a role in rendering the end-organ more susceptible to the damage caused by the actions of Pathway 1 and 2 genes. The cumulative effect of the interactions between genes belonging to different pathways can result in fatal autoimmunity. This suggests that understanding the mechanisms that are dysregulated in Pathway 1 genes, such as the *Sle1* genes, could provide insight into preventing the entire sequence of pathogenic events from unfolding.

What is also emerging from the various analyses of genetic susceptibility to SLE and other autoimmune diseases is that many of the causal variants of genetic predisposition are actually common alleles that *per se* are non-deleterious. HLA polymorphisms that are associated with predisposition to autoimmunity are the best example of this type of genetic element. In this regard, recent genomic analyses indicate that several other genes and gene families with immunoregulatory functions are highly diversified, presumably in response to pathogen-driven selection mechanisms. How then do these common variants elicit systemic autoimmunity? The answer to this question, which can be clearly demonstrated in murine models, appears to be that epistatic interactions between different combinations of polymorphic genes can lead to imbalances in immune regulation that may potentiate the development and progression of autoimmunity.

In this overview, we illustrate the importance of epistatic interactions between separate loci in the development of autoimmunity. In addition, we will demonstrate the ability of common alleles to mediate autoimmunity in specific genomic contexts, using data from our work and others. We postulate that susceptibility to autoimmunity may be a consequence of imbalances in immune regulation, elicited by certain combinations of specific alleles at multiple immunoregulatory loci.

Sle1b: common alleles that mediate a loss in tolerance to chromatin

As mentioned earlier, identification of a Pathway 1 gene, such as the *Sle1b* gene, could provide insight into the mechanisms responsible for the initial step of losing tolerance to chromatin. We have recently completed a detailed genomic analysis of the 940 kb congenic *Sle1b* interval, which links extensive polymorphisms in the SLAM/CD2 family of genes with the autoimmune phenotypes of B6.*Sle1b* (Wandstrat et al 2004). This family of immune receptor genes has been shown to transmit either stimulatory or inhibitory signals during cell–cell interactions between T, B, NK and monocyte cell lineages (Tangye et al 2000, Sidorenko & Clark 2003). Interestingly, they appear to be involved in the modulation of both innate and acquired immune responses due to their expression in a wide variety of cell lineages (reviewed in Veillette & Latour 2003).

A variety of studies were undertaken to look for functional polymorphisms between the B6 and B6.*Sle1b* strains, which differ solely at the *Sle1b* interval (Wandstrat et al 2004). As illustrated in Fig.1A, four of the SLAM/CD2 family genes (*Cd229*, *Cd84*, *Cs1* and *Cd48*) have non-synonymous mutations in exons encoding either ligand binding or cytoplasmic domains while *Cd244* is expanded in B6.*Sle1b* mice to a four locus cluster of genes that encode molecules with significant structural variations from the one gene product found in B6. In terms of expression level differences in splenic B or T cells, four SLAM/CD2 family genes, *Cd48*, *Ly108*, *Cd84* and *Cs1*, show differential gene expression. Interestingly, both *Ly108* and *Ly9* also show differential isoform usage between the two strains (Fig.1A). These changes are detectable well before overt signs of

EPISTATIC INTERACTIONS 79

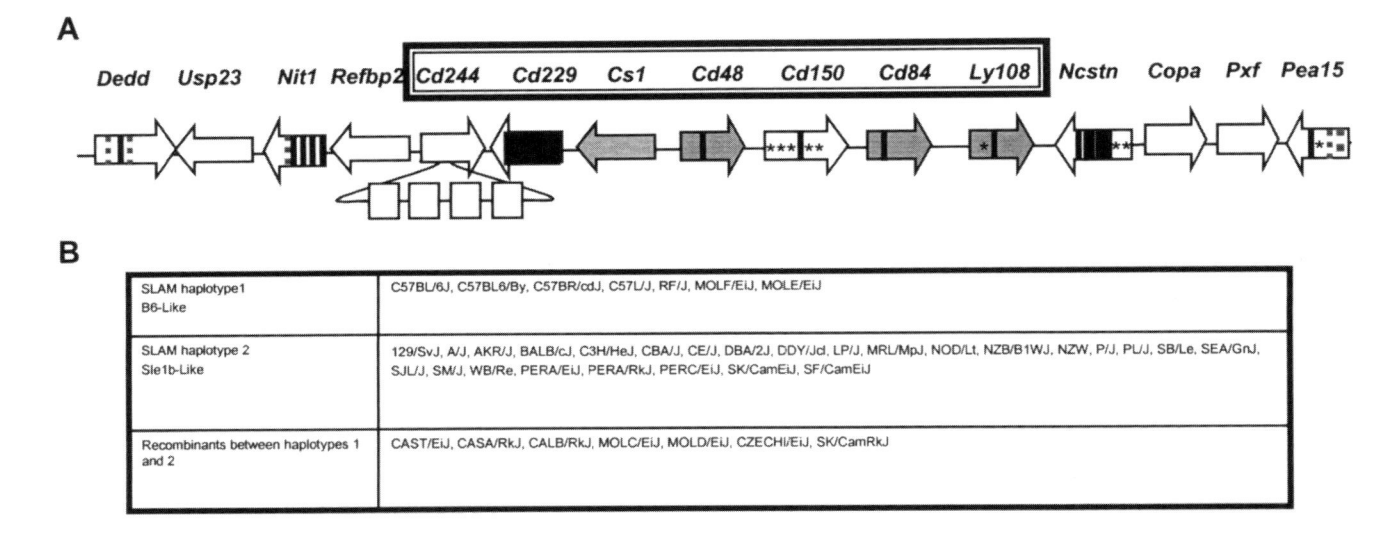

SLAM haplotype 1 B6-Like	C57BL/6J, C57BL/6/By, C57BR/cdJ, C57L/J, RF/J, MOLF/EiJ, MOLE/EiJ
SLAM haplotype 2 Sle1b-Like	129/SvJ, A/J, AKR/J, BALB/cJ, C3H/HeJ, CBA/J, CEJ/J, DBA/2J, DDY/Jcl, LP/J, MRL/MpJ, NOD/Lt, NZB/B1WJ, NZW, P/J, PL/J, SB/Le, SEA/GnJ, SJL/J, SM/J, WB/Re, PERA/EiJ, PERC/EiJ, SK/CamEiJ, SF/CamEiJ
Recombinants between haplotypes 1 and 2	CAST/EiJ, CASA/RkJ, CALB/RkJ, MOLC/EiJ, MOLD/EiJ, CZECHI/EiJ, SK/CamRkJ

FIG. 1. Functional polymorphisms in the SLAM/CD2 family distinguish two haplotypes in inbred strains. (A) SLAM/CD2 family members are the strongest candidates based on structural and expression polymorphisms. The indicated genes are considered candidates based on their expression in splenic lymphocytes. Arrows denote transcriptional direction. The Ig regions of the SLAM/CD2 family and a panel of single nucleotide polymorphisms (SNPs) in flanking genes were sequenced in 34 inbred, laboratory strains. Boxed genes indicate the seven members of the SLAM/CD2 family. Solid lines indicate SNPs that distinguish between the two haplotypes. $Cd244$ is expanded to a four-gene locus in haplotype 2. Asterisks denote SNPs found in a single strain and dotted grey lines indicate SNPs that do not follow a specific haplotype pattern. Grey shading designates those genes that show differential gene expression between the B6 and B6.$Sle1b$ strains in splenic B220$^+$ B cells and/or CD4$^+$ T cells at 2 months of age. (B) SNPs in the SLAM/CD2 family distinguish two haplotypes in inbred laboratory strains. This table describes the various inbred strains analysed and which of the two different SLAM/CD2 family haplotypes they share. In addition, analyses of 14 wild-derived, inbred strains identified recombinant versions of these two haplotypes.

autoimmunity or any other immunological phenotypes are detected in B6.*Sle1b* mice.

These analyses for *Sle1b* candidacy indicated that polymorphisms in gene(s) of the SLAM/CD2 family could be responsible for the various phenotypes observed in B6.*Sle1b* mice. It is interesting to note that all of the observed functional polymorphisms involve only moderate changes between the alleles of the two strains, with no immediately obvious functional consequences, such as the complete lack of a protein product. These data present two questions: are the *Sle1b* SLAM/CD2 family alleles, derived from the autoimmune prone NZM2410, unique in nature? Regardless, how could these functional polymorphisms affect the immune system such that these mice develop a loss in tolerance to chromatin and chronic lymphocyte activation?

To address the first question, the *Sle1b* alleles of these candidate genes were compared with those of other inbred laboratory strains to determine whether the observed structural changes are unique to *Sle1b* or other autoimmune strains in general. This approach has also been used in similar analyses of other disease susceptibility genes (Ueda et al 2003, Lee et al 2001, Lyons et al 2000, Chesnut et al 1993). Interestingly, this analysis revealed that this region forms essentially two haplotypes in standard laboratory mouse strains and that 29 of the 34 strains examined share the *Sle1b* alleles, henceforth referred to as SLAM/CD2 haplotype 2 (Fig. 1B). If this haplotype is responsible for autoimmunity in *Sle1b*, why then do all the normal, non-autoimmune strains, such as 129/SvJ, carrying this haplotype fail to breach tolerance to chromatin? One explanation is that the causal functional polymorphism was not detected in the original analyses. Another is that the ability of the SLAM/CD2 haplotype 2 to render susceptibility to autoimmunity is dependent on the background genome, in this case B6, due to unidentified epistatic interactions. The latter explanation suggests that regardless of the origin of the SLAM/CD2 haplotype 2, tolerance will be broken if moved onto the B6 background. To test this hypothesis, the corresponding interval from 129/SvJ was moved onto the B6 background (B6.*129c1*) and assessed for ANA production. Aged B6.*129c1* mice also develop significant levels of ANA production (Wandstrat et al 2004, Bygrave et al 2004). These data clearly indicate that the origin of the SLAM/CD2 haplotype 2 is irrelevant, and that it is its interaction with its genomic context that can drive autoimmunity. Such background-dependent allelic effects are becoming a paradigm in genetic studies of autoimmunity and have added a layer of further complexity to such analyses.

SLAM/CD2 family receptors and their association with autoimmunity

These data implicate functional polymorphisms in the SLAM/CD2 family as causative of the breach in tolerance to chromatin seen in B6.*Sle1b* mice. The mechanism(s) by which this is achieved remaining to be elucidated. This family of immune receptors and their related adaptor molecules, SAP and EAT2, have been the subject of intense investigation during the past few years. Each family member is expressed in a specific set of immune cell lineages, and their expression is altered by a variety of stimuli, including activation by antigen receptor systems, Toll receptors and cytokines. Their co-stimulatory functions during cognate antigen recognition between effector cells and antigen-presenting cells (APCs)/ targets are triggered via phosphorylation of ITSMs (immunoreceptor-based tyrosine switch motif) in their cytoplasmic domains and allows these receptors to modulate a variety of immune functions (for review, see Shlapatska et al 2001). These ITSM motifs, located in the intracellular region of all but one of the receptors, can interact with both activating and inhibitory signal transduction pathways by binding with SAP, EAT-2, SH-2 and SHIP-1 (reviewed in Veillette & Latour 2003, Engel et al 2003, Tangye et al 2000). Furthermore, certain members of this family express distinct isoforms that differ in their cytoplasmic tails, allowing for differential signalling capacities (Tovar et al 2002, Peck & Ruley 2000, Schatzle et al 1999). A variety of studies have demonstrated that triggering of this family can impact numerous immune functions, including macrophage and T cell activation, cytokine secretion and cytotoxicity (Mooney et al 2004, Wang et al 2004, Howie et al 2002, Martin et al 2001). Altogether, these data strongly indicate that the SLAM/CD2 family has the ability to modulate immune responses in a highly flexible fashion and hence may function as 'fine-tuners' of the immune response.

In the context of their association with autoimmunity, these analyses suggest that polymorphisms affecting both structure and expression of SLAM/CD2 family members may cause subtle shifts in the capacity and nature of the immune response to stimuli produced by pathogens and possibly self-antigens. The extensive polymorphisms distinguishing the haplotypes of B6 and B6.*Sle1b* may impact a variety of functional properties, including binding affinity, expression levels during cellular interactions and the nature of signalling via the cytoplasmic domains. For example, our analyses identified variations in *Ly108* isoform expression levels between B6 and B6.*Sle1b*, consistent with differential expression of cytoplasmic signalling domains for this SLAM/CD2 family member (Wandstrat et al 2004). Polymorphisms in expression of different isoforms, due to differences in regulation or internal splice sequences, can have functional consequences, as has been recently described for CTLA4 within the *Idd5.1* locus (Ueda et al 2003, Vijayakrishnan et al 2004). Cumulatively, these genetic variations may modulate the signalling outcomes of these molecules during a variety of cellular interactions, possibly leading to variations in the differentiation of several immune cell lineages during normal lymphocyte ontogeny and immune system development.

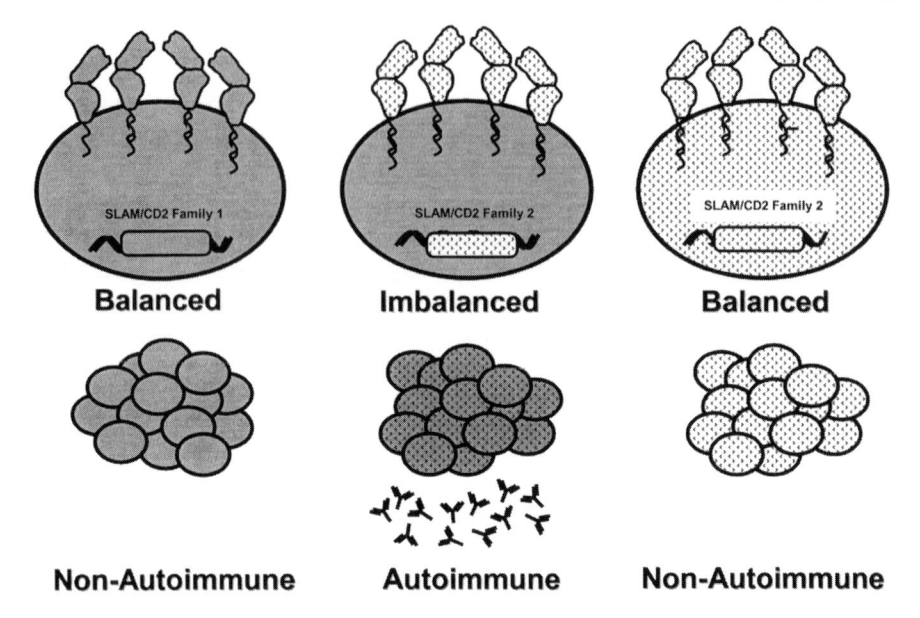

FIG. 2. SLAM/CD2 family haplotypes and the development of autoimmunity. The ability of SLAM/CD2 haplotype 2 to elicit autoimmunity is dependent upon interactions with the background genome. Epistatic interactions between the genetic variations in the background genome and the SLAM/CD2 haplotype could affect the development and possibly the nature of the immune system response. This may lead to an imbalance that culminates in the development of autoimmunity, as depicted in the centre panel.

Why then, does SLAM/CD2 haplotype 2 only cause autoimmunity when expressed on the B6 background? We postulate that B6-associated genetic variations in the downstream signalling pathways that transduce SLAM/CD2 family molecule signals lead to an imbalanced immune system in B6.*Sle1b* mice, which is responsible for the potent autoimmunity elicited by this locus, as illustrated in Fig. 2. The signalling properties of SLAM/CD2 family molecules can be dependent or independent of their interactions with the adaptor molecule SAP (Veillette 2004). A recent article has described that lack of SAP, due to genetic ablation, is in fact protective against pristane-induced lupus (Hron et al 2004). These data suggest that the observed polymorphisms in the SLAM/CD2 family may mediate their role by affecting the signalling properties of the cell types they are expressed in, and this in turn might be influenced by the signalling milieu expressed in the cells. Experiments are currently in progress to address these different questions.

Common alleles and autoimmunity

The nature of the genetic variants that underlie disease susceptibility for complex traits such as SLE is still under debate. Classic analyses of simple Mendelian diseases (for example, cystic fibrosis) have generally discovered that these are caused by collections of 'rare variants' that result in functionally defective alleles, which are incapable of performing critical cellular functions. Consistent with this model, one interpretation of the origins of genetic predisposition to autoimmunity would be that disease susceptibility results from the cumulative effects of many deleterious rare variants. This has been postulated as being probable for SLE based on the sheer number of reports describing lupus-like phenotypes in murine transgenic and knockout models, as well as from descriptions of rare variants in human SLE patients (reviewed in Vinuesa & Goodnow 2004). A second interpretation, termed the 'common variant/common disease' model, proposes that the additive and epistatic interactions occurring between combinations of common gene variants with individually weak effects are responsible for genetic predisposition to common diseases (Zwick et al 2000, Cargill et al 1999, Lander 1996, Chakravarti 1999, Reich & Lander 2001). In this model, the causative alleles are not necessarily deleterious loss-of-function mutations, but instead, are polymorphisms that modulate normal functions. Clearly, these two explanations are not mutually exclusive and it is likely that a combination of the above two scenarios impact disease susceptibility in human populations.

Our recent demonstration that the SLAM/CD2 family haplotype 2 is the more prevalent of the two haplotypes in standard inbred laboratory mouse strains supports the 'common variant/common disease' model. It could also be viewed as an artefact inherent to the original derivations of laboratory mice from a limited spectrum of the natural mouse population. However, further investigation of 15 fully inbred strains derived individually from wild mouse stocks, revealed that the SLAM/CD2 family is extensively diversified and does not fall into stable haplotypes in the wild. Some of these strains have recombinant versions of the haplotype that are comprised of different allelic combinations of B6 and *Sle1b*, in addition to some unique alleles (Wandstrat et al 2004). One of these SLAM/CD2 haplotypes, derived from CAST/Ei, also mediates autoimmunity when bred onto the B6 background, further supporting the common variant origin of the autoimmune phenotypes of *Sle1b*.

The extensive allelic variation in the SLAM/CD2 family discovered between B6 and B6.*Sle1b* is representative of the extensive diversity of this gene family in natural mouse populations. A detailed analysis of sequence variations in the SLAM/CD2 family among multiple *Mus* sub-species detected extensive additional polymorphisms in these genes, but also revealed that the SLAM/CD2 alleles in haplotype 2 are prevalent in natural mouse populations (N. Limaye,

K. Belobrajdic, A. Chan, F. Bonhomme, S. E. Edwards, E. K. Wakeland, unpublished results). These findings suggest that these are indeed common allelic variants that do not *per se* impair the ability of these animals to mount effective immune responses, and are hence being maintained via balancing selection. Additional evidence for the importance of allelic interactions comes from the many examples of attenuation or potentiation of knockout 'lupus-like' phenotypes that occur when these single-gene defects are moved to different genomic backgrounds (Shi et al 2002, Bolland et al 2002, Santiago-Raber et al 2001, Bickerstaff et al 1999, Mitchell et al 2002). In this regard, recent studies by Botto and co-workers strongly indicate that allelic interactions between the B6 and 129 genomes lead to potent lupus-like autoimmunity in the absence of any gene disruptions (Bygrave et al 2004). Taken together, these findings strongly support the importance of epistatic interactions among common allelic variants as a major contributing factor to susceptibility to autoimmunity.

The suppression of systemic autoimmunity as a consequence of epistatic interactions

In the previous sections, we described how functional polymorphisms in the SLAM/CD2 family are associated with the loss in tolerance seen in B6.*Sle1b* mice. However, these polymorphisms by themselves cannot elicit autoimmunity if the background genome does not support it. We have demonstrated earlier that suppressive modifier loci exist in the NZW genome, which prevent the development of pathogenic lupus despite the known ability of the *Sle1*, *Sle2* and *Sle3* loci to epistatically interact and mediate severe autoimmunity on the B6 background. These modifier loci, termed *Sles1–4*, cumulatively account for the lack of autoimmunity seen in NZW. These analyses also showed that *Sles1* specifically suppresses the break in tolerance to chromatin mediated by *Sle1*, but has no effect on the phenotypes of *Sle2* and *Sle3* on the B6 background (Morel et al 1999b).

The next question to address was how *Sles1* would affect the phenotypes of *Sle1* when an additional susceptibility locus was present. As previously mentioned, *Sle1* has been shown to be a necessary for severe disease initiation in our lupus models. Furthermore, the resulting systemic autoimmune phenotypes cannot be explained by additive effects alone and are indicative of strong epistatic interactions occurring between the *Sle1* genes and the additional susceptibility locus/loci. Interestingly, this is also true when *Sle1* is combined with susceptibility loci derived from other lupus models such as *Yaa* (*Y-autoimmune accelerator*), the *lpr* mutation and *FcRII* (Shi et al 2002, Bolland et al 2002, Morel et al 2000, Mohan et al 1999b). Male mice from the B6.*Sle1/yaa* strain develop a severe autoimmunity characterized by early onset and penetrant ANA production of various specificities, profound

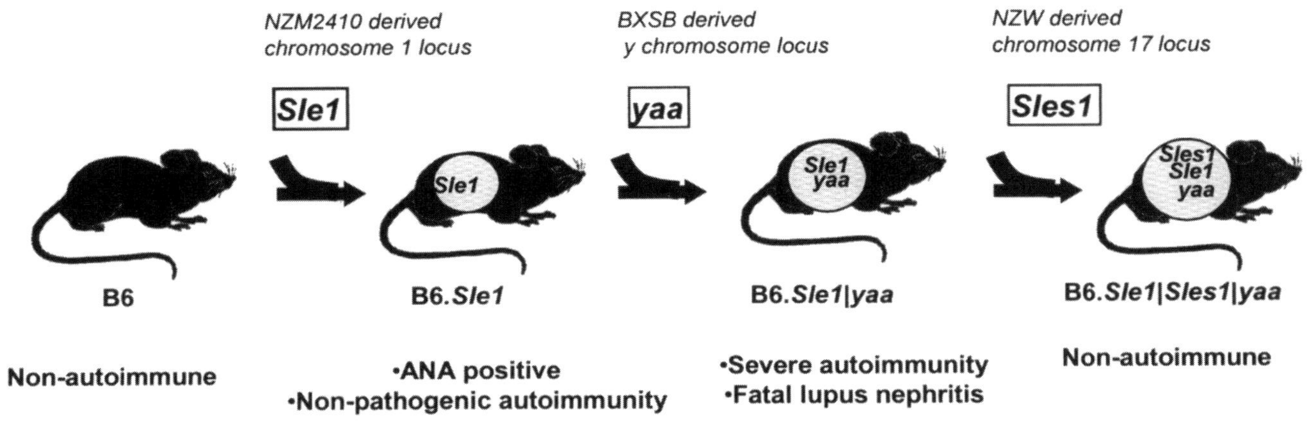

FIG. 3. Epistatic interactions modulate systemic autoimmunity. Introduction of the *Sle1* locus onto the B6 background results in non-pathogenic autoimmunity, characterized by a break in tolerance to chromatin and lymphocyte activation. Addition of the BXSB-derived *Yaa* locus leads to severe systemic autoimmunity culminating in fatal lupus nephritis, due to epistatic interactions between these two susceptibility loci. Introducing the NZW-derived *Sles1* suppressor locus, abrogates these phenotypes resulting in a non-autoimmune mouse, illustrating that there are many genetic paths leading to 'normal'.

splenomegaly and severe glomerulonephritis (GN), leading to a cumulative 9-month mortality of ~70%. Other phenotypes include a significant expansion in the percentage of splenic B and T lymphocytes that have activated/effector phenotypes (Croker et al 2003, Morel et al 2000). Introduction of *Sles1* onto this lupus model, comprised of susceptibility alleles derived from very different parental strains (NZM2410 and BXSB.*Yaa*) in epistatic interaction with each other, abrogates these phenotypes such that none of the mice die or develop any of the other phenotypes associated with this lupus model, as depicted in Fig. 3. The mechanism(s) behind this potent suppression is as yet unknown but it suggests that understanding it could provide great insight into how tolerance can be broken. Understanding the pathways that such suppressive modifiers impact to prevent autoimmunity might also illuminate key therapeutic targets.

References

Bickerstaff MC, Botto M, Hutchinson WL et al 1999 Serum amyloid P component controls chromatin degradation and prevents antinuclear autoimmunity. Nat Med 5:694–697

Bolland S, Yim YS, Tutter A, Wakeland EK, Ravetch JV 2002 Genetic modifiers of systemic lupus erythematosus in FcgammaRIIB-/- Mice. J Exp Med 195:1167–1174

Bygrave AE, Rose KL, Cortes-Hernandez J et al 2004 Spontaneous autoimmunity in 129 and C57BL/6 mice-implications for autoimmunity described in gene-targeted mice. PLoS Biol 2:E243

Cantor RM, Yuan J, Napier S et al 2004 Systemic lupus erythematosus genome scan: support for linkage at 1q23, 2q33, 16q12-13, and 17q21-23 and novel evidence at 3p24, 10q23-24, 13q32, and 18q22-23. Arthritis Rheum 50:3203–3210

Cargill M, Altshuler D, Ireland J et al 1999 Characterization of single-nucleotide polymorphisms in coding regions of human genes. Nat Genet 22:231–238

Chakravarti A 1999 Population genetics — making sense out of sequence. Nat Genet 21:56–60

Chesnut K, She J-X, Cheng I, Muralidharan K, Wakeland EK 1993 Characterizations of the candidate genes for IDD susceptibility from the diabetes-prone NOD mouse strain. Mamm Genome 4:549–554

Croker BP, Gilkeson G, Morel L 2003 Genetic interactions between susceptibility loci reveal epistatic pathogenic networks in murine lupus. Genes Immun 4:575–585

Engel P, Eck MJ, Terhorst C 2003 The SAP and SLAM families in immune responses and X-linked lymphoproliferative disease. Nat Rev Immunol 3:813–821

Howie D, Simarro M, Sayos J, Guirado M, Sancho J, Terhorst C 2002 Molecular dissection of the signaling and costimulatory functions of CD150 (SLAM): CD150/SAP binding and CD150-mediated costimulation. Blood 99:957–965

Hron JD, Caplan L, Gerth AJ, Schwartzberg PL, Peng SL 2004 SH2D1A regulates T-dependent humoral autoimmunity. J Exp Med 200:261–266

Lander ES 1996 The new genomics: global views of biology. Science 274:536–539

Lee SH, Gitas J, Zafer A et al 2001 Haplotype mapping indicates two independent origins for the Cmv1s susceptibility allele to cytomegalovirus infection and refines its localization within the Ly49 cluster. Immunogenetics 53:501–505

Lyons PA, Hancock WW, Denny P et al 2000 The NOD Idd9 genetic interval influences the pathogenicity of insulitis and contains molecular variants of Cd30, Tnfr2, and Cd137. Immun 13:107–115

Martin M, Romero X, de la Fuente MA et al 2001 CD84 functions as a homophilic adhesion molecule and enhances IFN-gamma secretion: adhesion is mediated by Ig-like domain 1. J Immunol 167:3668–3676

Mitchell DA, Pickering MC, Warren J et al 2002 C1q deficiency and autoimmunity: the effects of genetic background on disease expression. J Immunol 168:2538–2543

Mohan C, Morel L, Yang P, Wakeland EK 1997 Genetic dissection of SLE pathogenesis: *Sle2* on murine chromosome 4 leads to B-cell hyperactivity. J Immunol 159:454–465

Mohan C, Alas E, Morel L, Yang P, Wakeland EK 1998 Genetic dissection of SLE pathogenesis: *Sle1* on murine chromosome 1 leads to a selective loss of tolerance to H2A/H2B/DNA subnucelosomes. J Clin Invest 101:1362–1372

Mohan C, Yu Y, Morel L, Yang P, Wakeland EK 1999a Genetic dissection of SLE pathogenicity: *Sle3* on murine chromosome 7 impacts T cell activation, differentiation, and cell death. J Immunol 162:6492–6502

Mohan C, Morel L, Yang P, Watanabe H, Croker BP, Gilkeson GS, Wakeland EK 1999b Genetic dissection of lupus pathogenesis: a recipe for nephrophilic autoantibodies. J Clin Invest 103:1685–1695

Mooney JM, Klem J, Wulfing C et al 2004 The murine NK receptor 2B4 (CD244) exhibits inhibitory function independent of signaling lymphocytic activation molecule-associated protein expression. J Immunol 173:3953–3961

Morel L, Rudofsky UH, Longmate JA, Schiffenbauer J, Wakeland EK 1994 Polygenic control of susceptibility to murine systemic lupus erythematosus. Immunity 1:219–229

Morel L, Mohan C, Croker BP, Tian X-H, Wakeland EK 1997 Functional dissection of systemic lupus erythematosus using congenic mouse strains. J Immunol 158:6019–6028

Morel L, Mohan C, Schiffenbauer J et al 1999a Multiplex inheritance of component phenotypes in a murine model of lupus. Mamm Genome 10:176–181

Morel L, Tian X-H, Croker BP, Wakeland EK 1999b Epistatic modifiers of autoimmunity in a murine model of lupus nephritis. Immunity 11:131–139

Morel L, Croker BP, Blenman KR et al 2000 Genetic reconstitution of systemic lupus erythematosus immunopathology with polycongenic murine strains. Proc Natl Acad Sci USA 97:6670–6675

Morel L, Blenman KR, Croker BP, Wakeland EK 2001 The major murine systemic lupus erythematosus susceptibility locus, Sle1, is a cluster of functionally related genes. Proc Natl Acad Sci USA 98:1787–1792

Moser KL, Neas BR, Salmon JE et al 1998 Genome scan of human systemic lupus erythematosus: evidence for linkage on chromosome 1q in african-american pedigrees. Proc Natl Acad Sci USA 95:14869–14874

Peck SR, Ruley HE 2000 Ly108: a new member of the mouse CD2 family of cell surface proteins. Immunogenetics 52:63–72

Raman K, Mohan C 2003 Genetic underpinnings of autoimmunity — lessons from studies in arthritis, diabetes, lupus and multiple sclerosis. Curr Opin Immunol 15:651–659

Reich DE, Lander ES 2001 On the allelic spectrum of human disease. Trends Genet 17:502–510

Santiago-Raber M-L, Lawson BR, Dummer W et al 2001 Role of cyclin kinase inhibitor p21 in systemic autoimmunity. J Immunol 167:4067–4074

Schatzle JD, Sheu S, Stepp SE, Mathew PA, Bennett M, Kumar V 1999 Characterization of inhibitory and stimulatory forms of the murine natural killer cell receptor 2B4. Proc Natl Acad Sci USA 96:3870–3875

Shi X, Xie C, Kreska D, Richardson JA, Mohan C 2002 Genetic dissection of SLE: SLE1 and FAS impact alternate pathways leading to lymphoproliferative autoimmunity. J Exp Med 196:281–292

Shlapatska LM, Mikhalap SV, Berdova AG et al 2001 CD150 association with either the SH2-containing inositol phosphatase or the SH2-containing protein tyrosine phosphatase is regulated by the adaptor protein SH2D1A. J Immun 166:5480–5487

Sidorenko SP, Clark EA 2003 The dual-function CD150 receptor subfamily: the viral attraction. Nat Immunol 4:19–24

Tangye SG, Phillips JH, Lanier LL 2000 The CD2-subset of the Ig superfamily of cell surface molecules: receptor-ligand pairs expressed by NK cells and other immune cells. Semin Immunol 12:149–157

Tovar V, del Valle J, Zapater N et al 2002 Mouse novel Ly9: a new member of the expanding CD150 (SLAM) family of leukocyte cell-surface receptors. Immunogenetics 54:394–402

Tsao BP 2004 Update on human systemic lupus erythematosus genetics. Curr Opin Rheumatol 16:513–521

Ueda H, Howson JM, Esposito L et al 2003 Association of the T-cell regulatory gene CTLA4 with susceptibility to autoimmune disease. Nature 423:506–511

Veillette A 2004 SLAM family receptors regulate immunity with and without SAP-related adaptors. J Exp Med 199:1175–1178

Veillette A, Latour S 2003 The SLAM family of immune-cell receptors. Curr Opin Immunol 15:277–285

Vijayakrishnan L, Slavik JM, Illes Z et al 2004 An autoimmune disease-associated CTLA-4 splice variant lacking the B7 binding domain signals negatively in T cells. Immunity 20:563–575

Vinuesa CG, Goodnow CC 2004 Illuminating autoimmune regulators through controlled variation of the mouse genome sequence. Immunity 20:669–679

Vinuesa C, Angelucci C, Cook M, Goodnow C 2004 An ENU-based genome survey of autoimmunity alleles reveals a critical role for *Roqin* in the pathogenesis of a lupus-like syndrome with autoimmune thrombocytopenia. 12th International Congress of Immunology, July, Montreal, Canada (abstr)

Wakeland EK, Liu K, Graham RR, Behrens TW 2001 Delineating the genetic basis of systemic lupus erythematosus. Immunity 15:397–408

Wandstrat AE, Nguyen C, Limaye N et al 2004 Association of extensive polymorphisms in the SLAM/CD2 gene cluster with murine lupus. Immunity 21:769–780

Wang N, Satoskar A, Faubion W et al 2004 The cell surface receptor SLAM controls T cell and macrophage functions. J Exp Med 199:1255–1264

Zwick ME, Cutler DJ, Chakravarti A 2000 Patterns of genetic variation in Mendelian and complex traits. Annu Rev Genomics Hum Genet 1:387–407

DISCUSSION

Ting: Aside from *Sle1*, which you mentioned is an adhesion and co-stimulatory molecule, how much is known about the size of the genetic area that contains the other genes?

Wakeland: It varies depending on how far each fine mapping analysis has progressed. *Sles1* is localized to an interval of about 900 kb right now. This segment includes a portion of the MHC complex as well as a small segment centromeric to H2K. The MHC class II genes are included within the critical interval for *Sles1*, although we are pretty sure that they are not responsible for the phenotype. We currently have *Sle3* down to a segment of about 4 Mb, *Sle5* is localized to a segment of about 6 Mb, and *Sle1d* is located in a segment that contains about nine genes. At this point, our strategy for mapping autoimmune susceptibility genes in the mouse is evolving and I intend in the future to narrow the critical interval to a segment that contains less than five viable positional candidate genes. I'd like to be down to one gene, ideally. The reason for this is it is just too difficult to identify the causative gene in a definitive fashion when the critical interval contains many potential candidates. The identification of the causative gene is complicated by the fact that almost all of our intervals end up in regions that have extremely high SNP densities when the two parental genomes are compared. As a result, there is no shortage of variation to associate with the phenotype and the question generally ends up being about which of several possible variants is responsible for your phenotype? This is a difficult question to answer definitively, so our strategy is now to eliminate positional candidates via the generation of more recombinants.

Wijmenga: Is it fair to talk about modifiers? It seems that you have a group of genes that are more protective. Just as there are susceptible alleles, there might be protective alleles. It could be a balance between protection and susceptibility.

Wakeland: I agree that the terms 'protective' and 'susceptible' alleles are two views of the same genetic result. However, the term modifier in this context is used to emphasize the fact that *Sles1* specifically modifies the phenotype of *Sle1*, rather than *Sle2* or *Sle3*. We showed this in the original mapping study with congenic strains. At this point, it seems reasonable to propose that *Yaa*, *Sle1* and *Sles1* are all in the same pathway and that *Sles1* has the potential to shut down everything in that pathway. On the other hand, *Sles1* is unable to completely shutdown disease in other genetic combinations, such as the B6.*Sle1Sle2Sle3* triple congenic. Although *Sles1* completely abrogates disease in B6.*Sle1Yaa* mice, it only diminishes disease severity in the B6.*Sle1Sle2Sle3* triple congenic. Thus, *Sles1* is not an omnipotent suppressor, but instead appears to modify expression in the pathway that is affected by *Sle1*.

Goodnow: With autoimmune mutants it has been really helpful for us to see which things are primary and which are secondary. We do this by constructing mixed haemopoietic chimeras. You are in a great position to be able to do this. Have you taken the B6 LY5A mice which are wild-type (whatever that means) for all these loci and done mixed bone marrow chimeras?

Wakeland: Yes, we have done this for *Sle1*, *2* and *3*. This was done in collaboration with Eric Sobel (Sobel et al 1999, 2002a, 2002b). This was part of our strategy when we were looking for which other genes in our interval would be candidates. We knew on the basis of mixed bone marrow chimeras that *Sle1* was a T and B cell intrinsic gene. Only those cells would become activated in a mixed bone marrow chimera.

Goodnow: Have you looked at the effect of *Yaa* on top of this?

Wakeland: No.

Goodnow: In Mendelian autoimmune variants that are cell autonomous, autoimmunity caused by these variants in some cases is still suppressed by the presence of wild-type cells whereas in other cases even a subpopulation of leukocytes bearing the susceptibility gene is sufficient to break through and cause autoimmunity. To what extent do you see this or do you find that these are fully penetrant, even in the presence of wild-type cells?

Wakeland: In our case it is hard to say for sure because of issues concerning the relative engraftment of bone marrow from two distinct donors. Although mixed chimeras with *Sle1* express autoimmunity, is it expressed equivalently to the situation when *Sle1* bone marrow is used alone? We can't say for sure. Nonetheless, we can use this system to sort out which cells are involved in autoimmune interactions and it is a great strategy, although a technically challenging one.

Goodnow: Because you are on B6 you could use the LY5A marker. With *Yaa* on top of it where you have a robust, early T cell hyperactivation, the question is, is this a primary driving event or is it still reactive to dendritic cell (DC) hyperactivity?

Wakeland: That is a good question.

Kuchroo: Is *Sles1* on the B6 background inhibitory to the general immune responses, without any *Sle1* or *Yaa*? Or does it only work when *Sle1* is there?

Wakeland: We don't have a lot of data on *Sles1* on a B6 background by itself. But if you look at a B10.PL mouse, it would be fairly similar, because the *H2* region of PL is very similar to that of NZW. The point I was trying to make towards the end of my talk was that the B6.*Sles1Sle1Yaa* mouse doesn't have an unusual immunological phenotype and appears to respond normally to immunological stimulation. It is another genetic version of a 'normal' immune system.

Seed: I was curious about the CD150 expansion and the associated polymorphism. I am thinking about the connection with innate immunity. When there is a direct environmental driver one tends to see a lot of polymorphic diversification. In these various experimental syndromes, to what extent do you see germline VH utilization? Is it a CD5 T cell subset-driven phenomenon in most cases?

Wakeland: It is not a CD5 B1-type of B cell that produces the autoantibodies, but instead a normal B2-type antibody response using a variety of different V regions. Even when you look at the anti-nuclear antibody (ANA) production, you see indications of some somatic hypermutation, consistent with T dependent immune expansion. There is no preferential VH usage and the autoantibodies are not unusual, aside from the typical increased frequency of charged residues in the antibody binding sites. When we add *Yaa* or other susceptibility genes to *Sle1*, we drive the immune response further, resulting in autoantibodies to more nuclear antigens and higher titres of autoantibodies, although not the exact same V regions are utilized. We believe that the recruitment of B cells into the autoimmune response is somewhat stochastic, or just a chance process based on what receptors are available at the time that the chronic immune activation leads to a breach in tolerance.

Hafler: These are all naturally occurring haplotypes in the population. Could there have been a selective advantage in terms of an environmental event for them? If one exposed the native NZB mice to a variety of different infections that normally might be lethal, is there any situation in which the animals are protected? What is the selective advantage for these haplotypes?

Wakeland: We have been trying to persuade collaborators to try infecting B6.*Sle1b* mice versus B6 to see if the Cd150 polymorphism influences resistance to infectious disease. We haven't really found anything yet, but we continue to believe that there probably is an impact of this polymorphism on susceptibility to infection. Another tactic that we have employed to investigate this issue has been to analyse the evolutionary origins of the CD150 family polymorphisms, as well as *Tim1* and *Ctla4* in natural populations of wild mice. Our analyses indicate that most of the prevalent allelic lineages of these genes have long coalescence times, some of which go back through multiple *Mus* subspecies. This is similar to our results with the MHC, except that the MHC effect is much stronger. If balancing selection is impacting the diversity of these genes, then it is likely that it is in some way related to pathogen-driven selection for immune system diversity in natural populations of mice. You can make a similar argument for the prevalence in human populations of polymorphisms in HLA and other genes that are predisposing for autoimmunity. I think this will be commonly observed for genes that are predisposing for autoimmune susceptibility. They are diversified and this diversity is driven by the tremendous microbial and environmental diversity of natural ecosystems.

Cookson: Is *Yaa1* a gene or a locus?

Wakeland: That is a good question. It is actually a chromosome. It is the Y chromosome from a strain known as BXSB. The *Yaa* gene is remarkable in its ability to accelerate autoimmunity in the BSXB model. However, when it is introgressed onto B6 mice, it doesn't do anything, until you add a second gene such as *Sle1*, which results in the transition from a benign ANA-positive phenotype into pathogenic autoimmunity. Several groups have been trying to identify *Yaa*, but without success. Microarrays haven't worked thus far, although rumours of imminent breakthroughs have recently been circulating. Currently, *Yaa* is rather mysterious.

Abbas: For people who are not familiar with BSXB, it is the only mouse model of lupus where just the males get the disease. It violates all the so-called 'rules' of lupus.

Goodnow: How do you map when you have a Y chromosome that doesn't do meiosis?

Wakeland: Classical meiotic mapping can't be used. That has slowed things up considerably.

Vyse: Have you put *Yaa* with any other of your smaller *Sle1* subcongenic strains?

Wakeland: Laurence Morel has been doing this. This is one of the ways that we know that *Sle1c* doesn't drive the transition from ANA-positive to severe autoimmunity. If *Yaa* is crossed with *Sle1c*, there is no significant phenotypic amplification. For *Sle2* and *Sle3*, we don't know whether *Yaa* has a significant impact on the expression of their phenotypes.

Vyse: You might be getting at the nature of *Yaa* via this route.

Wakeland: I hope you are right.

Vyse: When you did your experiment of moving different segments from distal chromosome 1 on to B6, and you used *M. castaneous* because it had this recombination, it looked as if this congenic had a slightly milder phenotype. You suggested that you had already eliminated a bit of the *Slam* locus. Are you just nibbling away at it, and the phenotype is a result of inheriting the whole *Slam* haplotype?

Wakeland: That is a good question. However, the number of mice analysed for the CD150 families from 129 and CAST/Ei were small, only about 10 mice in each group. So, the slight difference in penetrance of ANA is not statistically significant, at least in this study.

Abbas: I have a question, comment and also a reflection of a personal bias. This is something that as a group we need to return to. How do you measure the effects of whatever gene or locus you are interested in? As a first approximation, many of us look at polyclonal T and B cell responses. But I feel that if we want to get answers, we need to measure responses to nuclear proteins or relevant autoantigens, and stop worrying about total B cell populations. This is true in people as well as in mice. The technology is getting better for looking at autoantigen-specific responses. To me, this has been a real failing in the field. We do what we can do, so we do experiments with anti-CD3 or LPS, but I am not sure this will give us the answers.

Hafler: I think that may be an over-simplification. It depends on the question being asked. These are complex assays. If one is looking at a haplotype that has a specific function, one has to carefully titrate the nature of the TCR signal. One can get insight into a pathway by doing this. The techniques for looking at the functionality of autoreactive T cells still remain problematic. The key may be to come up with better ways to interrogate cells.

Abbas: But if you start with the widespread appreciation that patients with diabetes get autoimmune attack against islets, for example, this is a restricted phenotype. The same is true for most other autoimmune diseases: there isn't widespread polyclonal dysregulation of all B cells. So we know that there is something unique about the responses to those autoantigens. It could be just the fact that the antigens are being released and although all the B cells are abnormal the responses are restricted to selected antigens, or it could be that lymphocytes with this specificity are somehow selectively affected. It is not an all-or-none situation. As a first approximation it is fine to do simpler polyclonal assays, but I think if gene mapping is going to get somewhere, we need to develop better assays as a community. We need surrogate measures for autoimmunity that can be picked up more easily.

Wakeland: We have worked very hard trying to find component autoimmune phenotypes that precede the initiation of autoimmunity in our congenic strains. It has been very difficult to identify an intrinsic defect prior to autoimmunity. What happens is that there is virtually nothing different between our congenic strain and a normal B6 mouse, and then hundreds of differences as they begin to develop autoimmunity. This is true whether you look at the bulk cell populations or global gene expression microarrays on isolated subsets. When we look early the only things we see in B6.*Sle1b* are the intrinsic variations in *Ly108* expression and a few other changes. There is no obvious defective pathway in these mice. However, once the mice start to become autoimmune, a variety of genes becoming dysregulated. It is a difficult situation to work on.

Wakeland: The *Sle1b* region doesn't show a lot of association with diabetes in crosses between NOD and B6. Alan Baxter did an induced lupus model of NOD that mapped a susceptibility gene to exactly the same region as *Sle1*. Beyond that, in MRL it doesn't appear to play a big role.

Seed: As a surrogate for using microbial pathogens to challenge the system, what about using some of the drugs that have been shown in humans to induce ANA-type reactive syndromes?

Wakeland: That is a good idea. We haven't done it.

Behrens: In regards to these SLAM molecules with lots of polymorphisms in the extracellular domain, can you demonstrate any difference in adhesion?

Wakeland: That particular assay is beyond our capabilities, but it would be interesting to know this.

References

Sobel ES, Mohan C, Morel L, Schiffenbauer J, Wakeland EK 1999 Genetic dissection of SLE pathogenesis: adoptive transfer of Sle1 mediates the loss of tolerance by bone marrow-derived B cells. J Immunol 162:2415–2421

Sobel ES, Morel L, Baert R, Mohan C, Schiffenbauer J, Wakeland EK 2002a Genetic dissection of systemic lupus erythematosus pathogenesis: evidence for functional expression of Sle3/5 by non-T cells. J Immunol 169:4025–4032

Sobel ES, Satoh M, Chen Y, Wakeland EK, Morel L 2002b The major murine systemic lupus erythematosus susceptibility locus Sle1 results in abnormal functions of both B and T cells. J Immunol 169:2694–2700

Mapping autoimmune disease genes in humans: lessons from IBD and SLE

Timothy J. Vyse, Angela M. Richardson*, Emily Walsh*, Lisa Farwell*, Mark J. Daly*, Cox Terhorst† and John D. Rioux*[1]

*Imperial College of London, Faculty of Medicine, Hammersmith Hospital, London W12 0NN, UK, *The Broad Institute of MIT and Harvard, Cambridge, MA 02139, USA and †Division of Immunology, Beth Israel Deaconess Medical Center, Harvard Medical School, Boston, MA 02115, USA*

Abstract. The inflammatory bowel diseases (IBD) and systemic lupus erythematosus (SLE) are common autoimmune diseases that affect 2–3 million people in the USA alone. Crohn's disease (CD) and ulcerative colitis (UC), the inflammatory bowel diseases, are idiopathic, chronic inflammatory disorders of the gastrointestinal tract. SLE is a chronic, multi-system autoimmune disease that generally presents in women of childbearing age as fatigue, arthralgia and rash. Although the aetiology of these two diseases is not fully known, it is believed that genetic, hormonal and environmental influences contribute to susceptibility. Genomewide linkage scans in IBD have revealed significant loci that, upon comprehensive association mapping strategies, yield what are believed to be causal susceptibility alleles. Human linkage studies performed to date in SLE have not been as informative, although genetic mapping in mouse models of SLE as well as candidate gene approaches have provided important clues to the genetic susceptibility in humans. We will examine how some of the recent advances in our understanding of genetic variation in the human genome are greatly improving our ability to map autoimmune disease genes in humans.

2005 The genetics of autoimmunity. Wiley, Chichester (Novartis Foundation Symposium 267) p 94–112

Complex traits

Autoimmune diseases, such as systemic lupus erythematosus (SLE) and inflammatory bowel disease (IBD), are complex human genetic traits. As such they do not follow the simple patterns of inheritance (e.g. dominant, recessive) characteristic of Mendelian diseases, such as cystic fibrosis or Duchenne's muscular dystrophy. Furthermore, the relationship between a causal genetic variant and its effect on an individual's risk of developing disease for a Mendelian

---

[1] This paper was presented at the symposium by John D. Rioux to whom correspondence should be addressed.

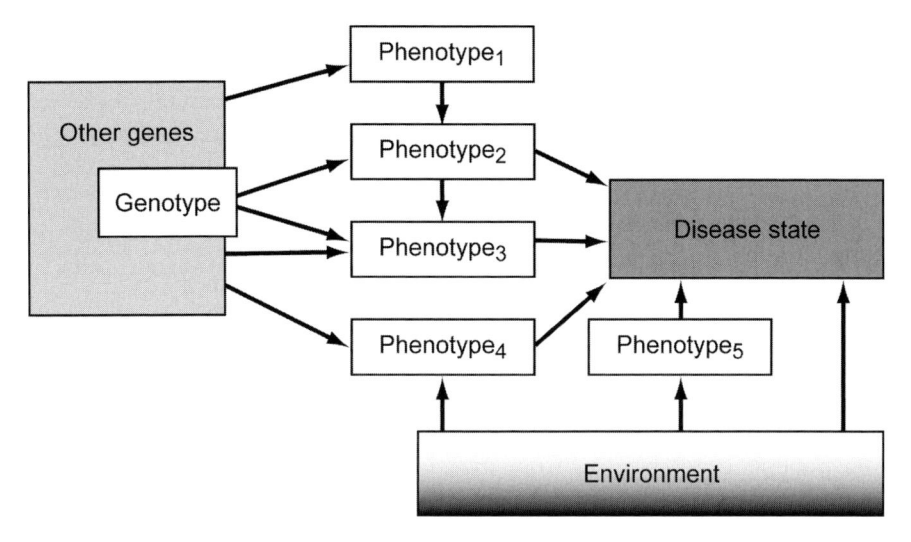

FIG. 1. In complex traits, the clinically recognized disease state is the result of interactions between multiple genotypes and the environment. The influence of any individual causal allele is modest and is likely to be more directly related to intermediate phenotypes (e.g. autoantibodies) than clinical disease.

trait is very different than for a complex trait. Specifically, the relationship in the former can be viewed as deterministic and the latter probabilistic.

Consequently, it is likely that any given genetic variant in a complex trait is likely to be more directly related to an intermediate phenotype (e.g. control of immune response). It is the combination of these intermediate phenotypes and environmental factors that leads to the complex phenotype recognized clinically as disease (Fig. 1). The genetic characteristics of common, complex diseases impact significantly on study design and interpretation. We will examine some of these issues in the context of the genetic studies that have been performed in the search for genes predisposing to IBD or SLE.

Inflammatory bowel disease (IBD)

The role of genetic risk factors in IBD is supported by the fact that siblings of Crohn's disease (CD) patients have a ~30-fold greater risk of developing IBD compared with unrelated individuals, while the relative risk to siblings for ulcerative colitis (UC) is 10–20-fold (Yang & Rotter 1994). Further evidence of genetic involvement is provided by twin studies demonstrating that monozygotic (MZ) twins are more concordant for disease than dizygotic (DZ) twins, a difference more pronounced in CD (50% vs. 3.8% and 18% vs. 4%, MZ vs. DZ in CD and UC, respectively) (Binder 1998).

In an effort to localize genetic variants predisposing to IBD, much effort has been spent performing genomewide searches for regions of linkage. To date, a dozen genomewide searches have been performed with more than 2000 affected relative pairs with IBD from ~1200 families. Six genomic regions show the most consistent evidence of linkage and have been designated *IBD1–IBD6* (MIM #s 266600, 601458, 604519, 606675, 606348 and 606674, respectively; *http://www.ncbi.nlm.nih.gov/entrez/query.fcgi?db=OMIM*). It should be noted that no single study identified all loci and, conversely, no single locus was identified in all studies. This apparent lack of consistency is explained by the modest power of individual family collections and the significant effect of sampling variance on the distribution of disease alleles between studies. The lack of power of individual studies is best illustrated by the first true replication of an IBD susceptibility locus (the *IBD1* locus on chromosome 16, LOD score=5.79) that resulted from pooling genotype data from over 613 families collected by 12 centres distributed throughout North America, Europe and Australia. It is striking that evidence for linkage in this study came from all 12 centres, including those that had not previously found convincing linkage to this locus (Cavanaugh 2001).

IBD1/CARD15

A genomewide search conducted by Hugot and co-workers in affected sibling pairs (Hugot et al 1996) provided the first evidence of linkage between the *IBD1* locus and IBD. This is the most consistently replicated finding in IBD and is specific to CD (Bonen & Cho 2003). Further work by Hugot et al (2001) utilized a positional mapping approach to identify an association between CD and mutations in an expressed sequence tag cluster representing *NOD2*, a gene located within the linkage peak of the *IBD1* locus. More specifically, three variants were identified as being associated with susceptibility to CD: SNP8 (Arg702Trp), SNP12 (Gly908Arg) and 'SNP13' (Leu10007fsinsC). *NOD2*, now known as *CARD15* (caspase recruitment domain 15), is a strong functional candidate for predisposition to IBD because it is homologous to plant proteins associated with pathogen resistance as well as playing a role in the expression of NF-κB in response to bacterial lipopolysaccharides (Bonen & Cho 2003). Using a candidate gene approach, Ogura et al (2001) and Hampe et al (2001) identified the Leu10007fsinsC mutation in *CARD15* as being associated with CD. One copy of the risk allele has been shown to increase risk for developing CD two- to fourfold, while two copies leads to a 20–40-fold increase in risk (Bonen & Cho 2003). Consistent with the linkage data, neither the Ogura nor Hampe study found an association between UC and this frameshift mutation.

In order to more extensively sample the variation in the *CARD15* region, 45 single nucleotide polymorphisms (SNPs) were typed in a cohort of CD cases and controls (Vermeire et al 2002). The haplotype structure of this 177 kb region was examined and four blocks containing little to no evidence of recombination were defined (Fig. 2A). The third block of 22 kb encompasses most of the *CARD15* coding sequence and has three haplotypes (A, B, C) accounting for most of the commonly seen variation. The results of a transmission disequilibrium test demonstrate that the C haplotype is overtransmitted from parents to affected offspring, while the A and B haplotypes are undertransmitted. Testing the three variant SNPs discovered by Hugot further separated the C haplotype into four subvariants (Fig. 2B): the wild-type haplotype, carrying the non-risk allele at all three SNPs, and three variants, each containing one risk allele. Statistical analysis shows that the wild-type C haplotype is undertransmitted from parents to affected offspring, while the three variants with risk alleles are each overtransmitted. Although the three subvariants are located on the same haplotype, that haplotype exists in a different genetic context as indicated by sequence differences in the flanking haplotype blocks, thus providing evidence that the three variations arose independently (Vermeire et al 2002).

Functional aspects of CARD15

The putative function of *CARD15* supports a role in susceptibility to IBD, although mice with this gene knocked-out do not exhibit microscopic or macroscopic disease (Pauleau & Murray 2003). The protein is composed of two CARD domains at the N-terminus, a central nucleotide-binding domain, and a leucine-rich repeat (LRR) domain at the C-terminus. *CARD15* is expressed in the cytoplasm of antigen-presenting cells and, via the LRR, is a receptor for muramyl dipeptide, a component of bacterial peptidoglycan. Paneth cells, located at the base of the crypts in the small intestine, have also been shown to express the *CARD15* gene product (Ogura et al 2003). An interesting hypothesis links *CARD15* with development of CD through the Paneth cell-mediated response to bacteria (Ogura et al 2003). The three variants associated with CD are located in or near the LRR, with the frameshift mutation truncating the LRR. When transfected into human embryonic kidney 293T cells, the CD-associated variants of this gene decrease the response of antigen-presenting cells to bacterial lipopolysaccharides as indicated by reduced production of cytokines (Ogura et al 2001). However, other studies have recently shown an increase in cytokine production via the TLR2 (toll-like receptor) pathway, mediated by reduced inhibition of NF-κB production (Watanabe et al 2004). Further work is required to fully delineate the function of the *CARD15* gene product.

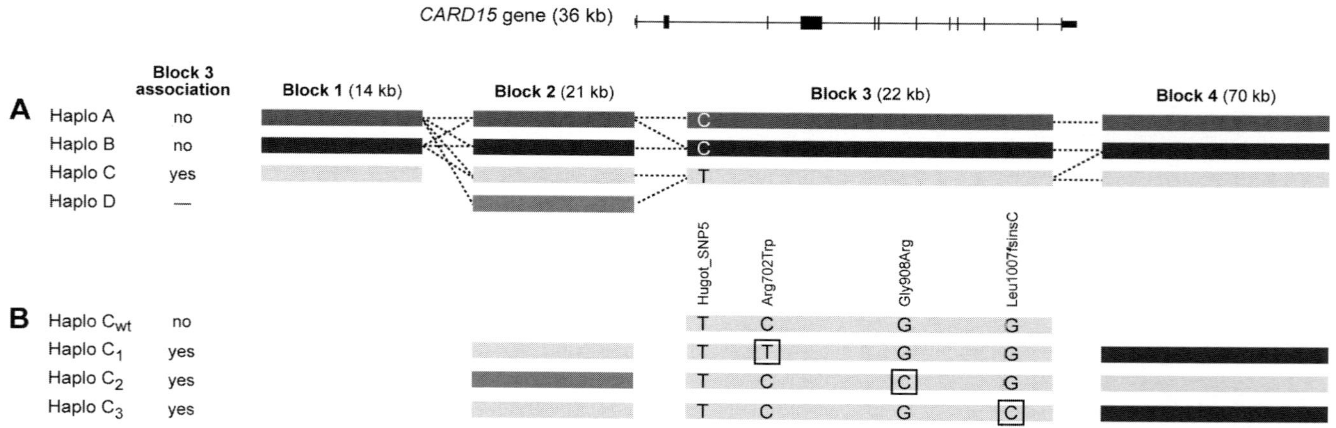

FIG. 2. *CARD15* variants are associated with Crohn's disease. (A) The association signal can be resolved to haplotype C of Block 3, tagged by allele T at Hugot_SNP5. (B) The three *CARD15* variants discovered by Hugot et al (Arg702Trp, Gly908Arg, Leu1007fsinsC) define three distinct haplotypes independently associated with CD.

IBD5

An 18 cM region on chromosome 5q31, later named *IBD5*, was shown to be significantly linked with CD in a genomewide scan (Rioux et al 2000). A hierarchical mapping project led to the identification of a 250 kb haplotype significantly associated with CD (Rioux et al 2001). This risk haplotype is very common — its estimated frequency in the general population is ∼37%, but it is carried by >75% of all CD patients studied. This association was replicated in a subsequent study of 555 German IBD trios ($\chi^2 = 12.7$, $P = 0.0002$). Three additional studies have since been published and a meta-analysis of all the replication studies provides overwhelming evidence of association ($P < 10^{-10}$). This meta-analysis estimates the strength of the effect as ∼1.30 [95% confidence interval 1.2, 1.4] (Daly & Rioux 2004), compared with the stronger effect estimated in the original study (∼2.25). This common phenomenon in genetic studies is termed the 'winner's curse'; i.e. the first study to report association of an allele will overestimate its effect.

A recent study reports the identification of two sequence variants on the risk haplotype highly associated with CD. The first (rs1050152) is a missense substitution in organic cation transporter, *OCTN1*, resulting in a leucine to phenylalanine substitution; the second (rs2631367) is a mutation in the promoter region of *OCTN2*. The investigators show that these genes are expressed in the gastrointestinal (GI) tract in epithelial cells, macrophages and T cells. Further analysis demonstrates that the variant forms of these proteins exhibit altered function: the mutation in *OCTN1* modifies cation transport, and the mutation in the promoter region disrupts activity (Peltekova et al 2004). Additional studies will be necessary to further elucidate the function of these variants on IBD pathogenesis. Finally, as these proposed causal alleles have not been proven to act independently of the other variants but are unique to the risk haplotype, the *IBD5* locus provides an example of the difficulties faced in proving causality in a large region of very strong linkage disequilibrium.

DLG5

A genomewide linkage study reported linkage (LOD = 2.3) of a region of chromosome 10 to IBD in a patient cohort from Germany and the United Kingdom (Hampe et al 1999). A comprehensive association mapping study performed in >500 German–British trios reported association between the haplotype block containing the *DLG5* gene and IBD. The association was then confirmed in an independent group of cases and controls. *DLG5* is an interesting functional candidate due to its expression in the GI tract and its putative function in scaffolding. The most frequently observed haplotype in the study (haplotype A; frequency = 34%) was undertransmitted from parents to IBD affected offspring and was hypothesized to exert a protective effect. The authors also demonstrated association signals originating from two missense mutations in the same gene, *R30Q* (frequency=10%), and the rare *P1371Q* (frequency=1%) These mutations are also known as *113A* and *4136C*, respectively.

We recently attempted to replicate this finding by performing an association study in a large cohort of European-derived cases ($n=249$) and controls ($n=247$). In our preliminary analysis, the data appears to confirm association of the minor allele of *R30Q* with IBD. However, we did not find evidence for the involvement of haplotype 'A' in IBD susceptibility. The variant form of *P1371Q* was not observed at a high enough frequency to allow for analysis (M. J. Daly, L. Farwell, A. Latiano et al, unpublished data).

Genotype–genotype and genotype–phenotype interactions

Genotype–genotype

CARD15 and IBD5. Several attempts have been made to determine if any of the genes predisposing to IBD act together in exerting their effect. In their study of *CARD15*, Vermeire et al (2002) found that 74% of all *CARD15*-positive cases also carried the *IBD5* risk haplotype. Stratification of the data indicated that *CARD15* and *IBD5* exert their effects independently (Vermeire et al 2002). Further support for this finding comes from a study performed by Armuzzi and co-workers who again found no evidence for epistasis between *IBD5* and *CARD15* (Armuzzi et al 2003).

Giallourakis and colleagues also examined the possibility of epistasis between *IBD5* and *CARD15*. There was no evidence of interaction in cases with CD; however, there was evidence of interaction between these two loci that conferred susceptibility to UC (Giallourakis et al 2003). A subsequent study (McGovern et al 2003) replicated the finding of an epistatic relationship between *IBD5* and *CARD15* in UC susceptibility.

CARD15 in UC susceptibility. In this study, the association was limited to the Arg702Trp variant of *CARD15*; the other two *CARD15* variants showed no evidence of epistatic interaction with *IBD5* predisposing to UC (McGovern et al 2003).

CARD15 and DLG5. In the *DLG5* study performed by Stoll et al (2004) stratification of the trios on the basis of the affected child's genotype suggests genetic interaction between the *DLG5* risk haplotype defined by *R30Q* and *CARD15* in CD susceptibility. However, this finding has yet to be replicated. Studies in large independent cohorts will be needed to achieve the required statistical power.

Genotype–phenotype

CARD15. IBD varies in its clinical presentations (localization, age of onset and disease behaviour, e.g. fistulization, stenosis and resection) and the connection between a given genotype and presentation of symptoms is not fully understood. Stratification of data based on genotype rather than linkage score is much more informative, since any true interaction must be with the underlying sequence variant and not family linkage status, which is only indirectly correlated with the underlying variation. Many investigations have been conducted to examine the role of *CARD15* in determining specific clinical subphenotypes of IBD with great consistency in the results. In one such study, univariate analysis of 239 CD patients for whom complete phenotype information was available demonstrated a significant association between *CARD15* and ileal involvement (OR=2.62, $P=0.0032$) rather than colonic involvement (OR=0.59, $P=0.02$). Further multivariate logistic regression analysis examining ileal involvement with the covariables of age at onset, gender, smoking, *CARD15* status and status at other genetic loci found that ileal phenotype is not correlated with any of these other variables (Vermeire et al 2002).

IBD5. Armuzzi et al (2003) reported an association between IBD5 and perianal CD in their study of genotype–phenotype interactions (relative risk, RR=1.7, $P=0.0005$). This risk was even more pronounced in individuals homozygous for the risk haplotype (RR=3.0, $P=0.0005$). No association was seen between patients without perianal disease and the IBD5 risk haplotype.

It is clear that we are at the very beginning of these types of explorations into genotype–phenotype relationships. Many more exciting discoveries should follow in the next several years.

Systemic lupus erythematosus (SLE)

SLE is a chronic, multisystem autoimmune disease with a worldwide incidence conservatively estimated at 12–104 cases per 100 000 individuals, with a 10:1 female gender bias (Hochberg 1997). There is a four- to fivefold higher incidence in many non-European populations (including African-American, East Asian and Southern Asian) compared with European populations (Samanta et al 1992, Johnson et al 1995, Molokhia et al 2003). That the prevalence of SLE in these high-risk groups is the same for individuals from these populations living in Europe or America indicates that genetic factors contribute to the differences in disease frequency.

Epidemiological studies reveal a significant genetic contribution to the pathogenesis of SLE. The relative risk to siblings of affected individuals is estimated to be 15–20-fold greater than that of the unrelated population

(Hochberg 1997). Although only limited numbers of studies have been published, twin concordance rates provide additional evidence for a genetic contribution in SLE: the concordance rate is 10-fold greater in monozygotic (MZ) than dizygotic (DZ) twins (24% vs. 2% and 57% vs. 5% in two independent studies) (Block et al 1975, Deapen et al 1992).

Genetics of SLE in mice and humans

Over the last several years, a number of groups have published genomewide and targeted linkage analyses in SLE (Moser et al 1998, Johanneson et al 1999, Shai et al 1999, Gaffney et al 2000). There is considerable heterogeneity across these linkage studies, no doubt reflecting small study sizes, genetic heterogeneity, and clinical heterogeneity in SLE. The most consistently mapped lupus susceptibility loci reside in the following regions: 1q23, 1q25-31, 1q41-42, 2q35-57, 4p16-15.2, 6p11-21 (MHC) and 16q12, all having been reported in two or more studies (Wakeland et al 2001, Tsao 2003).

In mice, genomewide linkage studies have implicated three susceptibility loci (*Sle1* on Chr 1, syntenic to human Chr 1q23; *Sle2* on Chr 4; and *Sle3* on Chr 7) in three different models of spontaneous lupus: the (NZB×NZW) F2 intercross, the NZM/Aeg2410 New Zealand mice, and the BXSB mice (Kono et al 1994, Rozzo et al 1996, Hogarth et al 1998). The phenotype of these mice is very similar to that in SLE patients, with the production of autoantibodies as well as multi-organ involvement, including severe nephritis. The creation of congenic strains on a non-lupus prone background demonstrates the different functions of these loci. *Sle1* mediates the loss of tolerance to nuclear antigens and is necessary for initiation of the pathogenic process of SLE; *Sle2* lowers the activation threshold of B cells; and *Sle3* mediates T cell dysregulation (Wakeland et al 2001). Interestingly, it has been shown that *Sle1* is necessary for the production of nephrophilic autoantibodies and clinical glomerulonephritis (Mohan et al 1999). Fine mapping of the *Sle1* locus in one mouse strain has demonstrated the presence of a cluster of functionally related genes that contribute to disease susceptibility (Morel et al 2001). This latter observation is very consistent with the human linkage data insofar as a cluster of disease susceptibility genes is likely to lead to a consistently observed linkage region, as is the case for 1q23 in human SLE.

The SLAM locus and SLE

Given the compelling evidence of linkage in human and mouse studies of SLE, we examined the chromosome 1q23 region for candidate genes having a function that could potentially be related to SLE pathogenesis. In doing so, we were struck by the presence of the *SLAM* cluster of genes in this region. Specifically, this region

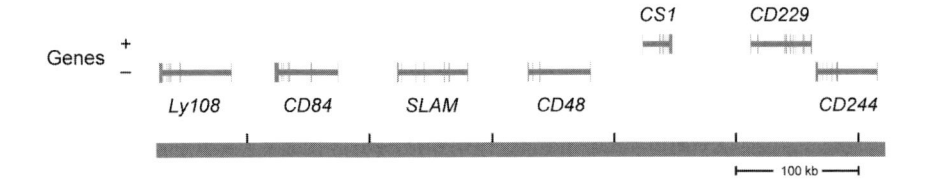

FIG. 3. Physical map of *SLAM* region located on human chromosome 1q23.

TABLE 1 Members of *SLAM* gene family cluster on human chromosome 1q23

Gene name	Synonyms	Binding to SAP/EAT
Ly108	*KALI, NTBA, SF2000, SLAMF6*	+
CD84	*LY9B, SLAMF5*	+
SLAM	*CD150, SLAMF1*	+
CD48	*SLAMF2*	−
CS1	*CRACC, 19A, SLAMF7, Novel Ly9*	−
CD229	*Ly9, SLAMF3*	+
CD244	*NAIL, SLAMF4, 2B4, Nmrk*	+

contains a cluster of functionally related genes (Fig. 3; Table 1) and is named after the *SLAM* (signalling lymphocytic activation molecule) gene. In addition to its location within the linkage region, emerging data provide strong arguments that the genes in the *SLAM* region have a crucial role in the key processes believed to lead to SLE. Specifically, the cluster of genes in the *SLAM* region belongs to the CD2 superfamily of molecules that regulate the responses of cells of the immune system. These genes are expressed in T cells, B cells, NK cells, dendritic cells, macrophages and monocytes; this broad pattern suggests that this family of genes is involved in the regulation of the immune response in a wide variety of cell types. Six genes of this cluster (*Ly108*, *CD84*, *SLAM*, *CS1*, *CD229*, *CD244*) recruit active Src kinases to their cytoplasmic tails using the adaptors of SAP (*SLAM*-associated protein) and EAT-2. The lipid-linked CD48 interacts with Src kinases in lipid rafts present in the plasma membrane of T cells and antigen-presenting cells. Furthermore, genetic manipulation of some of these genes has resulted in dramatic immunological abnormalities. For example, CD48-deficient mice have a pronounced defect in CD4$^+$ T cell activation (Gonzalez-Cabrero et al 1999).

To test this candidate region for association to SLE, we have started to create a haplotype map of this region. We then selected informative SNPs from this preliminary map and typed >400 SLE families. Our preliminary results show several peaks of association across the region (T. J. Vyse, A. M. Richards, L. Farwell, M. J. Daly, C. Terhorst, D. Rioux, unpublished data). The multiple association signals raise the interesting possibility that several genes in this region are associated with SLE susceptibility. However, further work is required to determine whether the signals are truly independent and to replicate the finding in an independent data set.

The major histocompatibility complex

The major histocompatibility complex (MHC) region has been implicated in IBD, SLE and most all other inflammatory and autoimmune diseases. Moreover, the MHC represents one of the most intensively studied regions in the human genome. Associations between autoimmune disease and alleles of genes in the region are among the most consistent findings in human genetics (Price et al 1999, Beck & Trowsdale 2000). Historically, attempts to characterize the region have focused on a handful of highly variable classical human leukocyte antigen (*HLA*) genes (Class I genes: *HLA-A, -B, -C*; and Class II genes: *HLA-DRB1, -DQA1, -DQB1, -DPA1, -DPB1*). These genes encode cell surface molecules that present antigenic peptides to T cells, thereby initiating an acquired immune response to invading pathogens and other foreign antigens. However, the classical *HLA* loci represent a minority of the genes found in the MHC region, since at least another 140 genes are present in this ~4 Mb region (Beck & Trowsdale 2000). By focusing on just the classical *HLA* genes, one may overlook other disease-influencing variation in the region. A more uniform, comprehensive haplotype map will help to discriminate between causal alleles and variation that is merely in linkage disequilibrium with them.

With this goal in mind, we set out to build an SNP haplotype map of the region. To integrate this map with the wealth of findings from association studies we typed 201 reliable, polymorphic, evenly spaced SNPs (target density, one SNP every 20 kb) in 136 independent chromosomes also typed for nine *HLA* genes, two *TAP* genes (involved in antigen processing), and 18 microsatellite markers. All markers were typed in families (18 multigenerational European pedigrees from the Centre d'Etude du Polymorphisme Humain [CEPH] collection) to allow direct assessment of phase and therefore simple reconstruction of haplotypes. Using these SNP data, we examined the haplotype patterns of the region and mapped these patterns relative to both genetic and physical distance (Walsh et al 2003), as assayed by an exceedingly high-resolution recombination map (Cullen et al 2002).

As it develops to its ultimate 1 kb density, this map should allow a thorough examination of the variation in the region. With this map of increased density and very large cohorts of patient and matched controls, it should be possible to localize the causal alleles for most autoimmune diseases.

Conclusions

Recently, significant advances have been made in mapping autoimmune disease genes in humans, especially in IBD. Linkage analyses have provided useful information and led to specific regions for follow-up studies. Some of these regions have been linked to multiple different diseases in multiple studies (e.g. MHC region). With the emerging data from the International HapMap Project regarding the common patterns of genetic variation and the increasing cost efficiency of typing technologies, comprehensive studies with large sample sizes are now becoming possible. These studies will focus on specific regions of the genome or the genome in its entirety and will undoubtedly lead to significant findings of association. The remaining challenges will be significant as identifying alleles with modest effect is only the first step. Much work will be necessary to replicate these association findings, demonstrate causality, establish the role of these associated variants in disease pathogenesis, elucidate the relationships between genotype and phenotype and identify the interactions between genotype and environment. There is no doubt, however, that comprehensive and powerful genetic studies will increase our knowledge surrounding autoimmune diseases.

Acknowledgements

The authors would like to thank the members of the Inflammatory Disease Research Group at the Broad Institute of MIT and Harvard. The authors would also like to thank L. Gaffney for help in the preparation of this manuscript. JDR is supported by the NIH/NIDDK (DK62432 and DK64869) and the Crohn's and Colitis Foundation of America. TJV is supported by the Wellcome Trust.

References

Armuzzi A, Ahmad T, Ling KL et al 2003 Genotype-phenotype analysis of the Crohn's disease susceptibility haplotype on chromosome 5q31. Gut 52:1133–1139

Beck S, Trowsdale J 2000 The human major histocompatability complex: lessons from the DNA sequence. Annu Rev Genomics Hum Genet 1:117–137

Binder V 1998 Genetic epidemiology in inflammatory bowel disease. Dig Dis 16:351–355

Block SR, Winfield JB, Lockshin MD, D'Angelo WA, Christian CL 1975 Studies of twins with systemic lupus erythematosus. A review of the literature and presentation of 12 additional sets. Am J Med 59:533–552

Bonen DK, Cho JH 2003 The genetics of inflammatory bowel disease. Gastroenterology 124:521–536

Cavanaugh J 2001 International collaboration provides convincing linkage replication in complex disease through analysis of a large pooled data set: Crohn disease and chromosome 16. Am J Hum Genet 68:1165–1171

Cullen M, Perfetto SP, Klitz W, Nelson G, Carrington M 2002 High-resolution patterns of meiotic recombination across the human major histocompatibility complex. Am J Hum Genet 71:759–776

Daly M, Rioux J 2004 New approaches to gene hunting in IBD. Inflamm Bowel Dis 21:111–115

Deapen D, Escalante A, Weinrib L et al 1992 A revised estimate of twin concordance in systemic lupus erythematosus. Arthritis Rheum 35:311–318

Gaffney PM, Ortmann WA, Selby SA et al 2000 Genome screening in human systemic lupus erythematosus: results from a second Minnesota cohort and combined analyses of 187 sib-pair families. Am J Hum Genet 66:547–556

Giallourakis C, Stoll M, Miller K et al 2003 IBD5 is a general risk factor for inflammatory bowel disease: replication of association with Crohn disease and identification of a novel association with ulcerative colitis. Am J Hum Genet 73:205–211

Gonzalez-Cabrero J, Wise CJ, Latchman Y et al 1999 CD48-deficient mice have a pronounced defect in CD4(+) T cell activation. Proc Natl Acad Sci USA 96:1019–1023

Hampe J, Schreiber S, Shaw SH et al 1999 A genomewide analysis provides evidence for novel linkages in inflammatory bowel disease in a large European cohort. Am J Hum Genet 64:808–816

Hampe J, Cuthbert A, Croucher PJ et al 2001 Association between insertion mutation in NOD2 gene and Crohn's disease in German and British populations. Lancet 357:1925–1928

Hochberg M 1997 The epidemiology of systemic lupus erythematosus. In: Wallace DJ, Hahn BH (eds) Dubois' Lupus Erythematosus, 5th edn, Williams & Wilkins, Baltimore, p 49–65

Hogarth MB, Slingsby JH, Allen PJ et al 1998 Multiple lupus susceptibility loci map to chromosome 1 in BXSB mice. J Immunol 161:2753–2761

Hugot JP, Laurent-Puig P, Gower-Rousseau C et al 1996 Mapping of a susceptibility locus for Crohn's disease on chromosome 16. Nature 379:821–823

Hugot JP, Chamaillard M, Zouali H et al 2001 Association of NOD2 leucine-rich repeat variants with susceptibility to Crohn's disease. Nature 411:599–603

Johanneson B, Steinsson K, Lindqvist AK et al 1999 A comparison of genome-scans performed in multicase families with systemic lupus erythematosus from different population groups. J Autoimmun 13:137–141

Johnson AE, Gordon C, Palmer RG, Bacon PA 1995 The prevalence and incidence of systemic lupus erythematosus in Birmingham, England. Relationship to ethnicity and country of birth. Arthritis Rheum 38:551–558

Kono DH, Burlingame RW, Owens DG et al 1994 Lupus susceptibility loci in New Zealand mice. Proc Natl Acad Sci USA 91:10168–10172

McGovern D, van Heel D, Negoro K, Ahmad T, Jewell D 2003 Further evidence of IBD5/CARD15 (NOD2) epistasis in the susceptibility to ulcerative colitis. Am J Hum Genet 73:1465–1466

Mohan C, Morel L, Yang P et al 1999 Genetic dissection of lupus pathogenesis: a recipe for nephrophilic autoantibodies. J Clin Invest 103:1685–1695

Molokhia M, Hoggart C, Patrick AL et al 2003 Relation of risk of systemic lupus erythematosus to west African admixture in a Caribbean population. Hum Genet 112:310–318

Morel L, Blenman KR, Croker BP, Wakeland EK 2001 The major murine systemic lupus erythematosus susceptibility locus, Sle1, is a cluster of functionally related genes. Proc Natl Acad Sci USA 98:1787–1792

Moser KL, Neas BR, Salmon JE et al 1998 Genome scan of human systemic lupus erythematosus: evidence for linkage on chromosome 1q in African-American pedigrees. Proc Natl Acad Sci USA 95:14869–14874

Ogura Y, Bonen DK, Inohara N et al 2001 A frameshift mutation in NOD2 associated with susceptibility to Crohn's disease. Nature 411:603–606

Ogura Y, Lala S, Xin W et al 2003 Expression of NOD2 in Paneth cells: a possible link to Chron's ileitis. Gut 52:1591–1597

Pauleau AL, Murray PJ 2003 Role of nod2 in the response of macrophages to toll-like receptor agonists. Mol Cell Biol 23:7531–7539

Peltekova VD, Wintle RF, Rubin LA et al 2004 Functional variants of OCTN cation transporter genes are associated with Crohn disease. Nat Genet 36:471–475

Price P, Witt C, Allcock R et al 1999 The genetic basis for the association of the 8.1 ancestral haplotype (A1, B8, DR3) with multiple immunopathological diseases. Immunol Rev 167:257–274

Rioux JD, Silverberg MS, Daly MJ et al 2000 Genomewide search in Canadian families with inflammatory bowel disease reveals two novel susceptibility loci. Am J Hum Genet 66:1863–1870

Rioux JD, Daly MJ, Silverberg MS et al 2001 Genetic variation in the 5q31 cytokine gene cluster confers susceptibility to Crohn disease. Nat Genet 29:223–228

Rozzo SJ, Vyse TJ, Drake CG, Kotzin BL 1996 Effect of genetic background on the contribution of New Zealand black loci to autoimmune lupus nephritis. Proc Natl Acad Sci USA 93:15164–15168

Samanta A, Roy S, Feehally J, Symmons DP 1992 The prevalence of diagnosed systemic lupus erythematosus in whites and Indian Asian immigrants in Leicester city, UK. Br J Rheumatol 31:679–682

Shai R, Quismorio FP Jr, Li L et al 1999 Genome-wide screen for systemic lupus erythematosus susceptibility genes in multiplex families. Hum Mol Genet 8:639–644

Stoll M, Corneliussen B, Costello CM et al 2004 Genetic variation in DLG5 is associated with inflammatory bowel disease. Nat Genet 36:476–480

Tsao BP 2003 The genetics of human systemic lupus erythematosus. Trends Immunol 24:595–602

Vermeire S, Wild G, Kocher K et al 2002 CARD15 genetic variation in a Quebec population: prevalence, genotype-phenotype relationship, and haplotype structure. Am J Hum Genet 71:74–83

Wakeland EK, Liu K, Graham RR, Behrens TW 2001 Delineating the genetic basis of systemic lupus erythematosus. Immunity 15:397–408

Walsh EC, Mather KA, Schaffner SF et al 2003 An integrated haplotype map of the human major histocompatibility complex. Am J Hum Genet 73:580–590

Watanabe T, Kitani A, Murray PJ, Strober W 2004 NOD2 is a negative regulator of Toll-like receptor 2-mediated T helper type 1 responses. Nat Immunol 5:800–808

Yang H, Rotter J 1994 Genetics of inflammatory bowel disease. In: Targan SR, Shanahan F (eds) Inflammatory bowel disease: from bench to bedside. Williams & Wilkins, Baltimore, MD, p 32–64

DISCUSSION

Cookson: I don't think you should be worried about the idea that there are multiple alleles within the gene-rich region that you described. There are precedents in yeast and all sorts of model organisms for quantitative trait loci

(QTLs) to have concentrations of variants with multiple alleles in genes which together contribute to the phenotype. We shouldn't be surprised to see this with immune loci in humans.

Rioux: I don't have proof that there are three independent loci in the SLAM region conferring risk to SLE, but it shows that since there is sufficient recombination, with a large enough sample size we should be able to answer that specific question. It certainly would be interesting if there were to be more than one independent locus in this region.

Cookson: Perhaps the way to investigate this is using a sort of regressive approach, such as David Clayton suggested. Breaking things down to haplotypes certainly gives you the information, but every time you make a haplotype, some of the time you are making mistakes and you are losing information.

Rioux: I don't think we need to do this analysis using haplotypes. This is just a way to look at the genomic region: first to verify that we are exploring all of the genetic variation in the region, and second in this case it shows that there is uncoupling of the genes in this region due to recombination events that have recurred in history. Unlike having a long haplotype that is associated like we saw for the chromosome 5 region (Rioux et al 2001), we do have a chance in this region to narrow it down to a single gene or a couple of genes.

Cookson: You can do this with regression more easily than you can by making haplotypes.

Rioux: I am not arguing with you about that. I simply don't want to give the impression that there is only one way to analyse these data. Having said that, if no recombination existed between this set of genes, regression wouldn't help you.

Wijmenga: Could it be linkage disequilibrium (LD) across blocks that you are picking up?

Rioux: These are preliminary data so we haven't yet proven that these are independent loci. It certainly is possible that these different association signals are related by LD; but it is unlikely given the extent of recombination. Regardless, I wanted to present these data since I think that it can illustrate the scenario where multiple genes in a genomic region could potentially contribute to disease phenotype. Such a scenario could explain the strong linkage results for some disease loci.

Ting: There are two groups who have looked at *NOD2* knockouts and have not seen the effect you described. This is a typical case where a knock-in would be helpful; I think they are doing this. A measurement of NF-κB is always paradoxical because it is most frequently associated with proinflammatory responses, but also has been linked to the resolution of inflammation. You pointed out that this is performed in an HEK cell line, and a question is whether you will get a different answer with macrophages/monocytes.

Rioux: The point I wanted to try to make is that we are sort of pulling on the tail of the elephant. We haven't got to the whole body of the question, which is how these alleles are leading to the disease. Each different assay or experiment can tell us a different piece of the puzzle but it might take a while to get the entire picture.

Abbas: Have the knockout mice been challenged by microbes?

Ting: They have been challenged with lipopolysaccharide, and there is somewhat of a change in endotoxin tolerance.

Rioux: In the publication reporting the knockout in the mouse (Pauleau & Murray 2003), I don't recall seeing evidence that they challenged the mice with dextran sodium sulphate (DSS) to see if there was a difference in the susceptibility to induction of mouse colitis.

Abbas: Or a bacterial challenge in the gut, which is the right experiment.

Ting: Not just with bacteria, but the specific bacteria associated with CD. This would be even nicer.

Abbas: If we know the correct ones.

Kuchroo: You made a comment that probably applies to many other genome scans. Different people have done genome scans and have come up with entirely different loci. You made the comment that this is because each of the studies is underpowered. We have undertaken a genome scan for experimental autoimmune encephalitis (EAE) and compared this to other genomewide scans undertaken for EAE. Each one of them in different strain combinations resulted in entirely different loci, and very few loci actually overlapped. One explanation is that the studies are underpowered. Alternatively because it is a polygenic disease and you don't need all the same genes to get the disease, is it possible that each family has a different set of genes that are playing a role to get to the same phenotype? If you combine them together you are left with very little overlap. This may not be because the studies are underpowered.

Rioux: That is similar to what I was saying. Any given disease study is essentially a group of different families, as opposed to a mouse study which is essentially looking at one family of identical individuals. If you take the UK as a population of interest, if you were to sample all CD patients, you would have the representation of all the different loci and have sufficient power to identify those loci. But if you only study a small sampling of perhaps 100 families, by definition you are not going to be evenly sampling all loci. The collection that you are studying over-represents certain loci and under-represents others. By putting data from the different studies together, you can show that this is the case — one good example is that for *IBD1* in CD (Cavanaugh 2001). These are underpowered studies that are not consistently representative of all loci.

Kuchroo: Another way of looking at this would be that if you put all these studies together, then the peaks that you get in one population will be lost. They will be evened out.

Rioux: The *IBD1/CARD15* locus demonstrates that is not the case. Meta-analysis studies in IBD also demonstrate that combining data can reveal real loci (Williams et al 2002, van Heel et al 2004). There is a consistency in the IBD studies that a lot of the loci that are identifiable by linkage are actually common to the different population.

Abbas: You are implying that the 'important' loci are the ones that will show up when you combine the data. Is that accurate?

Rioux: If by 'important' you mean it is common across populations and has a substantial relative risk to be found by linkage, then yes. This doesn't mean that there aren't other loci that are less common. For example, the chromosome 10 locus in IBD was a blip in two studies and wasn't seen in the meta-analysis, yet a susceptibility gene has recently been identified (Stoll et al 2004). There are loci that you won't be able to find by linkage but that you will be able find by association because this is a more powerful approach.

Abbas: Are the available studies done in such a way that you can take the raw data and combine them?

Rioux: The raw data are messy. But if you do a meta-analysis across studies, it looks cleaner.

Umetsu: The prevalence of CD has increased significantly over recent decades. What are the environmental factors that could be fuelling this rise, and are there known gene–environment interactions? Can the environment explain some of the differences between the different population studies where there are different environmental effects in one population that are not seen in another?

Rioux: There are two answers to that question. If we look at the three variants of *CARD15* there is a substantial difference in their frequency between populations. They are all found in Caucasian populations, but for example the *CARD15* variants appear to be less common in Northern Europe than in the USA. Both chromosome 5 and *CARD15* are not having any effect in Asian and African-derived populations. To answer your question about environmental factors, these haven't been well studied yet with respect to interactions with genes. It has been clearly shown that smoking has an effect on disease susceptibility. There is mouse work showing that bacterial flora are necessary for developing disease. People are just beginning to look at how some of these microflora may interact with disease phenotype.

Foote: How common are the *CARD15* mutations?

Rioux: In a general population they are in the 5–10% range, whereas in the CD population they are in the 20–30% range. The chromosome 5 locus is about 30% in normal populations and 60% in CD populations.

Wijmenga: I have a question about your meta-analysis. Did you identify new loci?

Rioux: We definitely saw other loci coming up. Whether they are real or not will require some experimental work.

Foote: Does *Mucin 2* come up at all?

Rioux: These are genomic regions of about 20 cM, so they don't identify particular genes.

Bowcock: I wanted to discuss the overlap between regions obtained in different genomewide linkage scans with families with different autoimmune diseases, since there are several examples. You could imagine that there are genes for immune cell activation, where susceptibility loci are the same, and genes for target organ specificity where there is no overlap. In CD and many other Th2-driven diseases, there is a 5q31 association. The Japanese group reported an association of a gain of a RUNX1 site in SLC22A4 that maps to 5q31. Have you looked at that site in CD and can you say that it is associated with this disease also?

Rioux: Just for the benefit of the audience, I'd like to remind people that OCTN1 and OCTN2 also have the SLC nomenclature. SLC22A4 is OCTN1 and SLC22A5 is OCTN2. They are both cation transporters. They appear to be general cation transporters although the literature would suggest that OCTN2 is more specific to carnitine, but recent data suggest that it is a more general transporter. There is a known Mendelian trait for an *OCTN2* defect which leads to a primary carnitine deficiency. I have looked at the variant the Japanese group reported for rheumatoid arthritis (RA). It is not on the *IBD5* risk haplotype for CD, it is actually on another haplotype which is under-transmitted in IBD studies. This variant is not associated with CD. I have not yet seen replication of that finding in an independent RA study.

Abbas: 5q31 is also one of the old asthma loci.

Rioux: We have looked at this particular haplotype in asthma and have not found evidence of association.

Kere: This was looked at for asthma in the Finnish population. It didn't show any associations there. Joint analysis in several pooled samples concluded that it has moderate effects.

Cookson: Interleukin (IL)13 plainly has effects on asthma susceptibility and association with IgE levels. So does SPINK5 which is at the other end of the cluster. There is debate about IL9 in the middle.

Rioux: IL13 is just a few kilobases away from this *IBD5* risk haplotype. There is correlation between the haplotype blocks but in the CD study the association did not extend out to IL13.

Kere: As an aside, the IL9 receptor has been repeatedly associated with asthma.

Abbas: It is worth pointing out that CD is thought to be a Th1-mediated disease. It could still be associated with that locus.

Rioux: I would be interested in hearing from the immunologists as to whether they believe it is such a clear-cut issue in humans.

Abbas: The statement has been made that CD is a Th1-mediated disease and that UC is a Th2-mediated disease. My sense of the phenotypes, lesions and literature is that the first half is probably correct: CD looks like a Th1-mediated disease, but there is zero evidence that UC, as classically defined in humans, has anything to do with Th2 cells. There are a couple of mouse models with adoptive transfers that have led to lesions that look like ulcerated lesions, and this has led to the notion that UC is a Th2-mediated disease. I don't think this is justified at the moment.

Rioux: The vast majority of animal models are colitic models, rather than having ileitis.

Worthington: We have attempted to replicate the Japanese finding in RA and have not found the same thing. I believe the Americans have done the same. We should be cautious about this.

Rioux: Were you able to combine your data with the American data?

Worthington: We haven't done this yet.

References

Cavanaugh J 2001 International collaboration provides convincing linkage replication in complex disease through analysis of a large pooled data set: Crohn disease and chromosome 16. Am J Hum Genet 68:1165–1171

Pauleau AL, Murray PJ 2003 Role of nod2 in the response of macrophages to toll-like receptor agonists. Mol Cell Biol 23:7531–7539

Rioux JD, Daly MJ, Silverberg MS et al 2001 Genetic variation in the 5q31 cytokine gene cluster confers susceptibility to Crohn disease. Nat Genet 29:223–228

Stoll M, Corneliussen B, Costello CM, Waetzig GH et al 2004 Genetic variation in DLG5 is associated with inflammatory bowel disease. Nat Genet 36:476–480

van Heel DA, Fisher SA, Kirby A, Daly MJ, Rioux JD, Lewis CM 2004 Inflammatory bowel disease susceptibility loci defined by genome scan meta-analysis of 1952 affected relative pairs. Hum Mol Genet 13:763–770

Williams CN, Kocher K, Lander ES, Daly MJ, Rioux JD 2002 Using a genome-wide scan and meta-analysis to identify a novel IBD locus and confirm previously identified IBD loci. Inflamm Bowel Dis 8:375–381

A combined genetics and genomics approach to unravelling molecular pathways in coeliac disease

Martin C. Wapenaar and Cisca Wijmenga[1]

Complex Genetics Group, Department of Biomedical Genetics, University Medical Centre Utrecht, Universiteitsweg 100, 3584 CG Utrecht, The Netherlands

> *Abstract.* Coeliac disease (CD) is a complex, inflammatory disorder of the small intestine induced by gluten. It is common and has a prevalence of $\sim$ 1:200 in Western populations. A major known susceptibility locus for CD is the HLA-DQ locus. However, the genetic contribution of this region is limited to $\sim$ 40%, so non-HLA genes must also be involved in the disease aetiology. Genetic studies have so far identified multiple loci that may potentially be involved in disease aetiology, although the majority of these loci are expected to point to genes with a small effect. A major CD locus on chromosome 19 was recently identified in the Dutch population. Interestingly, there is some marked overlap when comparing genetic linkage studies conducted in different autoimmune disorders, suggesting that common pathways contribute to these diseases. This knowledge may eventually help in identifying some of the disease genes. To identify the true disease-causing genes, linkage analysis needs to be followed by genetic association. Because of the nature of the probable mutations, it is to be expected that the investigation of gene expression data can assist in selecting candidate genes from linkage regions. Furthermore, expression data will point to the molecular pathways involved in the disease pathogenesis.
>
> *2005 The genetics of autoimmunity. Wiley, Chichester (Novartis Foundation Symposium 267) p 113–144*

Coeliac disease (CD; MIM 212750) is a chronic disorder caused by an inflammatory response to gluten, a dietary product present in wheat, barley and rye. Ingestion of gluten by CD patients leads to flattening of the duodenal mucosa, a gradual process classified according to Marsh (Fig. 1). CD occurs largely in Caucasians. The disease is less common in men, with a male to female ratio of 1:3. Recent studies revealed that the prevalence of CD is 1 in 100–300, which is much higher than previously thought. Although CD is one of the most

---

[1]This paper was presented at the symposium by Cisca Wijmenga to whom all correspondence should be addressed.

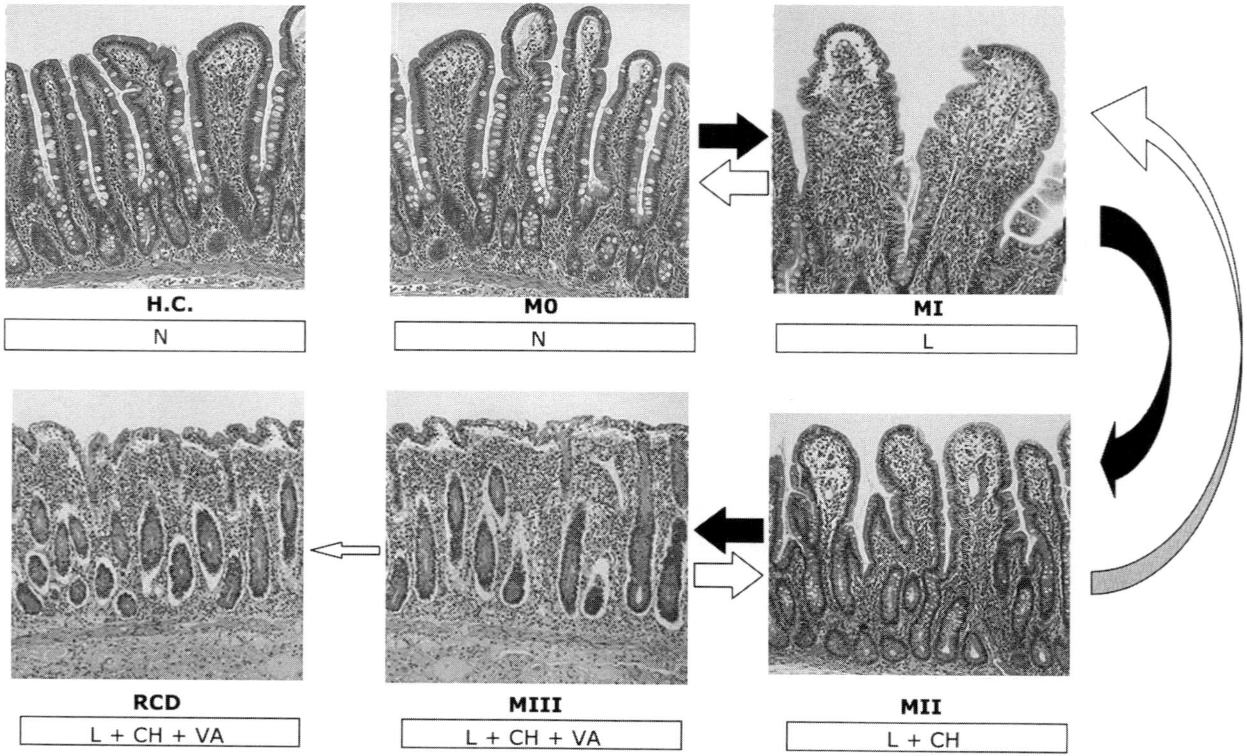

FIG. 1. Ingestion of gluten (black arrows) by CD patients (M0) results in lesions of the proximal small intestine. The range of abnormalities can be classified according to the Marsh classification. Marsh I (MI) comprises normal mucosal architecture with marked lymphocytosis (L). MII includes intraepithelial lymphocytes and crypt hyperplasia (CH) with branching and elongation of crypts. MIII comprises additional villous atrophy (VA). Upon treatment with a gluten-free diet (white arrows), the majority of patients undergo complete remission (M0), comparable to healthy controls (HC). A small percentage of patients become refractory (RCD) to the diet.

common forms of food intolerance in the world, approximately 85% of affected individuals go unrecognized.

Clinical presentation

The clinical presentation of CD comprises a wide spectrum of symptoms, most of them related to the malabsorption of nutrients from food. Typical symptoms of childhood CD include chronic diarrhoea, abdominal distension and a failure to thrive. Recurrent aphthous lesions in the mouth, dental enamel defects, fatigue, or an isolated iron-deficiency (anaemia) may also be manifestations of CD, both in children and adults. Other manifestations of CD may be dermatitis herpetiformis and osteoporosis. Moreover, infertility or recurrent abortions have also been observed in women with CD. Besides the paucisymptomatic presentation, some patients are even asymptomatic. Strict adherence to a gluten-free diet results in complete restoration of the small intestine and disappearance of the clinical symptoms.

CD is diagnosed in ∼4.5% of patients with type 1 diabetes mellitus (T1D) and autoimmune thyroid disease (ATD). Similarly, approximately 5% of patients with ATD are found to be positive for CD. This co-morbidity may suggest a common disease aetiology.

In recent years, serological tests have become available to screen for CD. However, the standard for CD diagnosis is still an intestinal biopsy sampling, an invasive procedure that requires general anaesthesia.

CD is a multifactorial disorder

CD is a typical example of a multifactorial disorder, i.e. a disease caused by the combined action of several genes and environmental factors. A recent Italian twin study found higher concordance rates for CD in monozygous (MZ) twins (86%) than in dizygous (DZ) twins (20%), indicating a strong genetic component in the development of CD (Greco et al 2002). CD aggregates in families with an approximate 10% recurrence risk for siblings of CD patients. So, based on a population prevalence of 0.5%, the sibling relative risk (λ_s) for development of CD is 20. There is, however, no Mendelian inheritance of the disease in families, suggesting that the genetic predisposition is derived from more than one gene. An important role for environmental factors is evident from the less than 100% concordance rate in MZ twins. So far, gluten is the only proven risk factor; it is also the major environmental risk factor for CD.

A strong association between HLA-DW3 and CD was identified as far back as 1976 (Keuning et al 1976). We now know that the primary association is with the genes encoding the HLA-DQα1 and HLA-DQβ1 peptides of the HLA-DQ2 heterodimer, localized in the major histocompatibility complex (MHC) on chromosome region 6p21.3. The HLA-DQ2 molecule, encoded by the *HLA-DQA1*05* and *HLA-DQB1*02* alleles in either the *cis* or the *trans* configuration, is expressed by more than 90% of CD patients. This is in strong contrast to the frequency of HLA-DQ2 carriers in the general population, which is 20–30%. A causal role for HLA-DQ2 has been demonstrated as this molecule can present the gluten-derived peptides to T cells.

Although HLA-DQ2 seems to be necessary for CD development, it is certainly not sufficient in itself. HLA-DQ2 alone can explain some 40% of the genetic variation underlying CD, implying that there are other non-HLA genes which are also important determinants of disease aetiology. A full understanding of the molecular events involved in the disease pathogenesis involves identification of the full repertoire of disease susceptibility genes.

Genetic studies conducted in CD

Both family-based linkage studies and population-based association studies have been performed to identify non-HLA genes (Fig. 2).

Genomewide linkage studies

Genomewide linkage studies have identified a number of putative loci across different populations (table 1), apart from the well-established HLA association. A locus on 5q31–q33 (*CELIAC2*) has been repeatedly identified in various genomewide linkage screens as well as in a meta- and mega-analysis by a large EU consortium, albeit with only suggestive evidence in most of the studies, implying a locus of modest effect. Interestingly, this same region has been implicated in inflammatory bowel disease (IBD) (IBD5; Rioux et al 2001), ATD (Sakai et al 2001), asthma (Xu et al 2001) and rheumatoid arthritis (RA) (Tokuhiro et al 2003), suggesting common inflammation and/or autoimmunity genes. The 5q31–q33 region contains a number of cytokine genes, none of which has so far shown association to CD (Ryan et al 2004) or to any of the other diseases in this region. Furthermore, the *CELIAC3* locus encompassing the *cytotoxic T-lymphocyte-associated antigen 4* (*CTLA4*) gene on chromosome 2q33 has been identified by both linkage and association studies in several different populations. However, this locus is considered to confer only a very modest risk for susceptibility to CD pathogenesis. *CTLA4* is an interesting functional candidate gene for T cell-mediated disorders. This is also in concordance with the identification of strong association between single nucleotide polymorphisms (SNPs) in *CTLA4* and type 1 diabetes (T1D), Graves' disease (Ueda et al 2003) and asthma. More recently a significant locus on chromosome 19 (*CELIAC4*) was identified in the Dutch population (van Belzen et al 2003), which awaits formal replication. The EU meta-analysis also suggested this locus, although the lod score was modest (Babron et al 2003). Surprisingly, this same region showed suggestive evidence for linkage in a recent meta-analysis of Crohn's disease (van Heel et al 2004). Ten additional genetic loci have been identified for CD that await formal replication (Table 1). Amongst these, the 9p21–p13 locus is of interest since this region has now been implicated in three different studies. Apart from the suggestive linkage with a lod score of 2.61 found by van Belzen et al (2004), studies in the Swedish/Norwegian (Naluai et al 2001) and the Finnish population (Liu et al 2002) showed lod scores of 1.78 and 1.11, respectively, with markers from the same region. Another interesting locus is on 6q21 (van Belzen et al 2003) since this region may also contain loci for T1D (*IDDM15*; Cox et al 2001), multiple sclerosis (MS) (Akesson et al 2002) and RA (Jawaheer et al 2003). It cannot be excluded that some of the CD genes actually predispose to a general susceptibility to autoimmunity and/or inflammation. Given the high co-morbidity of CD with other autoimmune disorders, common pathways may be involved in the destruction of the target tissues. Such a hypothesis, alluded to as the 'common variants/multiple disease' model, implies that many disease genes may not be disease-specific. Interestingly, this hypothesis might be correct as a comparison of a large number of linkage screens for autoimmune disorders showed substantial non-random clustering (Becker et al 1998).

So far 10 different genomewide linkage scans have been performed for CD. There is growing evidence that at least some of the regions identified will contain true susceptibility genes. Why has it been so difficult to identify these loci and why are there so many differences found by the various studies? There are a number of remarks we can make:

- In general, each of the samples studied is relatively small, ranging from a single large family to 102 families consisting only of affected pairs of relatives. Hence, each study has limited power in detecting new loci and even less power to replicate findings obtained in other studies.
- A large number of different populations have been studied, ranging from genetically homogeneous populations such as the Finns, to rather outbred populations such as the Americans. Therefore, it cannot be excluded that population-based differences are present in the magnitude to which the different loci contribute to disease susceptibility. This is actually already evident for both the *CELIAC2* and *CELIAC3* loci. For example, the Italian population shows strong linkage to *CELIAC2* on 5q31–q33 whereas most other populations show only modest lod scores that usually do not exceed the level of suggestive evidence for linkage.

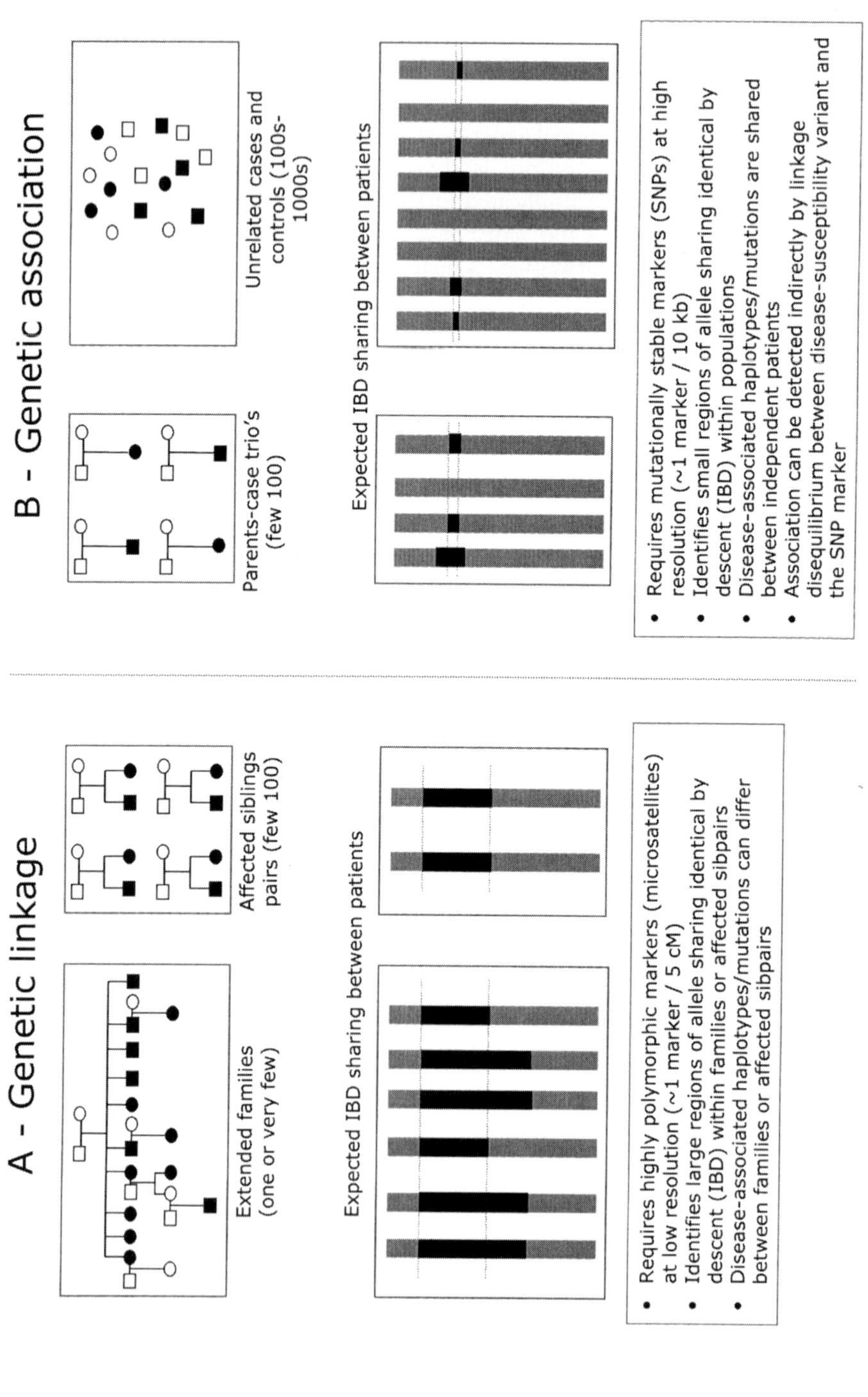

B - Genetic association

Unrelated cases and controls (100s-1000s)

Parents-case trio's (few 100)

Expected IBD sharing between patients

- Requires mutationally stable markers (SNPs) at high resolution (~1 marker / 10 kb)
- Identifies small regions of allele sharing identical by descent (IBD) within populations
- Disease-associated haplotypes/mutations are shared between independent patients
- Association can be detected indirectly by linkage disequilibrium between disease-susceptibility variant and the SNP marker

A - Genetic linkage

Extended families (one or very few)

Affected siblings pairs (few 100)

Expected IBD sharing between patients

- Requires highly polymorphic markers (microsatellites) at low resolution (~1 marker / 5 cM)
- Identifies large regions of allele sharing identical by descent (IBD) within families or affected sibpairs
- Disease-associated haplotypes/mutations can differ between families or affected sibpairs

FIG. 2. Two common genetic approaches can be used to find genetic variants (alleles) involved in the aetiology of CD: genomewide scans using highly polymorphic markers to identify chromosome regions harbouring disease-risk genes, and association studies between the disease phenotype and sequence variants in defined candidate genes. (A) Linkage studies in complex diseases are mainly being performed using affected pairs of siblings by searching for regions of excess allele sharing between affected individuals from one family (depicted in black). Siblings share 50% of their DNA on average, so a large number of sibpairs is required to detect linkage. The use of extended families is less common. (B) Association studies make predictions about the nature of the genetic variation underlying the disease (the CD/CV model). As a consequence, the identity-by-descent (IBD) region shared between independent patients is expected to be small (depicted in black). Association studies require many patients and can be both family-based (using the transmission disequilibrium test, TDT) or population-based (using case-control design). TDT can be used to avoid effects due to population stratification.

TABLE 1 Genome-wide linkage studies performed in CD

CD locus	Chromosomal location	Genes and tested candidates	Locus relative risk	Mapping method[a]	Significance[b]	Population	References
CELIAC2	5q31-q33			GWS, SR	Sug	Italian	Greco et al 1998, 2001
				Meta/mega-analysis	Sug	EU CD consortium[c]	Babron et al 2003
CELIAC3	2q33	CTLA4, ICOS	Very modest	SR	Sug	Finnish	Holopainen et al 2001
				GWS-ASP	Sug	Swedish/Norwegian	Naluai et al 2001
CELIAC4	19p13.1		2.6	GWS-ASP	Sig	Dutch	Van Belzen et al 2003
—	4p15			GWS-ASP	Sug	Finnish	Liu et al 2002
—	6p23			GWS-ASP	Sig	Irish	Zhong et al 1996
—	6q21			GWS-ASP	Sug	Dutch	Van Belzen et al 2003
—	6q25.3			4-generation family	Sug	Dutch	Van Belzen et al 2004
—	9p21-p13			4-generation family	Sug	Dutch	Van Belzen et al 2004
—	10p			GWS-ASP	Sug	Finnish	Rioux et al 2004
—	11p11			GWS-ASP	Sig	Irish	Zhong et al 1996
—	15q11-q13			GWS-IP	Sig	Finnish	Woolley et al 2002
—	15q26			GWS-ASP	Sug	Irish	Zhong et al 1996
—	22 cen			GWS-ASP	Sug	Irish	Zhong et al 1996

[a]GA genetic association, GWS genomewide scan, MMA meta/mega-analysis, SR selected regions based on previous genomewide scan data, GWS in ASP genomewide scan in affected sibpairs; GWS in IP genomewide scan in isolated populations.
[b]Sig = significant linkage: $P < 2.2 \times 10^{-5}$ (lod score >3.6); Sug = suggestive linkage: $P < 7.4 \times 10^{-4}$ (lod score >1.9). According to Lander and Kruglyak. The level of significance was based on multipoint values if available.
[c]The EU consortium consists of CD families from Finland, Sweden, Norway, UK, France and Italy.

- Although the gold standard for diagnosing CD is an intestinal biopsy, it is also clear that not every patient included in the published studies has been subjected to the same stringent diagnostic criteria. A study in the Netherlands in which all initial biopsies were re-evaluated by the same pathologist who specialized in CD, revealed some 20% misclassified samples, which were then excluded from the genomewide screen (van Belzen et al 2003). Inclusion of these samples might have seriously jeopardized finding significant linkage.

Functional candidate gene studies

Based on our limited knowledge of the disease process underlying CD, a number of pathways have been implicated, and hence genes from these pathways have been tested for their possible involvement in CD by genetic association studies. The most studied genes include those from immunological and inflammatory response pathways, including *CTLA4*, interferon gamma (*IFNγ*), interleukin 12B (*IL12B*) and interleukin 6 (*IL6*). In addition, transglutaminase 2 (*TG2*) has been studied because of its role in gluten modification. So far, none of these studies have shown evidence for involvement in CD pathogenesis, apart from inconsistent results obtained for *CTLA4* (see Table 2), both with respect to genetic association with SNPs in *CTLA4* as well as with markers covering the *CELIAC2* region (for an overview see Holopainen et al 2004). These results might suggest that the true susceptibility CD gene from this region has not yet been identified since rather strong association was observed for a region 2 Mb away from *CTLA4*. For the other functional candidate genes that were tested, it is probably still too early to truly exclude them since they might not always have been studied in a proper way. As the risk associated with most of the functional candidate genes is probably extremely modest — since the chromosomal regions to which they map usually do not show up in linkage studies — most studies might have been underpowered. Moreover, the incorrect gene variant might have been studied due to a lack of knowledge on the linkage disequilibrium structure of the gene.

How to go from a linkage region to a disease gene?

There are a number of promising linkage regions to investigate further for true CD susceptibility genes, including *CELIAC2* (5q31–q33), *CELIAC4* (19p13.1), and the regions on 9p21–p13 and 6q21. Unfortunately, each of these regions is several megabases in size and contains at least 100 different genes. None of the regions harbour obvious candidate genes, requiring the entire candidate regions to be scrutinized for the true disease susceptibility gene. The general strategy is to perform association studies across the entire region with SNPs tagged towards all the haplotypes spanning the locus. Once positive association is observed this

TABLE 2 Association studies of the *CELIAC 3* region encompassing *CD28/CTLA4/ICOS*

Population	Associated locus	P-value	Map location (Ensemble v20.34c.1)	Distance to CTLA4	Reference
French	CTLA4 (+49*A)	<0.0001	204941 kb	–	Popat et al 2002a[a]
Finnish	D2S116	0.0001	201870 kb	3071 kb	Popat et al 2002a[a]
Swedish/	D2S2392	0.037	199913 kb	5028 kb	Popat et al 2002a[a]
Norwegian	D2S2214	0.044	202933 kb	2008 kb	
	CTLA4 (+49*A)	0.012	204941 kb	–	
UK	D2S2214	0.007	202933 kb	2008 kb	King et al 2002
Italian	CTLA4 (+49*A)	0.003	204941 kb	–	Mora et al 2003
Swedish	CTLA4 (+49*A)	0.02	204941 kb	–	Popat et al 2002b
Finnish	ICOS haplotype	0.0006	205011 kb	70 kb	Haimila et al 2004
Meta-analysis[b]	D2S116	0.0006	201870 kb	3071 kb	Popat et al 2002a
	D2S2214	0.0014	202933 kb	2008 kb	
	CTLA4 (+49*A)	0.019	204941 kb	–	
Meta-analysis	D2S72	0.017	204962 kb	21 kb	Holopainen et al
EU-CD consortium[c]	D2S2214	<0.05	202933 kb	2008 kb	2204

[a]This reference summarizes seven different studies.
[b]The meta-analysis consist of CD families from Italy, Tunisia, Finland, Sweden, Norway, the Netherlands, UK, France and northern Europe.
[c]The EU consortium consists of CD families from Finland, Sweden, Norway, UK, France and Italy.

should be replicated in independent populations that also show linkage to the same region. This strategy however assumes that the underlying disease mutation or variation is a common variant—this is generally alluded to as the common variant/common disease (CV/CD) theory. There is ample evidence that this CV/CD theory is indeed correct. Well-known examples include the factor V Leiden mutation in relation to venous thrombosis, and the *ApoE4* allele in Alzheimer's disease. There is, however, also evidence to the contrary. Many different mutations have been identified in the *NOD2* gene that plays a role in the aetiology of IBD (Hugot et al 2001).

In Mendelian diseases the majority (59%) of mutations involve in-frame amino acid substitutions. For non-Mendelian multifactorial disorders we might however expect a quite different distribution of the types of mutations, such as regulatory mutations—these account for only 0.8% of the total in Mendelian disorders. The net effect of such mutations might be a change in the level of gene expression, as described recently for *CTLA4* (Ueda et al 2003). Another example includes psoriasis, where a disease-associated SNP leads to the loss of a RUNX1 binding site and might be responsible for the three- to fivefold down-regulation of *SLC4 3R1* in activated T cells (Helms et al 2003). Interestingly, regulation of *SLC22A4* expression by RUNX1 is associated with susceptibility to RA (Tokuhiro et al 2003). These examples suggest that studies aimed at genomewide expression profiling might actually aid in identifying those disease susceptibility genes that are associated with changes in transcription levels.

Gene expression profiling

Identification of genes with altered expression due to their involvement in disease aetiology and/or pathology is facilitated by microarray hybridizations or quantitative real time polymerase chain reaction (qRT-PCR). Microarray hybridization allows genomewide probing of transcriptional activity, although the currently available arrays are incomplete with respect to genome coverage. qRT-PCR is superior in sensitivity and accuracy compared to microarrays, but allows only a smaller number of genes to be tested in a single assay (10–400 genes). The type of biological sample selected for testing may also have a significant impact on the expression profile obtained. Tissue samples provide an overall insight into expression dynamics but transcriptional changes in a specific cell type may be too diluted and go undetected in this cumulative expression profile. Although specific cell types can be isolated by cell sorting or laser capture microdissection, they may lead to a biased approach that fails to observe relevant changes in cell types not tested for. For CD, two microarray studies on whole mucosal biopsy samples have been published (Diosdado et al 2004, Juuti-Uusitalo et al 2004). While both studies identified gene sets that showed little overlapping, when combined they pointed towards changes in similar processes: activated Th1 response, enhanced cell proliferation, reduced epithelial differentiation, recruitment of $\gamma\delta$T cells, B cells and macrophages, and the lack of changes in matrix metalloproteinases (Table 3). The unexpected finding of up-regulated genes involved in cholesterol and lipid metabolism (Diosdado et al 2004) was previously also observed in a microarray study on murine $\gamma\delta$T intraepithelial lymphocytes (Fahrer et al 2001), thereby revealing the increase of this cell type in the CD lesion. This also demonstrates the added power of comparing expression studies on whole tissue samples with their constituent cell types or a subset of them.

The ability to distinguish the healthy from the CD mucosa based on the expression profile opens the possibility of assembling a panel of marker genes for molecular phenotyping to assist in diagnosis and prognosis, similar to that for breast cancer, for example. Further dissemination of the CD pathological processes can be obtained by profiling biopsy samples from patients on a gluten-

TABLE 3 Microarray studies performed on CD duodenal biopsy samples

Reference	Diosdado et al 2004	Juuti-Uusitalo et al 2004	Diosdado et al ongoing work
No. of genes on microarray	19200	5184	21000
Patient groups tested[a]	HC (7), CD MIII UT (7), CD MIII T (4), RCD MIII T (4)	HC (4), CD MIII UT (4), CD M0 T (4)	HC (21), M0 T (11), MI T (8), MII T (10), CD MIII T (3), CD MIII UT (12), RCD MIII T (4)
No. of diff. expressed genes	229 (109: MIII vs HC; 120 CD MIII T vs CD MIII UT)	263 (156 CD MIII UT vs HC; 60 CD M0 T vs HC)	169 (over all categories)
Statistical analysis	Welch t-test	Manual inspection	MAANOVA
Pathways involved			
Th1 response	+	+	+
Role for $\gamma\delta$T cells	+	−	+
B cell maturation	−	+	−
Role for macrophages	+	−	−
Cell proliferation	+	−	+
Cell differentiation	+	+	+
Genes under linkage peaks	$P < 0.05$	Manual inspection	$P < 0.05$
2q33 karyoband	2	2	0
5q33 karyoband	8	3	2
6p21 (HLA region)	25	n.d.	10
6q21 locus	8	n.d.	0
9p13-p21 haplotype	6	n.d.	1
15q11-q13 locus	4	0	0
19p13 Lod-1 region	3	n.d.	3

[a]HC healthy control; CD MIII UT biopsy of CD patient with MIII lesion not treated by gluten-free diet; CD MIII T biopsy of CD patient with MIII lesion treated by gluten-free diet; CD MII T biopsy of CD patient with MII lesion treated by gluten-free diet; CD MI T biopsy of CD patient with MI lesion treated by gluten-free diet; CD M0 T biopsy of CD patient with M0 lesion treated by gluten-free diet; RCD MIII T biopsy of refractory CD patient with MIII lesion treated but unresponsive to gluten-free diet.
n.d. not determined.

free diet as they go through the successive stages into remission, or become refractory to the diet (Fig. 1). Molecular pathways may be identified, apart from those affected in patients, through RNAi knockouts of candidate genes in selected cell lines, or by data-mining the numerous microarray experiments that have been performed worldwide (Fig. 3).

Can identification of the perturbed molecular pathways lead us to the causative mutated gene(s)? Yes, because of the nature of the anticipated mutations, a major role is to be expected from gene expression studies. For this we have to combine the data on differential gene expression and pathway knowledge with the positional information from the genetic studies. This can in part be achieved by integrating data from genomewide linkage analyses and microarray expression studies. Alternatively, qRT-PCR can be applied on candidate genes that have been selected through linkage and subsequent association analysis. Moreover, genes that do not show differential expression themselves might be located in relevant genetic intervals and be constituents of disturbed molecular pathways, and therefore make excellent candidate genes. We have integrated both these genetic and expression data sets in TEAM (Fig. 4), a database developed in-house with a viewing interface (Franke et al 2004).

Looking towards the future

The current status on the genetics of CD reveals a small number of interesting regions that need further investigation, including the *CELIAC2* and *CELIAC4* loci. Since these regions are rather large, verifying an allele's contribution to the disease will be a daunting task, as has become clear from the *CELIAC4* locus (Fig. 5). A systematic approach to finding all sequence variants is impractical for small research laboratories. However, much work is currently being done in the field of functional genomics. Genetic studies should try to maximize their potential by incorporating data from protein interaction networks, gene expression, binding sites for transcription factors, large-scale RNA interference studies, and gene annotation to prioritize candidate genes. Moreover, for us to take full advantage of gene expression profiles, a comprehensive understanding of the complexities of gene networks is required, as well as their transcriptional regulation. However, to finally prove the involvement of a promising candidate gene, single gene studies will remain essential.

It is expected that the total genetic risk of CD can be attributed to only one — or a few — genes with large effect (such as *HLA-DQ2*), and many genes with very modest effect (such as *CTLA4*). More robust strategies such as genomewide association may be required to identify all CD susceptibility genes with a small effect. However, these strategies require rather different study designs including 100s to 1000s of samples, and SNPs that cover the entire genome and capture all haplotype blocks. It has been estimated that whole-genome association requires at least 200 000 SNPs. It is evident that such studies come at a high price, both with respect to statistical issues (the problem of multiple testing), the large amounts of DNA required, and the high costs of genotyping. Lately, there have been great improvements in high-throughput technology, lowering costs, and improved statistics. Since disease susceptibility alleles are expected to have additive and

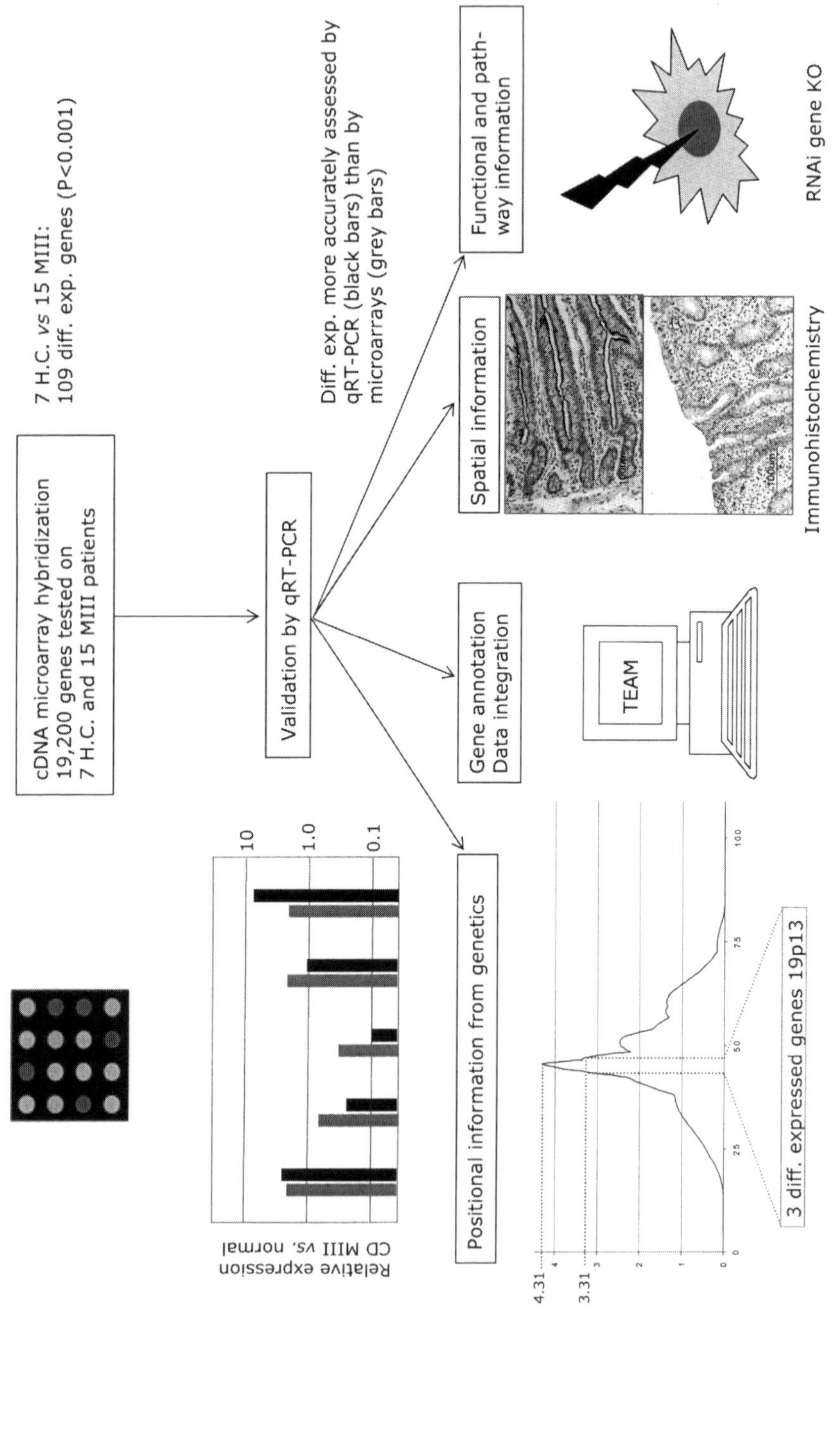
cDNA microarray hybridization
19,200 genes tested on
7 H.C. and 15 MIII patients
7 H.C. vs 15 MIII:
109 diff. exp. genes (P<0.001)
Validation by qRT-PCR
Diff. exp. more accurately assessed by
qRT-PCR (black bars) than by
microarrays (grey bars)
Relative expression
CD MIII vs. normal
10
1.0
0.1
Positional information from genetics
Gene annotation
Data integration
Spatial information
Functional and path-
way information
TEAM
Immunohistochemistry
RNAi gene KO
4.31
3.31
3 diff. expressed genes 19p13

FIG. 3. Selection strategy for candidate genes based on gene expression profiling. Starting from genomewide expression analysis using microarrays, Diosdado et al (2004) identified a number of differentially expressed genes when comparing 7 healthy controls (HC) to 15 MIII biopsies from CD patients. Initial validation of differentially expressed genes should be conducted by qRT-PCR. Follow-up experiments may comprise different experimental approaches. Genetic association can be used to further investigate positional candidate genes that show differential expression and mapping to known linkage intervals. For example, the *CELIAC4* region shows three differentially expressed genes. This selection procedure is facilitated by TEAM, which permits identification of candidate genes based on the known gene functions available in public data repositories. To gain insight into the underlying disease process the behaviour of differentially expressed genes in normal, pathogenic and experimentally manipulated tissues and cells can be evaluated. For example, immunohistochemistry provides direct insight into spatial and temporal expression patterns, whereas gene knockdowns using RNAi may help identify relevant disease pathways.

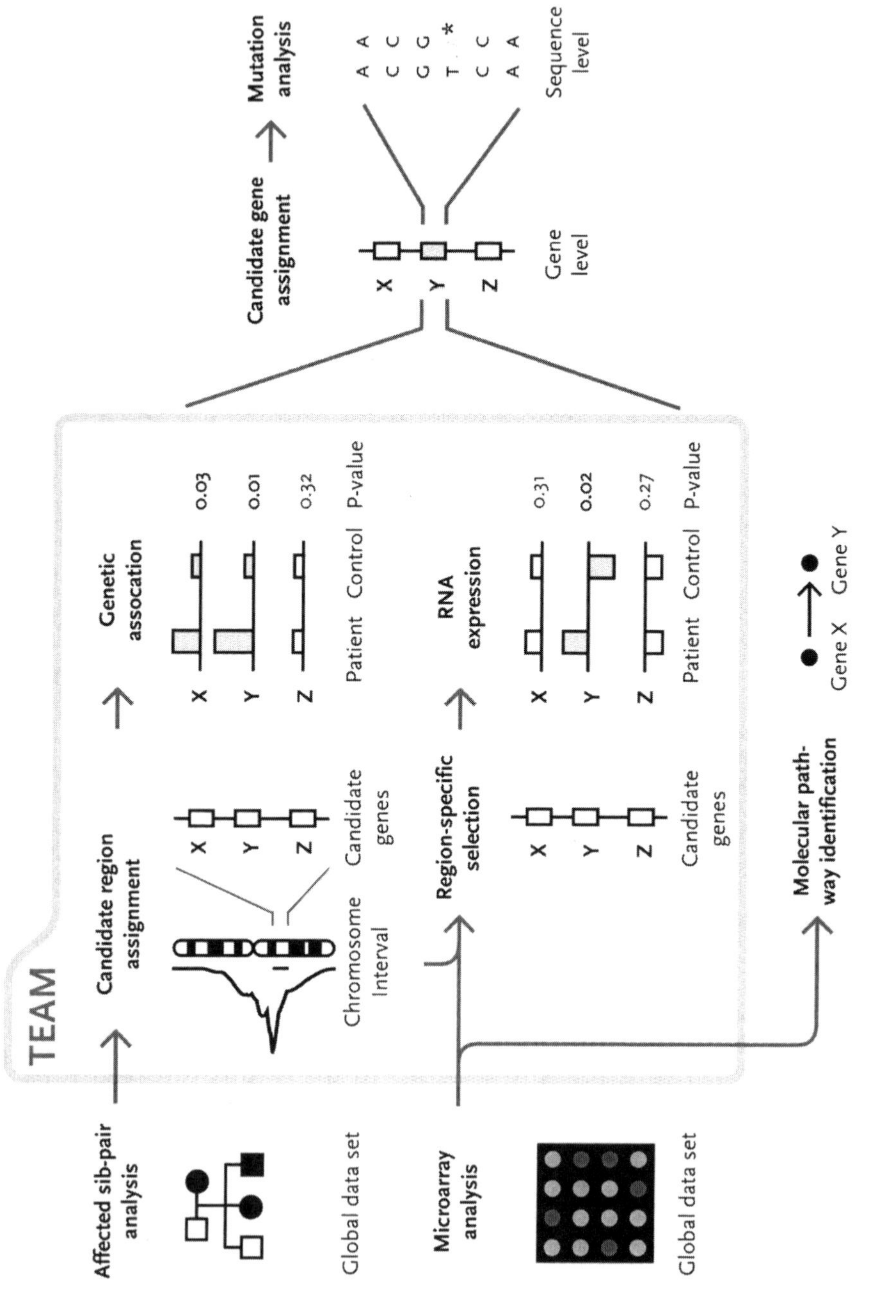
TEAM
Affected sib-pair analysis
Global data set
Microarray analysis
Global data set
Candidate region assignment
Chromosome Interval
Candidate genes
Genetic assocation
Patient Control P-value
0.03
0.01
0.32
Region-specific selection
Candidate genes
RNA expression
Patient Control P-value
0.31
0.02
0.27
Molecular pathway identification
Gene X Gene Y
Candidate gene assignment
Gene level
Mutation analysis
Sequence level

FIG. 4. TEAM is a database program that incorporates functionality for the integrated analysis of expression data, genetic data and annotation data. TEAM can be used in two ways: (1) By linking to online repositories such as Ensembl, Unigene and NCBI, we can use TEAM to help annotate genes and thereby facilitate the construction of molecular pathways; (2) by simultaneously viewing genetic linkage peaks and differentially expressed genes, we can use TEAM to facilitate selection of causative candidate genes, regardless of the availability of any functional annotation.

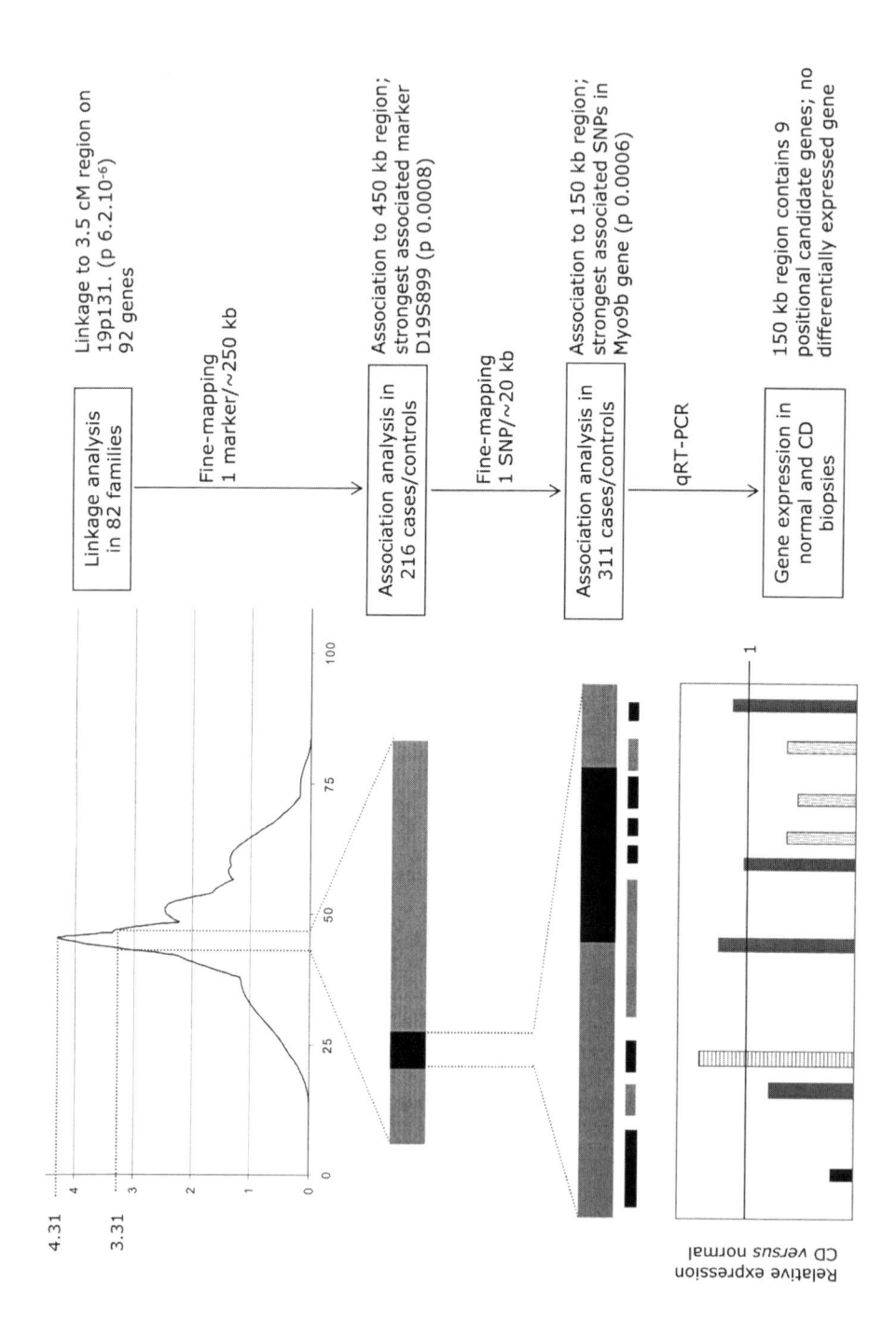

Linkage analysis in 82 families → Linkage to 3.5 cM region on 19p13.1. (p 6.2.10^{-6}) 92 genes

Fine-mapping 1 marker/~250 kb

Association analysis in 216 cases/controls → Association to 450 kb region; strongest associated marker D19S899 (p 0.0008)

Fine-mapping 1 SNP/~20 kb

Association analysis in 311 cases/controls → Association to 150 kb region; strongest associated SNPs in Myo9b gene (p 0.0006)

qRT-PCR

Gene expression in normal and CD biopsies → 150 kb region contains 9 positional candidate genes; no differentially expressed gene

FIG. 5. The *CELIAC4* locus was mapped to chromosome 19 by linkage analysis in affected pairs of siblings. The 95% confidence interval (maximum lodscore-1) measured 3.5 cM and harboured 92 genes. Subsequent association analysis using a higher density of simple tandem repeat markers (STRPs) revealed association to a 450 kb region, which was further investigated with a high resolution of SNPs. The SNP mapping narrowed the region down to 150 kb, which encompasses nine genes. These nine genes were analysed by qRT-PCR and none of the genes showed significant differences in expression levels on comparing RNA from small intestinal biopsies of CD patients with a MIII lesion to those of healthy controls, although the levels of expression showed some variation. One gene was slightly overexpressed (indicated by horizontal stripes) and three genes were slightly down-regulated (indicated by dots). Future experiments will focus on replication studies in additional populations and the identification of a haplotype shared by CD patients form different populations. To identify additional SNPs and putative disease-causing mutations, the 150 kb region will be subjected to sequence analysis.

epistatic interactions we also need statistical tools to analyse interactions between different genes, and between genes and environmental factors.

It is anticipated that newly identified CD susceptibility genes will lead to the development of easy applicable and non-invasive molecular diagnostic tools. These tools may vastly improve the diagnosis of CD particularly as, to date, some 85% of all CD patients go undiagnosed. Better diagnostic tools are obviously only part of the solution and should be coupled with increasing awareness among general practitioners and other health care professionals. Insight into the molecular pathways involved in CD aetiology may eventually provide new targets for therapeutic intervention.

Acknowledgements

The work described in this manuscript has been made possible by grants from the Dutch Digestive Disease Foundation (WS97-44, WS00-13and WS03-06) and the Netherlands Organisation for Scientific Research (902-22-204 and 912-02-028). We thank the members of the Dutch Celiac Disease Consortium and the Complex Genetics Group at the UMC Utrecht for helpful discussions. We thank Jackie Senior for improving the manuscript.

References

Akesson E, Oturai A, Berg J et al 2002 A genome-wide screen for linkage in Nordic sib-pairs with multiple sclerosis. Genes Immun 3:279–285

Babron MC, Nilsson S, Adamovic S et al (European Genetics Cluster on Coeliac Disease) 2003 Meta and pooled analysis of European coeliac disease data. Eur J Hum Genet 11:828–834

Becker KG, Simon RM, Bailey-Wilson JE et al 1998 Clustering of non-major histocompatibility complex susceptibility candidate loci in human autoimmune diseases. Proc Natl Acad Sci USA 95:9979–9984

Cox NJ, Wapelhorst B, Morrison VA et al 2001 Seven regions of the genome show evidence of linkage to type 1 diabetes in a consensus analysis of 767 multiplex families. Am J Hum Genet 69:820–830

Diosdado B, Wapenaar MC, Franke L et al 2004 A microarray screen for novel candidate genes in coeliac disease pathogenesis. Gut 59:944–951

Fahrer AM, Konigshofer Y, Kerr EM et al 2001 Attributes of gammadelta intraepithelial lymphocytes as suggested by their transcriptional profile. Proc Natl Acad Sci USA 98:10261–10266

Franke L, van Bakel H, Diosdado B, van Belzen M, Wapenaar M, Wijmenga C 2004 TEAM: a tool for the integration of expression, and linkage and association maps. Eur J Hum Genet 12:633–638

Greco L, Corazza G, Babron MC et al 1998 Genome search in celiac disease. Am J Hum Genet 62:669–675

Greco L, Babron MC, Corazza GR et al 2001 Existence of a genetic risk factor on chromosome 5q in Italian coeliac disease families. Ann Hum Genet 65:35–41

Greco L, Romino R, Coto I et al 2002 The first large population based twin study of coeliac disease. Gut 50:624–628

Haimila K, Smedberg T, Mustalahti K, Maki M, Partanen J, Holopainen P 2004 Genetic association of coeliac disease susceptibility to polymorphisms in the ICOS gene on chromosome 2q33. Genes Immun 5:85–92

Helms C, Cao L, Krueger JG et al 2003 A putative RUNX1 binding site variant between SLC9A3R1 and NAT9 is associated with susceptibility to psoriasis. Nat Genet 35:349–356

Holopainen P, Mustalahti K, Uimari P, Collin P, Maki M, Partanen J 2001 Candidate gene regions and genetic heterogeneity in gluten sensitivity. Gut 48:696–701

Holopainen P, Naluai AT, Moodie S et al (Members of the European Genetics Cluster on Coeliac Disease) 2004 Candidate gene region 2q33 in European families with coeliac disease. Tissue Antigens 63:212–222

Hugot JP, Chamaillard M, Zouali H et al 2001 Association of NOD2 leucine-rich repeat variants with susceptibility to Crohn's disease. Nature 411:599–603

Jawaheer D, Seldin MF, Amos CI et al (North American Rheumatoid Arthritis Consortium) 2003 Screening the genome for rheumatoid arthritis susceptibility genes: a replication study and combined analysis of 512 multicase families. Arthritis Rheum 48:906–916

Juuti-Uusitalo K, Maki M, Kaukinen K et al 2004 cDNA microarray analysis of gene expression in coeliac disease jejunal biopsy samples. J Autoimmun 22:249–265

Keuning JJ, Pena AS, van Leeuwen A, van Hooff JP, van Rood JJ 1976 HLA-DW3 associated with coeliac disease. Lancet 1:506–508

King AL, Moodie SJ, Fraser JS et al 2002 CTLA-4/CD28 gene region is associated with genetic susceptibility to coeliac disease in UK families. J Med Genet 39:51–54

Liu J, Juo SH, Holopainen P et al 2002 Genomewide linkage analysis of celiac disease in Finnish families. Am J Hum Genet 70:51–59

Mora B, Bonamico M, Indovina P et al 2003 CTLA-4 +49 A/G dimorphism in Italian patients with celiac disease. Hum Immunol 64:297–301

Naluai AT, Nilsson S, Gudjonsdottir AH et al 2001 Genome-wide linkage analysis of Scandinavian affected sib-pairs supports presence of susceptibility loci for celiac disease on chromosomes 5 and 11. Eur J Hum Genet 9:938–944

Popat S, Bevan S, Braegger CP et al 2002a Genome screening of coeliac disease. J Med Genet 39:328–331

Popat S, Hearle N, Wixey J et al 2002b Analysis of the CTLA4 gene in Swedish coeliac disease patients. Scand J Gastroenterol 37:28–31

Rioux JD, Daly MJ, Silverberg MS et al 2001 Genetic variation in the 5q31 cytokine gene cluster confers susceptibility to Crohn disease. Nat Genet 29:223–228

Ryan AW, Thornton JM, Brophy K et al 2004 A directed candidate gene analysis of coeliac disease susceptibility on chromosome 5. In abstract book of 11th ISCD, Belfast, April 2004 (abstract no. P41).

Sakai K, Shirasawa S, Ishikawa N et al 2001 Identification of susceptibility loci for autoimmune thyroid disease to 5q31-q33 and Hashimoto's thyroiditis to 8q23-q24 by multipoint affected sib-pair linkage analysis in Japanese. Hum Mol Genet 10:1379–1386

Tokuhiro S, Yamada R, Chang X et al 2003 An intronic SNP in a RUNX1 binding site of SLC22A4, encoding an organic cation transporter, is associated with rheumatoid arthritis. Nat Genet 35:341–348

Ueda H, Howson JM, Esposito L et al 2003 Association of the T-cell regulatory gene CTLA4 with susceptibility to autoimmune disease. Nature 423:506–511

van Belzen MJ, Meijer JWR, Sandkuijl LA et al 2003 A major non-HLA locus in celiac disease maps to chromosome 19. Gastroenterology 125:1032–1041

Van Belzen MJ, Vrolijk M, Meijer JWR et al 2004 A genomewide screen in a four-generation Dutch family with celiac disease: evidence for linkage to chromosomes 6 and 9. Am J Gastroenterol 99:461–477 van Heel DA, Fisher SA, Kirby A, Daly MJ, Rioux JD, Lewis CM; Genome Scan Meta-Analysis Group of the IBD International Genetics Consortium 2004 Inflammatory bowel disease susceptibility loci defined by genome scan meta-analysis of 1952 affected relative pairs. Hum Mol Genet 13:763–770

Woolley N, Holopainen P, Ollikainen V et al 2002 A new locus for coeliac disease mapped to chromosome 15 in a population isolate. Hum Genet 111:40–45

Xu J, Meyers DA, Ober C, Blumenthal MN et al (Collaborative Study on the Genetics of Asthma) 2001 Genomewide screen and identification of gene-gene interactions for asthma-susceptibility loci in three U.S. populations: collaborative study on the genetics of asthma. Am J Hum Genet 68:1437–1446

Zhong F, McCombs CC, Olson JM et al 1996 An autosomal screen for genes that predispose to celiac disease in the western counties of Ireland. Nat Genet 14:329–333

DISCUSSION

Abbas: I have a question about your array experiments. This will be relevant to other stories we will hear about. If you are looking for coeliac disease-specific changes, it doesn't seem appropriate to compare with a normal; you need to compare with another inflammatory disease of the bowel. There must be Crohn's disease arrays that have been published.

Wijmenga: In coeliac disease the small intestine is involved. There isn't another good inflammatory model you could use as a control.

Rioux: There have been a couple of gene expression studies but they have mostly been using surgical resection samples and not biopsy material from colonoscopy procedures. This might potentially be different.

Abbas: It is predictable that you are going to pick up inflammatory patterns.

Wijmenga: I didn't explain the big experiment we did: we started with severe villous atrophy and then took biopsies of people who had been treated with a gluten-free diet and were recovering. We also included biopsies from people who had completely recovered. Their intestine looked normal. By comparing these to normal controls we hoped to find some causally related genes. We still see a few differences between normal controls, who don't have the genetic susceptibility, and successfully treated coeliac disease patients. This is the best we can do. The only other small intestine inflammatory disease I am aware of is giardiasis. But we only have a sample from one patient.

Seed: Where do the glutamine-rich peptides end up when tissue transglutaminase cross-links into something else? Normally, isn't the function of the transglutaminase to cross-link glutamine on peptide with lycine? This could create autoantigens galore. Could the myosin be a target for cross-links?

Wijmenga: This Myo9B is not a typical myosin. It is a single-headed myosin molecule (O'Connell & Mooseker 2003).

Abbas: Someone from my department has a recent paper showing that it localizes to the T cell synapse (Jacobelli et al 2004). MyoH9 is not a contractile myosin; it is in T cells and localizes when T cells recognize antigens. There is some evidence that if you use dominant negatives against MyoH9 it messes up T cell responses.

Cookson: The question is, why gluten? Out of all the proteins why should there be a response to gluten? Is gluten an enzyme or is it toxic in any way to enterocytes in culture, or enterocytes from susceptible individuals?

Wijmenga: No. It is a storage protein in the grain that has to do with the elasticity of the dough in bread baking.

Cookson: The analogy is with allergens. People talk about allergens as proteins, but they are quite potent enzymes and they damage epithelial surfaces.

Wijmenga: Normally you wouldn't end up with those big peptides. This seems to be a problem. It is normally cut down into smaller units and it can't be presented any more.

Abbas: I don't think anyone has demonstrated enzymatic activity for gluten. I am sure people must have added it to epithelial cultures, though.

Rioux: In bread it has been baked so it won't still have enzymatic activity.

Wijmenga: We are going to be doing a test in the Netherlands where we will feed patients who have been on a diet for many years with what we think is the dominant peptide.

Cookson: The concept is that you don't get an immune reaction in the absence of danger signals. Something needs to tell the immune system that there is damage. Is there any evidence for this happening with gluten? Are the peptides toxic?

Wijmenga: I don't think the peptides themselves are toxic.

Rioux: It is an interesting question that hasn't been answered. Here the transglutaminase is having this function in cross-linking, yet at the same time it seems to be one of the primary targets for autoantibody production. It seems like a pretty big coincidence.

Wijmenga: You have so much tissue there, and it is normally intracellular. There could be a huge release of tissue transglutaminase upon tissue damage, which then becomes a target for autoantibody production.

Rioux: Wouldn't you expect then to have a broad range of auto-antibodies?

Seed: Factor XIII is a transglutaminase, too. The gluten peptides are very glutamine rich. If you add in an enzyme that cleaves glutamines you might be able to ameliorate the condition. Perhaps these iso-peptides are formed through modifying something local. The acidic peptide is presented via HLA to T cells that activate B cells that recognize these glutamine-rich peptides. It is like penicillin allergy: there is modification of endogenous proteins to generate the allergen.

Rioux: Do you think it would actually be modification, or formation of a complex?

Goodnow: You could get a hapten, tissue transglutaminase, and then the foreign helper peptide conjugated to it.

Seed: The hapten is the glutamine-containing peptide which goes on to various proteins via transglutaminase. Transglutaminase is the closest protein and the most likely to get haptenated. You could get an autoimmune response there by proxy.

Rioux: Do you think that there are other antigens or antibodies in this disease that perhaps we are not recognizing because we haven't done a comprehensive screen?

Wijmenga: There could be.

Kere: Is the tissue transglutaminase that you are referring to the same as transglutaminase 1?

Wijmenga: No, it is transglutaminase number 2. There is a family of 5.

Kere: There is a human knockout for transglutaminase 1, which causes recessive ichthyosis, a skin disorder.

Abbas: Can I ask a speculative question? Taking all the data together there is a relatively small number of loci that have been identified so far. Is this a reflection of the relative mechanistic simplicity of the disease? It is really a disease because of a Th1 response to one peptide. It is not multiple autoantigens and multiple immune responses. Can we be optimists and relate the pathogenic complexity of diseases with genetic association?

Rioux: To be honest, if you look at the numbers of families per coeliac disease genetic study (including our own), these studies are very underpowered. There is great potential, given the relatively high frequency of the disease to be able to do very powerful studies, but this hasn't been achieved yet.

Bowcock: I wanted to come back to the immune synapse. One psoriasis gene we found on chromosome 17 is *EBP50*. It is supposedly a negative regulator of immune synapse formation. Then there is the Zap70 mouse variant which develops rheumatoid arthritis. Zap70 is also a regulator of the immune synapse. If MyoH9 is also involved in autoimmunity, this would really point to synapse formation as being an important pathway.

Abbas: I am not sure that immunologists would call Zap70 a regulator of the immune synapse. There are many molecules that regulate signalling, much of which happens through the synapse. Some is positive and some is negative. It is a general concept that is very interesting. What puzzles me is why it just affects rheumatoid arthritis (RA): why not every other autoimmune manifestation? This genotype–phenotype correlation is intriguing. I think Chris Goodnow will specifically mention the Sakaguchi paper describing that mutation and the arthritis phenotype in his paper.

Goodnow: To add to what you just said, the Sakaguchi mouse doesn't just have RA. This was particularly emphasized in the paper, but it has inflammation all over the place.

Bowcock: Can I also bring into play the MHC? The question is, where is this acting? In the periphery, or the thymus?

Goodnow: The other thing that I am wary about is that synapses are just one of the fashions. This is where the candidate business comes unstuck. We get into circular logic. We get stuck on this all the time when we start mapping new ENU mutants. You can make a story of every gene in the locus for any given phenotype.

Umetsu: Coeliac disease seems to be a very common phenotype, present in up to 1% of the general population. Is there a selective advantage to having this predisposition?

Wijmenga: That's a question I have asked myself many times. No one knows. Wheat has been around as a food for many thousands of years.

Hafler: How long have humans been cultivating wheat?

Kuchroo: At least 10 000 years.

Hafler: That is after the development of who we are genetically.

Wakeland: It was the beginning of population expansion.

Kere: So there is strong selection against the phenotype. 10 000 years should have been enough to eliminate the variant.

Hafler: There must have been some positive selection for it, then. What about the heterozygote? There could be some selective advantage.

Abbas: What is the geographic distribution of the disease, and does this correlate with dietary habits?

Wijmenga: It is mainly in Caucasians.

Hafler: What about Asia?

Wijmenga: They eat rice there.

Lindgren: Couldn't that be because there is a selection towards heterozygosity in this disease? The parental genotype of the disease would be heterozygous and the children would have a more severe, homozygous form, of the disease which would affect the survival. Sickle cell anaemia and malarial infections are an example of this.

Wijmenga: There is definitely a dosage effect (Vader et al 2003). If there are two DQ2 molecules then the chance of getting the disease is increased fivefold. I don't think you get a more severe disease, though.

Wakeland: The DQ2 and DQ8 involvement in the disease may also operate against trying to select it out from the population. Those alleles are probably being maintained by their own selective advantage in some circumstances.

Hafler: Is there some defence against a microbe that is taken in orally?

Seed: My guess would be parasites, i.e. that heterozygotes would have more defence against a parasite. It is more likely to be a parasite than a bacterium. Let's assume that the parasite has some proteinaceous component to it. Most bacteria have membranes that aren't predominantly composed of protein. Parasites often cloak themselves in proteins that change frequently.

Cookson: I have a question about the interesting extended pedigree. The middle generation had 10 affected individuals. Were there any unaffected individuals?

Wijmenga: About 10 as well. I think both parents are affected. The mother has villous atrophy. The father refuses a biopsy but he cannot stand bread. It could be a more penetrant gene that is rare, but there also might be a higher genetic load because both parents are affected.

Cooskon: It almost looks Mendelian. You did the linkage analysis with a parametric model. What sort of figures did you put in for the unaffecteds?

Wijmenga: We left them out.

Cookson: 16 out of 17 is pretty dramatic.

Wijmenga: Although the lod score didn't reach significance.

Cookson: With 16 out of 17 you should get a lod score of 4.2 with the dominant model.

Wijmenga: We don't get this because of the penalty of the one recombinant (van Belzen et al 2004).

Goodnow: I am still struggling with why the peptides have to be modified, and how this fits in.

Wijmenga: They don't have to be modified. They also fit in the pocket if you don't modify them, but not as well. If you modify them they fit perfectly and the response is better. This is not true for all the peptides: some fit well without modification. If you isolate gluten-restricted T cells from patients you get a whole repertoire. They have T cells against a range of peptides, some modified some not (Vader et al 2002).

Goodnow: Is it a bit like thyroid disease, where tolerance can be thymically acquired to non-iodinated thyroglobulin peptides, but iodinated thyroglobulin peptides made in the thyroid gland represent a sufficiently different, potentially immunogenic type of epitope? Are the patients tolerant to the wild-type peptides they ingest, that are rendered immunogenic by the neo-epitope? Here, they are both non-self. Do the children immediately make a response when they are first exposed to gluten?

Wijmenga: Some do.

Goodnow: So there is no opportunity to become tolerant through dietary exposure?

Wijmenga: They are now doing studies in Sweden looking at this. If you introduce gluten slowly when the child is being breast fed, it seems that tolerance can develop (Ivarsson et al 2002). The question is what happens later in life.

Abbas: I read a couple of the reviews that you mentioned in your paper. Many of the people who write these articles make the statement you made: that the deamidated peptides have a much better fit for DQ2. Is that really based on structural information? Has anyone crystallized the DQ2 with the two different kinds of peptide?

Wijmenga: This is ongoing.

Abbas: I don't think they have even measured peptide binding in Biacor type assays.

Wijmenga: They just measure the activity of the T cells.

Abbas: That is the point I was leading up to. They don't even load purified DQ2 molecules; they load DQ2-expressing antigen presenting cells with either a native peptide or a deamidated peptide and look at T cell responses from these patients. They then make the assumption that what they are seeing is peptide binding to the MHC. It is a dangerous assumption to make unless someone gives you real structural information about binding data.

Hafler: There could be a lack of oral tolerance.

Abbas: It seems to be an important question that needs to be nailed down. It is doable with available technology.

Rioux: This is sort of analogous to what I was trying to raise with MDP and CARD15. Has anyone done binding studies with MDP and CARD15?

Ting: There is precisely the same problem.

Abbas: And then people make these assumptions that they are looking at physicochemical interactions. This is a poor assumption.

Goodnow: It can be difficult sometimes to measure receptor–ligand interactions. For a long time Mark Davis was gently criticized by biochemists for having cloned a 'receptor' (the T cell receptor) that had never been shown to receive anything, but ultimately that was shown.

Kere: I thought it would be interesting to remark here about the power of linkage studies. We have been discussing this power of linkage studies and the point made by several of us is that linkage studies have been underpowered for most complex diseases. Here we have seen a beautiful example of this with actual numbers. If you assume that a genetic effect has a relative risk of 2.5 you have a 92% power. If you go down to 2 you still have a 70% power. Your power for this study for 1.5 relative risk was 20%. In reality many of these genes have effects around 1.2 or 1.3. This is why it has been so problematic.

Abbas: What is the solution?

Rioux: Bigger studies.

Abbas: For some of these studies, such numbers may be difficult to reach.

Rioux: For inflammatory bowel disease (IBD), 10 studies have been published with 1200 families in all. If people worked together and did genomewide scans, this would be a good size. For something like coeliac disease with a frequency of 0.5% this should be possible.

Wijmenga: It seems to be a high frequency disorder but it is really hard to find families.

Kere: One thing is obvious here: the advantage that the isolated populations seem to have had in this respect. This is the skewed presentation of different genes in these isolated populations. You may have one gene by chance having a bigger effect in one population, and many other genes being downplayed. Then all of a sudden you have great power to find that one gene.

Cookson: Has this ever been proven to be the case with a complex disease? You told me yesterday that this wasn't the case with GRPA.

Goodnow: It's what Linda Wicker and John Todd depended on for their analysis of diabetes susceptibility in NOD. You fix *Idd1* before you map the other loci.

Wicker: But these are mice where particular genes can be held constant by experimental design.

Kere: If we take our asthma study as an example, it is not only because we have been so wonderful at doing the phenotype and the study altogether, but also because the H4 and H5 haplotypes that happen to be the risk causing alleles have relatively high frequencies in the final population.

Cookson: Are they different in frequency from other European populations?

Kere: They are slightly enriched. We don't need big changes in frequencies.

Rioux: It is fair to say that this is probably not the approach you would want to take for success. But what you are saying is that you can have these less frequent occurrences where there is a large skewing of one locus in a small study. I don't think this is going to be that common. When we did a similar sized study to Cisca Wijmenga for coeliac disease we saw something on chromosome 6 and didn't see any evidence for anything else.

Kere: That is basically the principle we tried to take advantage of, when we were looking at these families that seemed almost monogenic.

Cookson: That is not a population thing but a family thing. Another part of the success formula might be to look for big families, or families with more severe disease. You could make an argument that the more severe the phenotype is the more likely it is to be genetic. This is certainly the case with atopic dermatitis.

Wijmenga: If you have a family that is also a good argument.

Vyse: I wanted to bring the discussion round to B cells and the various antibodies that are associated with coeliac disease. Have you measured these in your patients and do they correlate with your biopsy samples? Secondly, have you looked in siblings or other supposed unaffected members of the family to see whether these individuals have a prevalence of these other antibodies? Could you use these phenotypes to inform your genetic and association studies?

Wijmenga: The tissue transglutaminase antibodies correlate perfectly well with the biopsies.

Vyse: Why, then, do you have to biopsy them? Why don't you measure the antibodies in the serum?

Wijmenga: This is a subject of debate. There are still patients who don't present antibodies yet still have coeliac disease. If you have antibodies against tissue transglutaminase you will have coeliac disease but you can still have coeliac disease without the antibodies. HLA typing plus looking at some other gene could bring the sensitivity close to 100%. Currently it isn't (Rostami et al 2003).

Abbas: Just to make a point for the geneticists, there is a common misconception that antibodies imply Th2 responses and not cellular inflammation. This is wrong. All high-affinity opsonizing and complement-fixing IgG antibodies in all species are Th1-dependent. Lupus is not a Th2-mediated disease, but this is often stated and widely accepted. When we start thinking about correlating pathogenetic mechanisms with genotypes, it is worth remembering that you are still looking a Th1 reaction in lupus.

Goodnow: I am still stuck on this issue of trying to fix some of the genotypes that are segregating in an outbred population to help tease out things. If you took all the mouse strains and bred them all together you would see nothing in terms of *Idd* susceptibility. Isn't there an example for hair colour in human genetics? It is much easier to see the epistasis between the loci in certain families where some of the loci are essentially fixed. It starts to behave like a Mendelian trait, whereas in the population at large it is very complex.

Cookson: There is a big gradient across Europe for polymorphisms in quite a few immune genes. Without making the population bottleneck argument, what you are saying is true. Something that is common in Sardinia might be completely absent in Scandinavia.

Rioux: What are the examples of this in complex traits?

Cookson: Delta CCR5, the complementary AIDS virus receptor. There is a big gradient across Europe for this.

Rioux: But there isn't a population where it is completely absent.

Cookson: It is down to 3% compared with 15%.

Kere: In hair colour genes we have a good example of drift, rather than selective advantage.

Goodnow: In certain families, particularly of Scottish descent, you can see powerful epistasis between some of the loci that you can't see in the population at large because the modifiers are so much more complicated.

Abbas: If it is true that loci or associations are going to vary across populations in Europe, then you have just made a mess of meta-analysis.

Wicker: No, because when you add it up you should still see these effects.

Rioux: We are talking about strength of association. But you will find the same association within population clades. If you take European-derived populations, for example, you may find differences in the strength of association between studies but the association will still be present. There may be differences say between European-, Asian- and African-derived populations. So I do not think that it is a mess as you suggest.

Wicker: I want to address Chris Goodnow's point. We are up to 4500 cases and controls, and we have started to condition the data based on susceptible genotypes. We are trying to do what we do with the mice. The problem is that we may have susceptibility alleles at say three of these loci (sometimes we can't use a homozygote category because it is too rare), and we might have a 20 to 1 odds ratio for cases versus controls for this combination, but we are now dealing with 40 patients with this particular genotype versus a couple of controls. It does follow the pattern of the congenic mice in the sense that combining certain genes appears to be leading to the observation of epistasis. Just a couple of the susceptibility alleles together gets you into a very susceptible range. Epistasis probably is happening, but it is not statistically significant yet.

Goodnow: It is just like *Idd1*. There are not many mice that have the I-A^{G7} major histocompatibility haplotype. If you were to look at the population at large and slice it on inheritance of I-A^{G7} the power dwindles to nothing.

Wicker: You actually do that when you collect your cases because they are highly enriched for the susceptible MHCs. It is quite dramatic. Then when you look at the medium-susceptibility MHCs you start seeing a big enrichment of non-MHC susceptibility alleles. It is much more obvious if you look at the medium-susceptibility MHC with these other genes coming in. It is exactly like mice, where if the mice are heterozygous for the susceptible allele at the MHC, susceptibility at the non-MHC genes is almost essential to get any disease penetrance.

Goodnow: That enrichment only works when you have one pathway to get to the disease. This is probably the case for MHC. Vijay Kuchroo is saying that if you have locus heterogeneity, you may not get that.

Wicker: If there is the statistical power to detect enrichment of a gene in the context of another disease locus in a case control study, I can imagine situations where this could be observed if the two loci either contribute to separate or to interacting pathways. It would not be possible to define the level at which disease genes interact or don't interact based on the level of enrichment observed.

Bowcock: In the case of autoimmune disease you have a nice example where you can throw out all your HLA-positive families and then do your linkage analysis. You came up with that locus on chromosome 18p, which had come up weakly in other genome scans. The question of HLA dependent and independent genes is very interesting.

Abbas: By 'dependent' do you mean if you eliminate the contribution of the HLA locus, what else pops up?

Bowcock: Yes.

Abbas: It would be tough to do in diabetes because a lot of the patients are DR3/4 heterozygotes.

Wicker: The problem with this conditioning is that you end up throwing away so many of your data.

Abbas: In some of these you would end up discarding a lot of your data.

Kere: The power within the remaining sample is then increased.

Wicker: We keep doing every combination, but although by eye it looks very encouraging, the statistics don't. The small sample size fights you every bit of the way.

Cookson: What is the value of finding something with a relative risk of 1.05 or 1.1? How heroic should we be?

Wicker: My previous comment was just in terms of looking for interactions or epistasis. Defining genes that have a relative risk of 1.05 or 1.1 in the entire population will fill in our knowledge of the pathways that are acting.

Hafler: It makes sense from a therapeutic point of view. Three or four such genes could increase the risk.

Vyse: Something with a very small risk in your whole population may confer a much higher risk in a subphenotype of that population.

Abbas: There is a lesson to be learned from HLA linkage in disease. 10–20 years ago when this was a growth industry there were many papers on the small relative risk of many diseases with various HLA alleles. Most of them have fallen by the wayside.

Hafler: You have to ask yourself why. Were these underpowered studies?

Abbas: Underpowered, of no demonstrated functional relevance, or not replicated in multiple studies. Bill's question is a little philosophical, but the experience with defined loci has been that weak relative risks have not withstood the test of time.

Hafler: Some of them have.

Rioux: The meta-analysis of the different HLA loci in the MHC region shows strong odds ratios. In this circumstance David Hafler is right: a lot of studies have been extremely underpowered. In our meta-analysis we threw out half the studies because they had less than 100 cases and controls.

Bowcock: In the *CTLA4* study the relative risk was very low, around 1.2.

Wicker: CTLA4 is an interesting example of a gene with a weak relative risk that has withstood the test of time. It was first studied predominantly within families but now with a very large case control study it has gotten stronger. One of the problems with family-based studies is the fact that, more often than in case control studies, there is a family history of the disease reflecting an aggregation of susceptibility genes, thereby losing power to detect the aggregated loci. In case controls, *CTLA4* comes out stronger. *CTLA4* is being seen in other case control studies of other autoimmune diseases.

Bowcock: What is it?

Wicker: In the families there was a relative risk of 1.15; we are now up to 1.4 in the case control study.

References

Ivarsson A, Hernell O, Stenlund H, Persson LA 2002 Breast-feeding protects against celiac disease. Am J Clin Nutr 75:914–921

Jacobelli J, Chmura SA, Buxton DB, Davis MM, Krummel MF 2004 A single class II myosin modulates T cell motility and stopping, but not synapse formation. Nat Immunol 5:531–538

O'Connell CB, Mooseker MS 2003 Native myosin-IXb is a plus-, not a minus-end-directed motor. Nat Cell Biol 5:171–172

Rostami K, Mulder CJ, Stapel S et al 2003 Autoantibodies and histogenesis of celiac disease. Rom J Gastroenterol 12:101–106

Vader W, Kooy Y, Van Veelen P et al 2002 The gluten response in children with celiac disease is directed toward multiple gliadin and glutenin peptides. Gastroenterology 122:1729–1737

Vader W, Stepniak D, Kooy Y et al 2003 The HLA-DQ2 gene dose effect in celiac disease is directly related to the magnitude and breadth of gluten-specific T cell responses. Proc Natl Acad Sci USA 100:12390–12395

van Belzen MJ, Vrolijk MM, Meijer JW et al 2004 A genomewide screen in a four-generation Dutch family with celiac disease: evidence for linkage to chromosomes 6 and 9. Am J Gastroenterol 99:466–471

Progress towards understanding the genetic pathogenesis of systemic lupus erythematosus

Timothy W. Behrens, Robert R. Graham, Chieko Kyogoku, Emily C. Baechler, Paula S. Ramos, Clarence Gillett, Jason Bauer, Ward A. Ortmann, Keli L. Hippen, Erik Peterson, Carl D. Langefeld*, Kathy L. Moser, Patrick M. Gaffney and Peter K. Gregersen†

Center for Immunology, University of Minnesota Medical School, Minneapolis, *Section on Biostatistics, Wake Forest University School of Medicine, Winston-Salem, NC, †Robert S. Boas Center for Genomics and Genetics, North Shore Long Island Jewish Research Institute, Manhasset, NY, USA

> *Abstract.* In order to better understand the genetic factors that initiate systemic lupus erythematosus (SLE), we are using both linkage and association approaches to identify susceptibility genes for the disease. Association studies have recently identified three HLA Class II haplotypes as well as a functional missense polymorphism in protein tyrosine phosphatase (PTP) PTPN22 as important risk alleles for SLE. Here, we will review these data, and explain how these findings contribute to an understanding of the genetic architecture of human SLE.
>
> *2005 The genetics of autoimmunity. Wiley, Chichester (Novartis Foundation Symposium 267) p 145–164*

Systemic lupus erythematosus (SLE) (OMIM 152700) is a chronic, systemic autoimmune disease that results in inflammation in a broad range of organ systems. While some patients have a milder form of the disease characterized by elevated titres of antinuclear antibodies (ANAs), arthritis and skin/mucosal membrane involvement, the majority of patients will suffer more severe clinical manifestations, which include renal inflammation (nephritis), cerebritis, pleuritis, pericarditis, haemolytic anaemia, clotting and thrombocytopaenia. Autoantibodies are found in virtually every patient, and many show an unusual specificity for nucleic acids (ssDNA, dsDNA) and nuclear antigens such as the Ro and La RNA-binding proteins, RNP and the U1 splicing protein. Approximately 90% of patients with SLE are female, suggesting that sex hormones have an important role in disease. Up to 5% of the general population show elevated titres of serum ANAs in the absence of disease, and it is estimated that the presence of ANAs increases the risk for the eventual development of SLE by about 40-fold (Arbuckle et al 2003). Interestingly, autoantibodies often predate the development of clinical symptoms by several years, and, in particular, antibodies to dsDNA, Sm and nRNP, when present, are harbingers of the onset of disease (Arbuckle et al 2003).

Many genes have been implicated in susceptibility to SLE (reviewed in Alarcon-Riquelme & Prokunina 2003, Gaffney et al 2002, Kelly et al 2002, Tsao 2003, Wakeland et al 2001). Convincing data suggests that polymorphisms in the following genes contribute to human lupus: Fc receptors (and in particular FcγRIIA, RIIIA, and RIIB); early components of the complement cascade (C1q, C2, C4); and more recently the *PD1* gene, a cell surface protein related to CD28 that is involved in down-regulation of T cell responses. Genetic mapping in SLE has identified a large number of linkage intervals that appear likely to harbour additional important susceptibility alleles for SLE (reviewed in Alarcon-Riquelme & Prokunina 2003, Gaffney et al 2002, Kelly et al 2002, Tsao 2003, Wakeland et al 2001). The strong linkage signal at 6p21 and the subsequent confirmation of association of HLA alleles with SLE (discussed below) is evidence that at least some of these linkage signals will result in the identification of relevant genes. However, there will also be important SLE susceptibility genes that do not fall in linkage peaks—the lymphoid phosphatase PTPN22 is a good example of this (discussed below). Given recent important advances in genotyping technology and progress on haplotype mapping of the human genome (Gabriel et al 2002), comprehensive association studies will soon become a reality, and are likely to identify many additional genomic regions and genes contributing to the SLE phenotype.

The HLA

The HLA region on human chromosome 6p21.3 spans approximately 3.6 Mb of DNA and contains over 200 genes, many with important roles in the immune system (Dawkins et al 1999, Rhodes & Trowsdale 1999). The telomeric Class I region contains the polymorphic HLA A, B, and C genes, which are expressed ubiquitously and function to present antigenic peptides to $CD8^+$ T cells. The centromeric Class II region encodes the highly polymorphic DR, DQ and DP genes. These are expressed on antigen presenting cells and serve to present peptides to $CD4^+$ helper T cells. The Class II region also contains genes important for antigen processing, including the TAP, LMP and DM genes. The Class III region lies between the Class I and II regions, and contains many genes important for the immune system, including the cytokines tumour necrosis factor (TNF)α and lymphotoxin A, and the complement components Factor B, C2 and C4. There are also many genes within the HLA region with no obvious function in the immune system.

GENETICS OF SLE   147

In addition to their role in determining transplantation tolerance (Snell 1948), HLA Class I and II alleles show genetic associations with many inflammatory and autoimmune disorders (reviewed in Vyse & Todd 1996). Examples include the association of Class I HLA B27 with ankylosing spondylitis, HLA Cw6 with psoriasis, and Class II DRB1*0401 (DR4) with rheumatoid arthritis (RA), DRB1*1501 (DR2) with multiple sclerosis, DRB1*0301 (DR3) with IgA deficiency, and both DRB1*0301 and DRB1*0401 with type 1 diabetes mellitus (T1D). Due to linkage disequilibrium within the HLA, it has often been difficult to determine whether the observed associations reflect the Class I or Class II alleles themselves, linked genes, or combinations of genes carried on a particular haplotype.

Previous case/control association studies have examined the potential role of HLA Class I and II alleles in genetic susceptibility to SLE (Arnett 1997, Harley et al 1998). The most consistent findings have been modest associations of DRB1*1501 (DR2) and DRB1*0301 (DR3) alleles in whites with SLE. However, these associations have, on balance, been less convincing than those observed in RA (DR4) or T1D (DR3). Furthermore, SLE Class II associations in non-white ethnic groups have shown little consensus.

Family-based association analysis of the HLA

Genetic mapping in 187 SLE sibpair families identified a lod score of 4.19 on the short arm of human chromosome 6 (Gaffney et al 1998, 2000). After genotyping an additional 31 microsatellite markers across 6p, including 6 markers within the HLA, the strongest evidence for allele sharing by affected siblings was within the HLA (Graham et al 2002). Using the pedigree disequilibrium test (PDT), a multi-allelic test for association in complex pedigrees (Martin et al 2000), the marker D6S2446 in the Class II region showed the strongest evidence for association ($P = 9 \times 10^{-4}$) (for additional details see Graham et al 2002). Interestingly, this marker is located in the 75 kb interval between the highly polymorphic DRB1 and DQB1 genes. To extend these findings, we genotyped the original cohort of 187 families, including an additional 34 sibpair families, with a dense panel of 56 microsatellite markers across the HLA region (average inter-marker distance 62 kb). Using the PDT, the strongest evidence for association was again found in the Class II region at D6S2446 ($P = 4 \times 10^{-5}$).

The same marker panel was then applied to an independent sample of 123 simplex families (single SLE patient with both parents). Once again, marker D6S2446 showed the best evidence for association in the simplex collection ($P = 2 \times 10^{-3}$). The results of the PDT at D6S2446 for the combined collection of sibpair and simplex pedigrees (total 334 families) was highly significant ($P = 3 \times 10^{-8}$). Other regions within the HLA also showed evidence for association, and it remains to be determined whether these signals represent independently contributing alleles.

Identification of three HLA risk haplotypes in SLE, containing DRB1*1501 (DR2), DRB1*0301 (DR3) and DRB1*0801 (DR8)

To determine whether the observed effect at Class II was due to a single, or multiple risk haplotypes, the individual alleles of D6S2446 and short haplotypes containing this marker were examined for association. Three individual alleles of D6S2446 and multimarker haplotypes containing these alleles showed significant transmission disequilibrium. Sequence-specific oligonucleotide typing of DRB1 and DQB1 alleles in founders carrying one of the risk alleles at D6S2446 revealed that the three risk haplotypes contained DRB1*1501/ DQB1*0602 (DR2/DQ6), DRB1*0301/ DQB1*0201 (DR3/DQ2), and DRB1*0801/ DQB1*0402 (DR8/DQ4), respectively. Of interest, families carrying one or more of the identified risk haplotypes accounted for nearly all of the evidence for association in the Class II region, and the 84 families lacking one of the identified Class II risk haplotypes showed no disequilibrium at D6S2446 by PDT analysis.

Visualizing ancestral recombinant Class II risk haplotypes

In order to visualize the recombinant Class II containing risk haplotypes, we first examined all founder haplotypes containing allele 6 at D6S2446. The consensus allele for each marker on the extended haplotype was determined, and founder haplotypes were colour-coded, with maroon indicating an exact match with consensus, and gold denoting a difference from consensus (Fig. 1A, reproduced here in greyscale). Missing data or alleles with ambiguous phase are highlighted in grey.

The D6S2446-6 founder haplotypes were sorted based on the number of contiguous marker alleles identical to the consensus extended haplotype. This revealed multiple ancestral recombinant DRB1*1501-containing haplotypes (with the size of the recombinant haplotypes decreasing from top to bottom, Fig.1A). Haplotypes were grouped based on length, and each group was tested for association using the TDT (Spielman et al 1993). Haplotype clusters showing overall significant transmission distortion are highlighted in blue (right side of the panel). The group of short recombinant haplotypes having a 22:11 T:NT (transmitted: not transmitted) ratio suggested a telomeric ancestral recombinant 'breakpoint' at approximately marker MN6S2468 (marked by left-most *). To determine the location of the centromeric ancestral 'breakpoint', we again sorted the founder haplotypes, first on identity centromeric to D6S2446, and then on

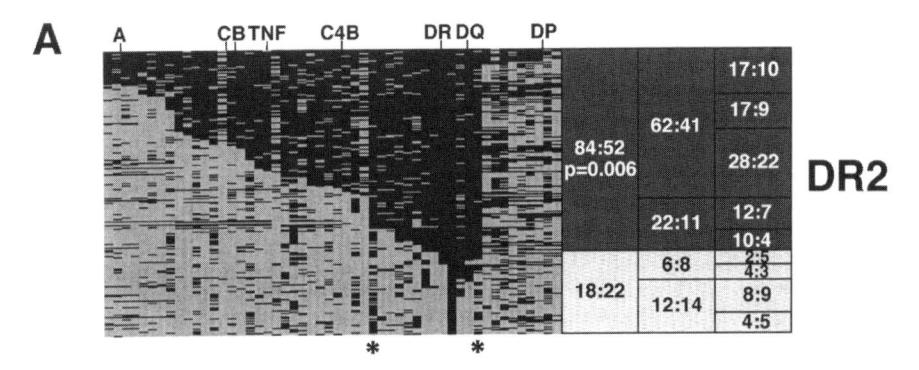

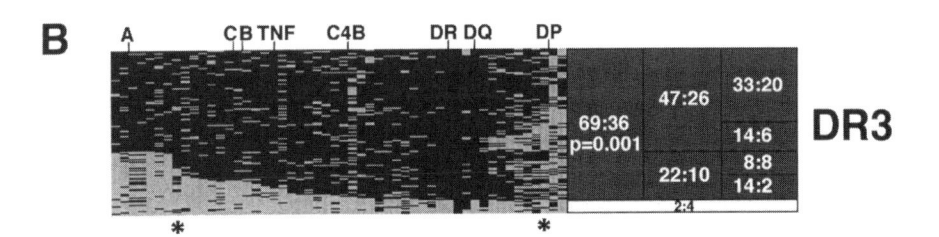

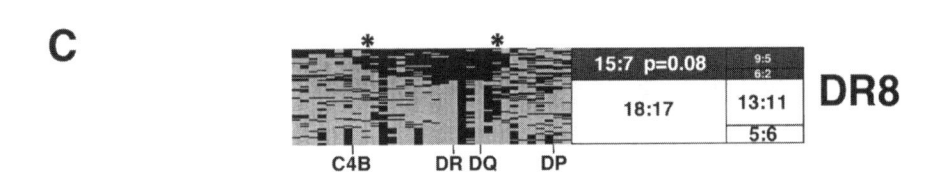

FIG. 1. Visualization of SLE HLA risk haplotypes. (A) Shown are founder haplotypes carrying allele 6 at marker D6S2446 (DRB1*1501/DR2 linked). The consensus ancestral haplotype containing D6S2446-6 was determined, and individual alleles colour-coded (here shown in greyscale): marker alleles identical to consensus in maroon (dark grey); alleles different from consensus in gold (mid grey); missing data or alleles with ambiguous phase in light grey. After sorting by telomeric length (left), groups of founder haplotypes (total $n=176$) were tested by TDT, with the numbers shown referring to the ratio of transmitted:non-transmitted (T:NT) haplotypes. The grey boxes on the right of the figure indicate significant transmission distortion ($P<0.05$) for the larger groups; white boxes indicate non-significant TDTs. (B) Founder haplotypes ($n=110$) carrying D6S2446-8 (DRB1*0301/DR3 linked) were sorted based on telomeric length, and TDT was performed. (C) Founder haplotypes ($n=68$) carrying D6S2446-5 (DRB1*0801/DR8 linked) were sorted based on overall length, and TDTs performed. Asterisks (*) represent the approximate boundaries of the haplotypes showing convincing evidence for transmission distortion.

extent of telomeric identity (not shown). This demonstrated that founder haplotypes extending centromeric to marker MN6S2944 (right-most *) had a similar level of transmission distortion as haplotypes that extended beyond. Thus, the estimated centromeric 'breakpoint' on this haplotype is ~60 kb centromeric to DQB1 (~66 kb centromeric of D6S2446), near marker MN6S2944, a known recombination hotspot within the HLA (Jeffreys et al 2001).

Founder haplotypes that contained allele 8 at D6S2446 (in strong disequilibrium with DRB1*0301) were then analysed using the same strategy (Fig. 1B). Based on the visualized ancestral haplotypes, it was clear that the level of linkage disequilibrium on this haplotype was much higher than observed for the DRB1*1501 haplotype. HLA A, B, and C typing confirmed that this haplotype corresponds to the HLA A1-B8-DR3 haplotype, which is known to have unusually extensive disequilibrium (Dawkins et al 1999). Due to the relative paucity of ancestral recombinants, the risk region within DRB1*0301-containing haplotypes could not be narrowed beyond a ~1 Mb region encompassing most of the Class III and Class II regions. Consensus alleles for the extended ancestral DRB1*0801 haplotype could only be identified up to the Class I/Class III boundary (Fig. 1C). Haplotypes containing DRB1*0801 were less common in this family collection, however the risk interval could be narrowed to a ~500 kb region.

Elevated HLA risk haplotype frequencies in SLE cases vs. controls

We next compared HLA risk allele frequencies in 280 female white SLE index cases from the family collection and 174 female white controls. The risk haplotypes were more common on SLE patient chromosomes than controls, with approximately a two-fold increased frequency (Graham et al 2002). DRB1*0301-containing haplotypes conferred the highest degree of risk (heterozygous genotypic relative risk [GRR]=2.6), followed by DRB1*0801-containing haplotypes (GRR=2.2) and DRB1*1501-containing haplotypes (GRR=1.9). We also noted that combinations of risk alleles provided higher relative risk for SLE than a single allele (Table 1). Strikingly, nearly two-thirds (64%) of the patients carried at least one of the risk haplotypes, as compared to 38.5% of controls ($P=1.3\ 10^{-7}$). We conclude that the identified Class II risk haplotypes are enriched in SLE patients, and show strong association in a case-control study design.

Thus, by visualizing recombinations on the ancestral haplotypes carrying DRB1*1501 and DRB1*0801, the major risk regions on these haplotypes could be narrowed to a ~500 kb region containing both *DRB1* and *DQB1*. The only other genes in this interval are two genes of unknown function — chromosome 6 open reading frame 10 (*C6orf10*, formerly known as testis specific basic protein), and butyrophilin-like family member II (*BTNL2*) — together with *DRA* (invariant), *DRB3* and *DRB5* (additional β chain genes present on the

TABLE 1 Class II susceptibility haplotypes provide dose-dependent risk for SLE

Risk haplotype[a]	SLE[b] n=280	Controls[c] n=174	P value	Relative risk
	Frequency (%)			
Heterozygote for 1 of 3 risk haplotypes	45.0	33.9	0.0190	1.3
Compound heterozygote	12.1	2.3	2.3×10^{-4}	5.2
Simple homozygote	6.8	2.3	0.0340	3.0
Any combination of risk haplotypes	63.9	38.5	1.3×10^{-7}	1.7

[a]Haplotypes containing the three DRB1/DQB1 risk alleles were determined by microsatellite genotypes for markers D6S2666/2665/2446.
[b]Index cases from white SLE families.
[c]Unrelated female white controls.
P values determined by Chi-square analysis.
Relative risk calculated as frequency SLE/frequency controls.

DRB1*0301 and DRB1*1501 haplotypes, respectively), and *DQA* (a different allele for each of the risk haplotypes). Further typing using SNPs across these various haplotypes should allow us to determine whether the genetic effect in this region is limited to the Class II *DRB1* and *DQB1* genes, or includes other linked genes, possibly acting in epistasis.

The extensive disequilibrium of the DRB1*0301 haplotype severely limits the ability to localize the genetic effect on this haplotype. It is important to note that the TNF-alpha and C4 'null' alleles, which have previously been suggested as risk factors for SLE (Arnett 1997, Harley et al 1998), are both carried on the extended A1/B8/DR3 haplotype. These data suggest that caution should be exercised before assigning risk to any individual gene on the DRB1*0301 haplotype, given the extensive disequilibrium observed. We cannot at this time rule out the possibility that other genes on the extended haplotype may also be contributing to risk. We have recently extended these studies by typing additional cases from two independent family collections, essentially tripling our effective sample size, and these new studies provide additional support for our conclusions (Graham et al, unpublished data). However, important work remains to be accomplished. The generation of a dense SNP map across the MHC (Walsh et al 2003), and the surprising finding that linkage disequilibrium patterns within the MHC may not be all that different from the rest of the genome, indicates that further studies in this region will be required to tease out additional genetic contributions to SLE.

PTPN22/PEP: a phosphatase that inhibits T cell signalling

Several recent studies indicate that *PTPN22* is an important susceptibility allele for many different autoimmune diseases (reviewed below). *PTPN22* (also referred to in the literature as Lyp, for the human gene) was originally cloned from human thymocytes during a search for PTPs involved in lymphocyte development (Cohen et al 1999). PTPN22 is a cytoplasmic PTP expressed in spleen, thymus, tonsil, and in peripheral B and T lymphocytes (Cohen et al 1999) as well as myeloid cells (Chien et al 2003). The primary PTPN22 amino acid sequence has an N-terminal phosphatase domain and four proline-rich SH3-domain binding sites at the C-terminus. In T cells, PTPN22 associates constitutively with signalling proteins Cbl and Grb2 (Cohen et al 1999, Hill et al 2002). In Jurkat T leukaemia cells, PTPN22 expression causes down-regulation of Cbl tyrosine phosphorylation after T cell receptor (TCR) stimulation (Cohen et al 1999). Furthermore, TCR and CD28 signalling to the interleukin (IL)2 promoter is diminished in the presence of overexpressed wild-type, but not catalytically inactive PTPN22 (Hill et al 2002). Thus, overexpression studies suggest that PTPN22 functions as a negative regulator of TCR signalling.

PEP, the mouse homologue of PTPN22, is expressed in spleen, thymus, lymph node, and bone marrow (Matthews et al 1992). Primary sequence analysis shows a 70% overall homology between PEP and PTPN22, and 89% homology within the catalytic domain. Overexpression studies indicate that PEP also acts as a strong repressor of TCR signalling (Cloutier & Veillette 1999). Like the human gene, PEP contains several proline-rich repeats at the C-terminus. The most proximal proline-rich repeat region in PEP, termed the P1 domain, interacts with the SH3 domain of Csk (Cloutier & Veillette 1996). Lck is also a substrate of PEP, and Csk and PEP function to inactivate Lck (Cloutier & Veillette 1999). One current model posits that Csk inhibits Lck by phosphorylating a negative regulatory tyrosine (Y505), while PEP reduces Lck function by dephosphorylating a positive regulatory tyrosine (Y394) (Gjorloff-Wingren et al 1999).

PEP deficiency results in disinhibition of TCR signalling

PEP deficient mice ($Pep^{-/-}$) were recently generated and characterized (Hasegawa et al 2004). Thymocyte numbers and subsets are similar in $Pep^{-/-}$ and wild-type animals. However, older $Pep^{-/-}$ mice have enlarged spleens and lymph nodes due to increased numbers of T cells within the effector/memory T cell subset. Also, $Pep^{-/-}$ effector T cells display increased proliferation and cytokine production when stimulated through antigen receptors. Enhanced T cell function correlates with augmented phosphorylation of the TCR-proximal activating kinase ZAP-70. The PEP-null mice also demonstrate that PEP is not involved in the regulation of all tyrosine kinase-associated receptors. Although the PEP substrate Lck regulates signal transduction through cytokine (IL2 and IL15) receptors (Hatakeyama et al 1991) as well as TCR signalling, cytokine signalling appears to be unaffected by loss of PEP (Hasegawa et al 2004). The *Pep* knockout mice also showed an excessive number of spontaneous germinal centres in spleen, and elevated levels of T-dependent Abs IgG1 and IgG2a, suggesting an excessive level of T cell help for antibody production. In summary, the $Pep^{-/-}$ mice demonstrate that PEP serves as a specific negative regulator of TCR signalling and T cell activation.

PTPN22 and human autoimmunity

Begovich et al (2004) recently showed that a missense polymorphism (rs2476601; 1858C→T) in PTPN22, a key molecule regulating TCR signalling in memory/ effector T lymphocytes (Hasegawa et al 2004), was strongly associated with human RA. The polymorphism occurs in the proximal proline-rich SH3 binding domain of PTPN22, resulting in substitution of a highly conserved arginine with tryptophan (R620W). As noted above, this proline-rich region is an important docking site for Csk (C-terminal Src tyrosine kinase) (Cloutier & Veillette 1996). *In vitro* experiments have now shown that the R620W polymorphism affects the ability of PTPN22 to bind Csk (Begovich et al 2004, Bottini et al 2004). Interestingly, this SNP was independently shown to be associated with T1D (Bottini et al 2004).

PTPN22 R620W is a risk allele for human SLE

In collaboration with Begovich and colleagues, we investigated the possible association of the R620W SNP with SLE (Kyogoku et al 2004). We compared PTPN22 R620W genotype frequencies in an initial cohort of 185 white SLE cases, where a single case was randomly selected from SLE sibpair families in the University of Minnesota collection (Gaffney et al 2000), to results generated from 926 white controls (Begovich et al 2004). The C/T genotype was observed in 38 of 185 SLE cases (20.5%) and the T/T genotype in 6 cases (3.2%). Compared with controls (C/T 15.4%, T/T 1.0%), the C/T and T/T genotypes were significantly overrepresented in the SLE cases ($P=0.0109$, Fisher's exact test). Similar results were obtained when genotypes from a second affected case from the families were examined and compared to the same controls ($n=180$, C/T 16.1%, T/T 4.4%, $P=0.0060$). We then confirmed this finding using independent replication cohorts: a collection of 201 SLE cases recruited at the University of Minnesota as part of a trio family collection, an independent collection of 139 SLE cases derived from the Hopkins Lupus Cohort (Petri 2000), and a second large group of controls ($n=1035$). Overall, these groups showed very comparable PTPN22 R620W

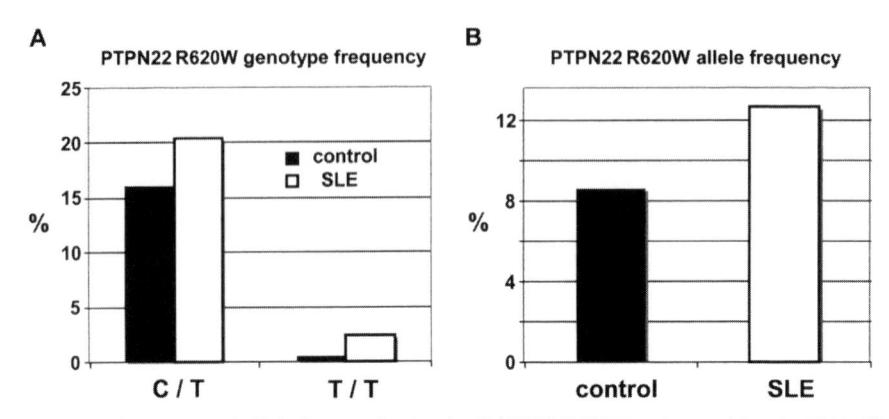

FIG. 2. Genotype and allele frequencies for the PTPN22 R620W polymorphism in SLE. (A) Shown are genotype frequencies of white controls ($n=1961$) and white SLE cases ($n=525$). The increased C/T genotype frequency in SLE had an odds ratio of 1.37 (95% confidence interval [CI] 1.07–1.75), while the T/T genotype had an odds ratio of 4.37 (CI 1.98–9.65) ($P=0.00009$). (B) Minor T allele frequency difference between SLE (12.67%, 1050 chromosomes) and controls (8.64%, 3922 chromosomes) was significant ($P<0.0001$).

genotype frequencies as observed in the multiplex family cases (Kyogoku et al 2004).

We next examined all the data together, and compared allele frequencies of the R20W SNP in 525 independent white SLE cases and 1961 matched white controls (Fig. 2). This analysis yielded the following estimates for SLE genotype frequencies: 20.4% C/T, 2.5% T/T ($P=0.00009$, compared to the combined control data: 16.1% C/T and 0.6% T/T). The odds ratios in the combined datasets suggested a dose effect, with heterozygotes at increased risk relative to C/C homozygotes [OR=1.37, 95% CI= (1.07,1.75)], and T/T homozygotes with greater than twice the risk of heterozyogotes [OR=4.37, 95% CI=(1.98,9.65)]. The overall risk allele frequency of R620W in 525 SLE cases was 12.67%, compared with an allele frequency of 8.64% in 1961 white controls ($P<0.0001$). The risk allele was present in 22.9% of SLE patients compared to 16.7% of controls.

There were no significant differences in frequencies of lupus sub-phenotypes in cases carrying one or more copies of the risk allele compared with cases lacking the risk allele (as defined by the criteria used to diagnose SLE), although our power to detect these effects was somewhat limited by sample size. The risk allele is less common within African–American and Hispanic/Latino populations than in North American whites (Begovich et al 2004), and our current collection was underpowered to assess the possible influence of the 620W allele in these populations.

These data, together with the recent evidence for association of R620W with T1D (Bottini et al 2004) and RA (Begovich et al 2004), suggest that PTPN22 R620W is a potent genetic risk factor for both organ specific (T1D) and systemic (RA and SLE) autoimmune syndromes. Additional typing in a large collection of families enriched for multiple autoimmune diseases confirms these data for T1D, RA and SLE (Criswell et al 2005). In addition, we found that individuals with Hashimoto's autoimmune thyroid disease also have an elevated allele frequency for the R620W SNP (Criswell et al 2005). Of interest, the SNP showed no association with psoriasis or multiple sclerosis in this collection. Two additional studies have now confirmed the association of the R620W SNP with diabetes in convincing fashion (Smyth et al 2004, Onengut-Gumuscu et al 2004), and one of these also found significant association with Graves' disease (Onengut-Gumuscu et al 2004).

Of interest, all of the human autoimmune diseases shown to date to be associated with PTPN22 R620W are characterized by the production of autoantibodies (e.g. anti-GAD Abs in T1D, anti-citrulline Abs and rheumatoid factor in RA, anti-TSHR antibodies in Graves', anti-microsomal and thyroglobulin antibodies in Hashimoto's, and a vast array of autoantibodies in SLE), and the appearance of these antibodies often pre-dates clinical disease (Arbuckle et al 2003, Rantapaa-Dahlqvist et al 2003). This is reminiscent of the phenotype of the $Pep^{-/-}$ mice, which show elevated levels of T-dependent antibodies. The data are consistent with the possibility that the 620W variant of PTPN22 may predispose individuals to autoimmunity by facilitating the generation of certain disease-associated autoantibodies, thereby contributing to disease onset and perhaps progression. The PTPN22 polymorphism may lead to excessive T cell help for antibody production, or alternatively may be associated with intrinsic abnormalities in B cells. The US Census Bureau estimates that there are currently 290 million people living in the USA, of which 234 million are white. Given a carrier frequency for PTPN22 R620W of about 16.7% in whites and a rough estimate of about half that in the other ethnic groups, we estimate that there are 44 million people in the USA alone that carry this SNP. Using a conservative estimate of a 5% carrier rate, there are likely to be at least 300 million carriers worldwide. Given this frequency of the PTPN22 R620W SNP in the population, it is important that we understand how this gene contributes to autoimmunity.

Modelling the initiation and pathogenesis of SLE

The available genetic data in SLE, based on the work of many investigators, allow us to outline a working model for the initiation and maintenance of SLE in humans. The model predicts that individuals carrying specific common polymorphic alleles or combinations of alleles are at significantly increased risk for the production of nuclear autoantibodies, which may be present for many years prior to diagnosis. HLA class II alleles, perhaps in concert with other genes in epistasis on the relevant haplotypes, predispose to SLE by facilitating presentation of antigens that lead to a break in tolerance. The fact that homozygosity or compound heterozygosity for HLA class II haplotypes increases risk for disease has at least two possible explanations. First, the risk class II alleles may present the relevant self-antigens, and individuals carrying two copies present higher amounts of potentially autoimmune peptides. Alternatively, there may be a paucity of regulatory T cells that are more efficiently selected and activated on non-risk class II alleles.

Genetic polymorphisms in proteins that regulate signalling thresholds in lymphocytes, and in particular negative regulatory proteins such as PTPN22, may result in the 'tuning' of the immune system, ever so slightly, towards a hyper-reactive state. We will eventually identify many additional gene products that together constitute the 'wiring' of the immune system, and this wiring will be somewhat different for every individual in the population. We envision a gradation of risk based on the number and combination of SLE risk alleles that a person inherits. Some individuals may be essentially 'hard-wired' for the development of SLE, and normal environmental encounters with enteric bacteria or sunlight may be all that is necessary to initiate disease. In other individuals, carrying fewer susceptibility alleles, or alternatively carrying protective alleles, may require a more serious environmental insult. These scenarios beg the question of the nature of such environmental factors. A reasonable argument has been made for Epstein-Barr virus as an initiating factor (James et al 1997), although the jury is still out given the nearly ubiquitous exposure to this virus. Certain drugs and solvents are suspected as being able to induce a lupus-like phenotype, and ultraviolet damage from sunlight can trigger flares of lupus. Other factors are suspected but not proven (Cooper & Parks 2004). The interface of the environment with the genetics of lupus remains a challenging, but important, area for further study.

A key event in the initiation of SLE is the production of nuclear autoantibodies. Given the large number of mouse knockout and transgenic models that develop an SLE-like phenotype with autoantibody production, the pathways contributing are likely to be complex and highly integrated. Once production of potentially pathogenic antibodies begins, there is likely the need for additional triggers or genetic factors to initiate disease. The intriguing data from Harley and colleagues, showing that autoantibodies appear in serum years before the first symptoms of SLE (Arbuckle et al 2003), suggest that the early initiation phase of disease can be quite prolonged. Indeed, healthy individuals may carry high titres of autoantibodies and never develop disease. The crossing-over from benign autoimmunity to disease is poorly understood, and longitudinal, prospective studies will be needed to fully address this issue.

The break in normal immune tolerance that leads to autoimmunity in SLE could be at essentially any level of the immune system — thymocyte selection, peripheral T cell tolerance, central B cell tolerance/receptor editing, peripheral B cell tolerance, or defects in innate immunity. Recent data indicate that as many as 75% of all newly made B cells have some specificity for cytoplasmic and/or nuclear antigens (Wardemann et al 2003) suggesting that receptor editing of B cells could be an Achilles' heel in SLE. Impaired efficiencies in receptor editing would result in the migration of increased numbers of potentially self-reactive B cells into the periphery, thereby providing a substrate for pathologic autoantibody production.

While certain autoantibodies directly cause disease by binding directly to target tissues (e.g. anti-platelet antibodies in thrombocytopenia, anti-red blood cell antibodies in haemolytic anaemia, and anti-phospholipid antibodies leading to thrombosis), others act indirectly through the formation of immune complexes (ICs) that deposit in tissues and cause end-organ damage. Polymorphisms in genes of the complement cascade and Ig Fc receptors likely exhibit their contributions to disease through handling of circulating ICs.

Some of the antigens targeted in lupus may be modified during apoptosis (Casciola-Rosen et al 1994, Utz et al 1997), and the disease is characterized by increased rates of lymphocyte apoptosis. Anti-nuclear antibodies with specificity for histones and DNA have the potential to form large ICs of nuclear material, released from either necrotic or apoptotic cells. Chromatin-containing ICs induce B cell hyperproliferation through co-ligation of the B cell receptor (BCR) and toll-like receptor 9 (TLR9) (Leadbetter et al 2002), and similarly dendritic cells exposed to chromatin ICs have accelerated and excessive production of interferon and other inflammatory mediators. Recent experiments have clearly shown that chromatin containing ICs are present in serum of humans with SLE (Ronnblom & Alm 2001), and these ICs have the ability to induce interferon (IFN)α production by plasmacytoid dendritic cells (Blanco et al 2001). A majority of SLE patients carry a prominent IFN gene expression signature in their peripheral blood cells (Bennett et al 2003, Baechler et al 2003), and this signature is a marker for increased disease activity and severity (unpublished data). These new findings suggest an important role for the IFN pathway in mediating disease in lupus, and perhaps other autoimmune disorders (e.g. myositis). IFN drives the differentiation of B cells into plasmablasts, and increases the differentiation of monocytes into highly efficient antigen-presenting dendritic cells; thus IFN may function to perpetuate and accelerate disease. Together, these data indicate that a variety of genetic factors may contribute to SLE at several distinct stages of disease development and progression. Further work will lead to a better understanding of human

SLE, and the eventual fruit of this effort will be improved diagnostics and the development of more rational therapies.

Acknowledgements

We are grateful to the patients and their referring physicians for their participation in these studies. We also thank all our laboratory members and staff, past and present, who have contributed to this work. These studies were supported by grants and contracts from NIAMS, NIAID, the Alliance for Lupus Research, the Mary Kirkland Center for Lupus Research, and the Minnesota Lupus Foundation.

References

Alarcon-Riquelme ME, Prokunina L 2003 Finding genes for SLE: complex interactions and complex populations. J Autoimmun 21:117–120

Arbuckle MR, McClain MT, Rubertone MV et al 2003 Development of autoantibodies before the clinical onset of systemic lupus erythematosus. N Engl J Med 349:1526–1533

Baechler EC, Batliwalla FM, Karypis G et al 2003 Interferon-inducible gene expression signature in peripheral blood cells of patients with severe lupus. Proc Natl Acad Sci USA 100:2610–2615

Begovich AB, Carlton VE, Honigberg LA et al 2004 A missense single-nucleotide polymorphism in a gene encoding a protein tyrosine phosphatase (PTPN22) is associated with rheumatoid arthritis. Am J Hum Genet 75:330–337

Bennett L, Palucka AK, Arce E et al 2003 Interferon and granulopoiesis signatures in systemic lupus erythematosus blood. J Exp Med 197:711–723

Blanco P, Palucka AK, Gill M, Pascual V, Banchereau J 2001 Induction of dendritic cell differentiation by IFN-alpha in systemic lupus erythematosus. Science 294:1540–1543

Bottini N, Musumeci L, Alonso A et al 2004 A functional variant of lymphoid tyrosine phosphatase is associated with type I diabetes. Nat Genet 36:337–338

Casciola-Rosen LA, Anhalt G, Rosen A 1994 Autoantigens targeted in systemic lupus erythematosus are clustered in two populations of surface structures on apoptotic keratinocytes. J Exp Med 179:1317–1330

Chien W, Tidow N, Williamson EA et al 2003 Characterization of a myeloid tyrosine phosphatase, Lyp, and its role in the Bcr-Abl signal transduction pathway. J Biol Chem 278:27413–27420

Cloutier JF, Veillette A 1996 Association of inhibitory tyrosine protein kinase p50csk with protein tyrosine phosphatase PEP in T cells and other hemopoietic cells. Embo J 15:4909–4918

Cloutier JF, Veillette A 1999 Cooperative inhibition of T-cell antigen receptor signaling by a complex between a kinase and a phosphatase. J Exp Med 189:111–121

Cohen S, Dadi H, Shaòul E, Sharfe N, Roifman CM 1999 Cloning and characterization of a lymphoid-specific, inducible human protein tyrosine phosphatase, Lyp. Blood 93:2013–2024

Cooper GS, Parks CG 2004 Occupational and environmental exposures as risk factors for systemic lupus erythematosus. Curr Rheumatol Rep 6:367–374

Criswell LA, Pfeiffer KA, Lum B et al 2005 Analysis of families in the Multiple Autoimmune Disease Genetics Consortium (MADGC) collection: the PTPN22 620W allele associates with multiple autoimmune phenotypes. Am J Hum Genet 76, in press

Dawkins R, Leelayuwat C, Gaudieri S et al 1999 Genomics of the major histocompatibility complex: haplotypes, duplication, retroviruses and disease. Immunol Rev 167:275–304

Gabriel SB, Schaffner SF, Nguyen H et al 2002 The structure of haplotype blocks in the human genome. Science 296:2225–2229

Gaffney PM, Moser KL, Graham RR, Behrens TW 2002 Recent advances in the genetics of systemic lupus erythematosus. Rheum Dis Clin North Am 28:111–126

Gaffney PM, Kearns GM, Shark KB et al 1998 A genome-wide search for susceptibility genes in human systemic lupus erythematosus sib-pair families. Proc Natl Acad Sci USA 95:14875–14879

Gaffney PM, Ortmann WA, Selby SA et al 2000 Genome screening in human systemic lupus erythematosus: results from a second Minnesota cohort and combined analyses of 187 sib-pair families. Am J Hum Genet 66:547–556

Gjorloff-Wingren A, Saxena M, Williams S, Hammi D, Mustelin T 1999 Characterization of TCR-induced receptor-proximal signaling events negatively regulated by the protein tyrosine phosphatase PEP. Eur J Immunol 29:3845–3854

Graham RR, Ortmann WA, Langefeld CD et al 2002 Visualizing human leukocyte antigen class II risk haplotypes in human systemic lupus erythematosus. Am J Hum Genet 71:543–553

Harley JB, Moser KL, Gaffney PM, Behrens TW 1998 The genetics of human systemic lupus erythematosus. Curr Opin Immunol 10:690–696

Hasegawa K, Martin F, Huang G et al 2004 PEST domain-enriched tyrosine phosphatase (PEP) regulation of effector/memory T cells. Science 303:685–689

Hatakeyama M, Kono T, Kobayashi N et al 1991 Interaction of the IL-2 receptor with the src-family kinase p56lck: identification of novel intermolecular association. Science 252:1523–1528

Hill RJ, Zozulya S, Lu YL et al 2002 The lymphoid protein tyrosine phosphatase Lyp interacts with the adaptor molecule Grb2 and functions as a negative regulator of T-cell activation. Exp Hematol 30:237–244

James JA, Kaufman KM, Farris AD et al 1997 An increased prevalence of Epstein-Barr virus infection in young patients suggests a possible etiology for systemic lupus erythematosus. J Clin Invest 100:3019–3026

Jeffreys AJ, Kauppi L, Neumann R 2001 Intensely punctate meiotic recombination in the class II region of the major histocompatibility complex. Nat Genet 29:217–222

Kelly JA, Moser KL, Harley JB 2002 The genetics of systemic lupus erythematosus: putting the pieces together. Genes Immun 3 (suppl 1):S71–S85

Kyogoku C, Langefeld CD, Ortmann WA et al 2004 Genetic association of the R620W polymorphism of protein tyrosine phosphatase PTPN22 with human SLE. Am J Hum Genet 75:504–507

Leadbetter EA, Rifkin IR, Hohlbaum AM et al 2002 Chromatin-IgG complexes activate B cells by dual engagement of IgM and Toll-like receptors. Nature 416:603–607

Martin ER, Monks SA, Warren LL, Kaplan NL 2000 A test for linkage and association in general pedigrees: the pedigree disequilibrium test. Am J Hum Genet 67:146–154

Matthews RJ, Bowne DB, Flores E, Thomas ML 1992 Characterization of hematopoietic intracellular protein tyrosine phosphatases: description of a phosphatase containing an SH2 domain and another enriched in proline-, glutamic acid-, serine-, and threonine-rich sequences. Mol Cell Biol 12:2396–2405

Onengut-Gumuscu S, Ewens KG, Spielman RS, Concannon P 2004 A functional polymorphism (1858C/T) in the PTPN22 gene is linked and associated with type I diabetes in multiplex families. Genes Immun 5:678–680

Petri M 2000 Hopkins lupus cohort. 1999 update. Rheum Dis Clin North Am 26:199–213, v

Rantapaa-Dahlqvist S, de Jong BA, Berglin E et al 2003 Antibodies against cyclic citrullinated peptide and IgA rheumatoid factor predict the development of rheumatoid arthritis. Arthritis Rheum 48:2741–2749

Rhodes DA, Trowsdale J 1999 Genetics and molecular genetics of the MHC. Rev Immunogenet 1:21–31
Ronnblom L, Alm GV 2001 A pivotal role for the natural interferon alpha-producing cells (plasmacytoid dendritic cells) in the pathogenesis of lupus. J Exp Med 194:F59–63
Smyth D, Cooper JD, Collins JE et al 2004 Replication of an association between the lymphoid tyrosine phosphatase locus (LYP/PTPN22) with type 1 Diabetes, and evidence for its role as a general autoimmunity locus. Diabetes 53:3020–3023
Snell GD 1948 Methods for the study of histocompatibility genes. J Genet 87–98
Spielman RS, McGinnis RE, Evans WJ 1993 Transmission test for linkage disequilibrium: the insulin gene region and insulin dependent diabetes mellitus (IDDM). Am J Hum Genet 52:506–516
Tsao B 2003 The genetics of human systemic lupus erythematosus. Trends Immunol 24:595–602
Utz PJ, Hottelet M, Schur PH, Anderson P 1997 Proteins phosphorylated during stress-induced apoptosis are common targets for autoantibody production in patients with systemic lupus erythematosus. J Exp Med 185:843–854
Vyse TJ, Todd JA 1996 Genetic analysis of autoimmune disease. Cell 85:311–318
Wakeland EK, Liu K, Graham RR, Behrens TW 2001 Delineating the genetic basis of systemic lupus erythematosus. Immunity 15:397–408
Walsh EC, Mather KA, Schaffner SF et al 2003 An integrated haplotype map of the human major histocompatibility complex. Am J Hum Genet 73:580–590
Wardemann H, Yurasov S, Schaefer A et al 2003 Predominant autoantibody production by early human B cell precursors. Science 301:1374–1377

DISCUSSION

Ting: In your SLE patients, are their plasmacytoid DCs different? With your larger numbers of patients do you see that correlation clearly?

Behrens: Jacques Banchereau has looked at this. He found lower numbers of plasmacytoid DCs in blood from SLE patients. But if you look at tissue biopsy of inflamed skin from lupus patients there are increased numbers of plasmacytoid DCs in the cutaneous tissues mediating some of the inflammation.

Wakeland: We have also seen a decrease in the plasmacytoid DCs in the peripheral blood of lupus patients, but we have not looked in tissue. We do not detect significant increases in α interferon in plasma from patients with active lupus, but we do see a similar molecular signature of type 1 interferons, as Tim just described quite nicely. The origin of this interferon signature is somewhat mysterious.

Abbas: I want to make a general point. Many of us intellectually and practically search for commonalities between autoimmune diseases and the existence of multiple autoimmune disease in patients or kindreds. Findings of one knockout giving rise to multiple autoimmune manifestations support that search. But to me, what is really striking looking at Tim Behrens' data, is that this seems not to be correct. Of all the autoimmune diseases, lupus seems to be an interferon α dominant disease. Conversely, the clinical trial data would suggest that rheumatoid arthritis (RA) is a tumour necrosis factor (TNF) dominant disease. If these turn out to be correct, then at the very least this says that in different autoimmune diseases there is something fundamentally different in the pathways that give rise to the clinical manifestations. I think no one would have predicted that lupus would have shown such a striking interferon signature. There is a general point to be made that not all autoimmunity is going to turn out to be the same at the effector stage. I don't know the implications of this in terms of hunting for genes.

Goodnow: It means buy Amgen stock!

Hafler: In terms of the effector stage (signalling) one thing I find striking clinically is that multiple sclerosis (MS) doesn't seem to segregate with lupus. It is surprising that MS does not seem to have that same allelic frequency, although there may be other related alleles, which are linked to MS. Clearly, these are different diseases and they have different manifestations. But there may be similar defects or allelic variation in signalling pathways related to the affector rather than the effector part. This is the converse of what you are saying. There is a commonality among autoimmune diseases.

Kuchroo: I would not have expected organ-specific autoimmune diseases such as MS and type 1 diabetes to have too much in common.

Hafler: They don't segregate together clinically. The only autoimmune disease associated with MS might be thyroid disease.

Behrens: There are very few data. In our MADGC families we see a cluster of MS, RA, lupus and autoimmune thyroid disease. At least half of these families have three or four of these diseases.

Rioux: But these families were ascertained to have multiple different autoimmune diseases.

Hafler: Specifically, a prospective study at the Mayo Clinic suggested that the only disease with a modest association with MS is thyroid disease.

Behrens: We reviewed all the data out there. There are lots of small studies, and no large ones. We have ascertained a lot of these families through lupus probands and RA probands. If there is any bias in this data set, we should be over-represented for RA and lupus. We are finding that these families are linked with MS.

Abbas: The reason I want to make this point is that in addition to, or perhaps instead of, searching for genes associated with autoimmunity, perhaps we need to make more of an effort to identify signatures that will classify different diseases, whatever they are. Then we should be looking for genes common to all the TNF disorders, or all the interferon disorders.

Wicker: The effector phase is very heterogeneous, too. With the clinical trials of anti-TNF, there are some wonder stories with 30% having a very significant response to anti-TNF but there are a lot of non-responders.

Behrens: If you talk to the rheumatologist on the street, TNF has worked for about 75% of patients. The people who go into these studies tend to be the most difficult to treat, who have failed multiple different therapies.

Abbas: It is impressive that in less than five years this is now the standard of practice. We are beginning to talk of RA as a TNF-mediated disorder, which is a complete change in conceptualizing the disease. If it really is a TNF-mediated disorder rather than or in addition to a T cell or antibody mediated disorder, this totally changes the way we should think about it. Crohn's disease may be the same, but MS is not. They are all T cell-mediated delayed-type hypersensitivity (DTH), Th1-like lesions on the surface, but the clinical trials say they aren't. If this turns out to be correct, the data available now have to make us think about this.

Wicker: In the long term, going after the effector phase is not as good as going after the cause, which would be a breakdown of tolerance. This should be the long-term goal. Suppressing the effector phase does increase the rate of infection.

Abbas: I am just saying that if this is correct, then the genetics may be different, as might the pathogenesis.

Foote: Is there any association between your signatures and your phosphatase or CD40?

Behrens: We haven't looked at that carefully. We will rapidly run into huge number problems because we are down to 12% allele frequency with PTP, and much less than that with CD40. This is an argument for bringing together large consortia.

Worthington: What treatments were the patients on? Were they treatment naïve?

Behrens: It was a mixed bag. The goal of the study is to look at 300 patients longitudinally over a year, getting serum, cells, RNA and DNA at each recorded time point. These are the baseline data. We will look at the effect of steroid treatment on interferon signature. In general, it appears that this is a marker for bad disease. People who have this interferon signature tend to be flaring and have bad lupus. Some are treatment naïve, some aren't.

Vyse: I want to understand the definition of the interferon signature. You put interferon on cells and looked at the genes that were upregulated. To characterize this, you really want to put a range of other cytokines on cells and look at the profiles there.

Behrens: We have done this with TNF, IL1, IL6, CPG and Toll 3, 4 and 7 ligands. We have analysed the signatures induced by these agents in normal peripheral blood cells. There are clearly genes that are up-regulated by TNF that are also up-regulated in the blood of lupus patients. However, when you perform correlation coefficients for the group of genes, and compare the global pattern in patients with IFN, TNF or IL pathway signatures, IFN is a strong winner. From this we conclude that TNF is probably playing a minor role, if any. Some additional data that make us think that interferon is the relevant cytokine come from a recent proteomics experiment. We looked at IFN high, low and control individuals, measuring 140 different anylates in their serum. The IFN high patients have a number of IFN-inducible chemokines and other soluble proteins in their blood whereas IFN-low patients don't. We think we have a protein marker of this IFN signature that we can measure by ELISA.

Abbas: You and Peter Gregersen were looking at RA patients to see whether there was a cytokine signature. What were the results?

Behrens: Some of these patients do have a TNF signature. This is what you might expect. Others have an interferon signature very similar to what is observed in lupus, although it's found in only a minority of patients.

Goldstein: Were the CD40 data only linkage or do you have any kind of association data?

Behrens: The linkage peak is right over the top of CD40. The only association data we have are minimal at this point. We are currently working with collaborators to type trios with Central and South American ancestry.

Goldstein: It is fortunate that you have trios, since one would worry about stratification in this case.

Behrens: I was surprised to learn that in the USA there is a 60% Caucasian admixture in Mexican Americans.

Goldstein: My other question concerns the at-risk haplotype for CD40. Did you check whether it is the ancestral or derived allele in that haplotype? Did you try to use this in any tests of selection?

Behrens: We see a large number of tightly linked SNPs that travel together on an ancestral haplotye, found in many populations.

Goldstein: There are seven sites that distinguish the haplotypes. For each of these sites does the at risk haplotype have the derived or the ancestral allele? This information might help you in a test of selection.

Behrens: We haven't looked at that.

Abbas: I want to plant an idea that we might be able to discuss later. This is to reemphasize a point that Vijay Kuchroo and Chris Goodnow were making from mouse studies and what their implications might be for the human studies. If you take all the loci that have been identified as being associated with susceptibility to EAE, for example, in different inbred strains, and then mix everything together in a meta-analysis, you would lose all the significance. Simply increasing the sample size will not make anything significant. If you take EAE susceptible loci in mice and combine all the information, this will not be productive. What is the implication of this for doing a similar thing in humans?

Hafler: That's a dumb experiment.

Rioux: Your whole discussion is going to be predicated on your initial statement saying that by putting these mice together you are going to lose a signal in meta-analysis.

Wicker: I don't agree with this either.

Kuchroo: There are five genomic scans for EAE using different strain combinantions. Two were done from the SJL B10.S mice, one was a backcross F1 analysis and the other was an F2 analysis. Thank goodness, in those two some of the loci overlap. But if you look at the whole genome scans there is more overlap with the loci that Linda Wicker has picked up in diabetes and EAE than all the EAE loci picked up for these five genomic crosses.. The best data we have is that many EAE loci overlap with diabetes.

Foote: Why would you do that? If you end up with significant linkage in a particular cross, using inbred mouse strains there is no reason to do a meta-analysis on them.

Kuchroo: This wasn't meta-analysis. We eyeball the data looking at how many of these turn up as common loci that are playing a role in EAE.

Abbas: It is really asking how many of these are susceptibility loci across strains. If you try to do this the answer is none.

Wicker: No, there is a fatal flaw in your logic. It is to do with restricted analysis when any two strains are used because in many cases they will share particular susceptibility alleles, so you can't directly compare one cross to another. If you put all of the strains in one big room and grew up 50 000 mice and then analysed them for their disease phenotype you could find most of the loci.

Kuchroo: In humans we assume these are different families with same loci affecting the disease phenotype but it could be that there are different genetic elements contributing to give you the same disease phenotype, and then we put them all together.

Kere: I may have this wrong, but it is really different diseases in these different strains. In humans it would be like taking one growth disorder and comparing it with another.

Abbas: They are not different diseases phenotypically.

Cookson: No, if you take 20 different strains of mice and breed them together over 20 generations, mapping their pedigree so you know where everything is coming from, you can use the mice you end up with to map diseases, and you will do that with a great degree of precision.

A molecular dissection of lymphocyte unresponsiveness induced by sustained calcium signalling

Vigo Heissmeyer*, Fernando Macián*[1], Rajat Varma†, Sin-Hyeog Im*[2], Francisco García-Cozar*[3], Heidi F. Horton‡, Michael C. Byrne‡, Stefan Feske*, K. Venuprasad§, Hua Gu¶, Yun-Cai Liu§, Michael L. Dustin† and Anjana Rao*[4]

*Department of Pathology, Harvard Medical School and the CBR Institute for Biomedical Research, 200 Longwood Avenue, Boston, Massachusetts 02115, †Program in Molecular Pathogenesis and Department of Pathology, Skirball Institute of Molecular Medicine, New York University School of Medicine, New York, NY10016, ‡Wyeth Research, 200 CambridgePark Drive, Cambridge, Massachusetts 02140, §Division of Cell Biology, La Jolla Institute for Allergy and Immunology, San Diego, CA 92121, and ¶Department of Microbiology, Columbia University, College of Physicians and Surgeons, 701 West 168th Street, HHSC, New York, NY 10032, USA

Abstract. In lymphocytes, integration of Ca^{2+} and other signalling pathways results in productive activation, while unopposed Ca^{2+} signalling leads to decreased responsiveness to subsequent stimulation (anergy). The Ca^{2+}-regulated transcription factor NFAT has an integral role in both aspects of lymphocyte function. NFAT cooperates with the transcription factor AP-1 (Fos/Jun) to up-regulate genes involved in productive activation of lymphocytes. However, in the absence of AP-1, NFAT imposes an opposing genetic programme that leads to lymphocyte anergy. Anergy is implemented at least partly through proteolytic degradation of the key signalling proteins PKCθ and PLCγ1. Sustained Ca^{2+}–calcineurin signalling increases mRNA and protein levels of the E3 ubiquitin ligases Itch, CblB and Grail and induces expression of Tsg101, the ubiquitin-binding component of the ESCRT1 endosomal sorting complex. Subsequent stimulation or homotypic cell adhesion promotes membrane translocation of Itch and the related protein Nedd4, resulting in PKCθ and PLCγ1 degradation. T cells from *Itch*- and *CblB*-deficient mice are resistant to anergy induction. Anergic T cells show

---

[1]Present address: Albert Einstein College of Medicine, Department of Pathology, 1300 Morris Park Ave, Bronx, NY 10461, USA.
[2]Present address: Department of Life Science, Kwangju Institute of Science and Technology, 1 Oryong-dong, Puk-ku, Kwangju 500-712, Korea.
[3]Present address: Hospital Universitario de Puerto Real, Unidad de Investigación, Carretera Nacional IV Km. 665, 11510 Puerto Real, Cádiz, Spain.
[4]This paper was presented at the symposium by Anjana Rao to whom correspondence should be addressed.

impaired calcium mobilization after TCR triggering and are unable to maintain a mature immunological synapse. Thus Ca^{2+}–calcineurin–NFAT signalling links gene transcription to a multi-step programme that leads to impaired signal transduction in anergic T cells.

2005 The genetics of autoimmunity. Wiley, Chichester (Novartis Foundation Symposium 267) p 165–179

In healthy people, self-antigens do not elicit a significant immune response. Rather, self-reactive lymphocytes are rendered non-functional by a combination of several mechanisms: clonal deletion in the thymus, tolerance induction in the periphery, and the actions of regulatory T cells (Kamradt & Mitchison 2001, Kruisbeek & Amsen 1996). Here we focus on the biochemical and transcriptional mechanisms underlying T cell 'anergy', a state in which T cell antigen receptors are uncoupled from their downstream signalling pathways and the T cells are unresponsive to stimulation through the T cell receptor (TCR) (Boussiotis et al 1997, Fields et al 1996, Li et al 1996).

Whether T cells become anergic or make a robust immune response depends on the conditions under which they recognise the antigen. If pathogens or 'danger' signals are sensed by the immune system, toll-like receptors which recognize pathogen-associated molecules are activated, the expression of major histocompatibility proteins and co-stimulatory molecules such as B7-1/CD80 and B7-2/CD86 on antigen-presenting cells (APCs) is increased, and T cells concurrently receive signals through the TCR and through co-stimulatory receptors such as CD28 which bind the B7 proteins. The combined activation of antigen and co-stimulatory receptors on T cells leads to full activation of several signalling pathways and culminates in a productive immune response. In contrast, in the absence of danger signals such as those evoked by infection with pathogens, T cells recognize antigens (e.g. self-antigens, orally ingested antigens or injected soluble antigens) without concomitant engagement of co-stimulatory receptors, and an anergic or self-tolerant state is imposed (Macian et al 2004, Lesage & Goodnow 2001).

The T cell anergy programme is imposed by NFAT

We have shown that T cell anergy is the result of a transcriptional programme induced by NFAT, a transcription factor regulated by calcium and the calcium/ calmodulin-dependent phosphatase calcineurin (Macian et al 2002, Heissmeyer et al 2004). NFAT-family proteins are highly phosphorylated and reside in the cytoplasm of resting cells (Crabtree 1999, Rao et al 1997, Crabtree & Olson 2002, Hogan et al 2003). In cells activated through a variety of cell-surface receptors including the TCR, elevation of intracellular calcium levels activates calcineurin, which dephosphorylates NFAT. This induces a conformational change which results in nuclear translocation, increased DNA binding and transcriptional activity (Okamura et al 2000).

Recent structural data emphasize the remarkable versatility of NFAT binding to DNA. NFAT can bind as a monomer to DNA, assuming a large variety of configurations in which the two domains of the DNA-binding domain — the N-terminal specificity domain and the C-terminal dimerization domain — adopt different positions relative to each other as a result of the fact that they are separated by a flexible linker region (Stroud & Chen 2003). At composite NFAT:AP-1 elements found in the regulatory regions of many target genes, NFAT proteins bind cooperatively with an unrelated transcription factor, AP-1 (Fos-Jun) (Chen et al 1998, Macian et al 2001). At DNA elements which resemble NF-κB sites, NFAT proteins bind DNA as dimers (Giffin et al 2003, Jin et al 2003). In cooperation with GATA proteins, NFAT activates transcription of the Th2 cytokine genes interleukin (IL)4, IL5 and IL13 (Avni et al 2002, Monticelli et al 2004, Hogan et al 2003). Each of these configurations appears to be associated with transcription of a different subset of target genes.

Depending on its DNA-binding configuration and the partner proteins available, NFAT mediates transcriptional programmes leading to productive activation or anergy in T cells. In T cells that have been stimulated through both the TCR and co-stimulatory receptors, several transcription factors including NFAT, NFκB and AP-1 are robustly activated, allowing NFAT proteins to bind cooperatively to DNA together with AP-1 (Chen et al 1998). The cooperation between NFAT and AP-1 leads to induction or repression of a very large number of effector cytokine, chemokine and other genes that are essential for the productive immune response (Macian et al 2000, Rao et al 1997). Recent transcriptional profiling of a T cell clone stimulated with PMA and ionomycin put the number of genes induced (up-regulated) under these conditions at $\sim$570 (Macian et al 2002). In contrast, in T cells that have been activated through the TCR alone, calcium signals predominate and NFAT activation is dominant over NF-κB and AP-1 activation. These conditions can be mimicked by treatment of T cells with ionomycin alone, which also leads to T cell anergy (Schwartz 2003). Transcriptional profiling of the ionomycin-treated D5 Th1 cell clone showed induction of a different, smaller set of genes ($\sim$165) encoding negative regulators of T cell signalling (Macian et al 2002). Among these were:

- genes encoding several tyrosine phosphatases which would be expected to down-regulate TCR signalling by opposing the effects of tyrosine kinases such as ZAP70, Lck and Itk

- genes encoding inhibitory cell surface receptors, particularly CD98, which influences integrin affinity via activation of the small G protein Rap1a
- the gene encoding diacylglycerol (DAG) kinase, which metabolizes the second messenger DAG, which would be expected to attenuate MAP kinase signalling and decrease AP-1 activation
- genes encoding various proteases and E3 ubiquitin ligases (Macian et al 2002).

The calcineurin inhibitor CsA abolished induction of almost all genes in either category, implicating calcineurin/NFAT signalling in both the activation and anergy programmes. These results are consistent with our previous findings using human T cells (Feske et al 2001).

We confirmed that the ionomycin-induced genes were strongly associated with T cell anergy and were transcriptional targets of NFAT in the absence of AP-1. The genes were up-regulated *in vivo* in T cells from orally tolerized mice. A constitutively-active NFAT1 protein that was engineered to be unable to interact with AP-1 induced T cell anergy as well as a large number of the anergy-associated genes; conversely, T cells lacking NFAT1 were resistant to anergy induction and showed much lower induction of the majority of anergy-associated genes.

The E3 ligases, Itch, CblB and GRAIL are transcriptional targets of the T cell anergy programme

We were intrigued by the possibility that the proteases and E3 ligases found among the anergy-associated genes might induce T cell anergy by promoting degradation of downstream signalling molecules. To test this hypothesis, we began by comparing the levels of several signalling molecules in untreated and anergic T cells. We found that several signalling molecules—PLCγ1, PKCθ and RasGAP—were indeed degraded in T cells in a calcium- and calcineurin-dependent manner (Heissmeyer et al 2004). Further analysis showed, however, that although calcium/calcineurin signalling was essential to prime the cells for the degradation step, the degradation was not actually implemented unless cell–cell contact or TCR stimulation occurred (Heissmeyer et al 2004). This suggested that degradation occurred in two steps: a calcineurin/NFAT-mediated transcriptional programme of anergy induction led to up-regulation of effector molecules which were activated to begin the degradation programme upon cell–cell contact. Because total levels of conjugated ubiquitin were increased in anergic T cells, we examined the potential involvement of E3 ubiquitin ligases in T cell anergy.

Notably, the three targets of the Ca^{2+}/calcineurin-dependent degradation programme, PLCγ1, PKCθ and RasGAP had one feature in common: they all possessed at least one C2 domain. C2 domains come in various forms: they can mediate Ca^{2+}-dependent binding of proteins to phospholipids, or they can serve as protein–protein interaction domains, which may be either Ca^{2+}-dependent or -independent (Nalefski & Falke 1996). Since C2 domains are also found in the Itch/Nedd4 family of E3 ubiquitin ligases, we asked whether these E3 ligases were involved in degradation of signalling proteins in anergic T cells. Itch was a particularly attractive candidate since the naturally-occurring mouse mutant, *Itch*, lacks the Itch protein and develops an autoimmune/inflammatory problem that is fatal on the C57BL/6 background and is characterized by massive lymphocyte infiltration into the skin and other organs (Perry et al 1998, Fang et al 2002), We showed that PLCγ1 co-immunoprecipitated with both Nedd4 and Itch, and was a substrate for ubiquitination and degradation by Itch. Moreover, PLCγ1 degradation was not observed in Itch-deficient T cells that had been subjected to sustained calcium signalling, strongly implicating Itch in the process of PLCγ1 degradation (Heissmeyer et al 2004).

We asked whether Itch and Nedd4 were targets of the anergy programme, i.e. whether they were up-regulated at the mRNA or protein levels or otherwise modified in anergic T cells. We found that *Itch* mRNA increased up to 10-fold after 6–10 h of ionomycin treatment, while Itch protein levels were increased by threefold after 16 h (Heissmeyer et al 2004). This increase was blocked by CsA. *Nedd4* mRNA and protein levels were not affected, but both Itch and Nedd4 moved to the 'detergent-insoluble' membrane fraction in a manner dependent on sustained calcium signalling as well as TCR stimulation or cell–cell contact. We also examined CblB and GRAIL, two other E3 ligases that have been implicated in T cell anergy and tolerance. CblB-deficiency is associated with spontaneous T cell activation, autoantibody production and enhanced susceptibility to experimental autoimmune encephalitis (Chiang et al 2000, Bachmaier et al 2000); moreover, CblB was shown to be a major susceptibility gene for autoimmune diabetes in rats (Yokoi et al 2002). The levels of *CblB* and *Grail* mRNAs, as well as CblB protein, increased by eight- to 11-fold in ionomycin-treated T cells, and this increase was largely blocked by CsA (Heissmeyer et al 2004). Genetic evidence for the involvement of Itch and CblB in the T cell anergy programme was obtained by showing that T cells from *Itch*- and *CblB*-deficient mice were resistant to anergy induction and showed little or no PLCγ1 degradation after being exposed to sustained calcium signalling followed by cell–cell contact (Heissmeyer et al 2004). These data suggest that at least one of the molecular mechanisms underlying autoimmunity in Itchy (Itch-deficient) and CblB-deficient mice is the inability to properly implement anergy. However these are not the only molecules involved: as described below, we favour the hypothesis that T cell anergy is a multigene programme in which a large number of negative regulatory signalling molecules cooperate to down-regulate T cell responses (Heissmeyer & Rao 2004).

Surprisingly, degradation of PLCγ1 and PKCθ in anergic T cells was not blocked by proteasome inhibitors. Moreover, the predominant form of PKCθ we observed in anergic T cells was a mono-ubiquitinated form (Heissmeyer et al 2004). This led us to suspect that degradation of signalling proteins in anergic T cells was not accomplished via the proteasome, which binds with high affinity only to proteins tagged with four or more ubiquitin moieties (Hershko & Ciechanover 1998). Rather, our results implicated the lysosomal pathway, in which mono- and di-ubiquitin-tagged proteins associated with the limiting membrane of endosomes are recognized by Tsg101, a ubiquitin receptor associated with the endosome-associated sorting complex ESCRT1 (Katzmann et al 2002). Ubiquinated proteins that bind Tsg101 are sorted into invaginating structures that form the internal vesicles of late endosomes/multivesicular bodies (Hicke 2001). The multivesicular bodies ultimately fuse with lysosomes and deliver their contents for lysosomal degradation (Seto et al 2002). Consistent with involvement of Tsg101 in the anergy programme, protein levels of Tsg101 were increased ∼threefold in T cells rendered anergic by ionomycin treatment, and this increase was blocked by CsA (Heissmeyer et al 2004).

Consequences of PLCγ1 and PKCθ degradation: instability of the immunological synapse in anergic T cells

Anergic cells showed one predictable consequence of PLCγ1 degradation: compared to untreated T cells, they mobilized calcium very poorly in response to TCR stimulation (Wells et al 2003, Heissmeyer et al 2004). This phenomenon was also observed in T cells from orally tolerized mice (Heissmeyer et al 2004). We also examined the formation and maintenance of the immunological synapse in anergic T cells. This structure, which forms at the interface between the T cell and the antigen-presenting cell (APC), is characterized by central TCR/MHC:peptide and peripheral LFA1/ICAM1 contacts and there is considerable evidence that it constitutes an important site for regulation of signalling (Monks et al 1998, Grakoui et al 1999). We showed that PLCγ1 function was essential for maintenance of the outer LFA1/ICAM1 contact ring of the immunological synapse (Heissmeyer et al 2004). When T cells were allowed to come into contact with a lipid bilayer containing labelled MHC-peptide and ICAM1 molecules, they formed a mature synapse within about 5 min. When such fully formed synapses were treated with PLC inhibitors, the outer LFA1/ICAM1 contact ring was observed to undergo rapid disintegration (Heissmeyer et al 2004). This was exactly the behaviour observed in anergic T cells in which we had shown PLCγ1 degradation after TCR stimulation: the kinetics of synapse formation were identical between untreated and anergic T cells, but whereas untreated T cells maintained synapse structure for over an hour, anergic T cells formed the mature synapse, the outer ring of which then disintegrated within the next few minutes (Heissmeyer et al 2004). These anergic cells displayed a 'migratory' phenotype, in which the cells began moving away from the disrupted LFA1/ICAM1 ring, dragging the central TCR–MHC clusters behind them. In this respect, the anergic T cells behave like cells that do not receive a TCR-mediated 'stop' signal (Negulescu et al 1996, Dustin et al 1997, Dustin 2002). Thus the anergy-inducing signal has a potent, dual inhibitory effect on T cell responses: T–APC contact is necessary for initial degradation of signalling molecules, but the subsequent disruption of intracellular signalling leads to disintegration of the contact interaction, loss of stable T cell–APC contact and migration of anergized T cells away from APC (Heissmeyer & Rao 2004).

Comparison of the kinetics of synapse disintegration in control and $CblB^{-/-}$ T cells confirmed that $CblB$ had a role in the anergy programme. Wild-type and $CblB^{-/-}$ T cells both formed stable synapses upon contact with lipid bilayers. However, whereas wild-type T cells that has been subjected to calcium-induced anergy showed rapid synapse disintegration, anergized $CblB$-deficient T cells were substantially protected from this effect, showing a decreased level of synapse disintegration only at late times. Thus $CblB$ is partly responsible for synapse instability in anergic T cells, but other factors contribute to synapse disintegration at later stages (Heissmeyer et al 2004).

The programme of T cell anergy

Our data suggest the following multistep model of T cell anergy. The programme is initiated by sustained Ca^{2+}–calcineurin–NFAT signalling, under conditions where AP-1 is not activated and so the AP-1-independent, anergy-associated gene expression programme is induced. The anergy-associated genes include several negative regulators, among which are three E3 ligases — Itch, CblB and GRAIL. Tsg101, the ubiquitin-binding component of the endosomal sorting complex is also up-regulated. Together, increased expression of the E3 ligases and Tsg101 primes the T cells for degradation of two critical signalling proteins, PLCγ1 and PKCθ. Degradation actually occurs during a second step of T cell–APC contact, during which the immunological synapse forms normally and the E3 ligases Itch, Nedd4 and CblB colocalize with activated substrate proteins in the detergent-insoluble membrane fraction. As a result, the active, membrane-proximal pool of signalling proteins becomes mono-ubiquitinated and capable of stable interaction with Tsg101, resulting in sorting of the mono-ubiquitinated proteins into multivesicular bodies where they are targeted for lysosomal degradation. In a third step, degradation of active PLCγ1 and PKCθ leads to diminished TCR/LFA1 signalling and disintegration of the outer LFA1-containing ring of the immunological synapse. The loss of stable APC contact further reduces the antigen responses of the anergic T cells. Thus the difference in gene expression profile between normal and anergic T cells is transformed through ubiquitin modification into a transient increase in turnover of activated signalling proteins, thereby altering the migration behaviour of T cells and establishing a persistent unresponsive state.

As we have pointed out previously, the attractive feature of this down-regulatory programme is that signalling molecules would be targets for degradation only when they are activated (Heissmeyer et al 2004). In a normally-activated T cell, PLCγ1-dependent production of second messengers continues for several hours (Huppa et al 2003). In an anergic T cell in which the Itch, CblB, Nedd4 and GRAIL E3 ligases are up-regulated or preactivated for membrane localization, PLCγ1 and PKCθ would be mono-ubiquitinated at 'raft'/endosomal membranes immediately upon activation. This would lead to Tsg101 binding, sequestration of the active enzymes within endosomes, and degradation. Thus, T cell anergy would be imposed through a localized and efficient process in which PLCγ1 and PKCθ would be eliminated only in the context of active, membrane-localized signalling complexes, and the bulk of cellular PLCγ1 would not necessarily be depleted.

Perspectives

We have outlined data in support of the hypothesis that NFAT mediates not only productive activation of T cells but also T cell anergy and peripheral tolerance. We propose that TCR stimulation without co-stimulation induced T cell anergy/tolerance because it was associated with calcium signalling without appreciable activation of PKC/IKK/Ras/MAP kinase signalling, which would lead to unbalanced activation of NFAT relative to AP-1. If this hypothesis is correct, it should be possible to induce a long-lasting tolerant state even in the presence of ongoing immune stimulation, simply by disrupting the NFAT:AP-1 interaction. This should disrupt transcription of genes involved in productive immunity and divert NFAT activity towards the transcription of anergy-inducing genes. We are currently engaged in testing this hypothesis by identifying peptide and small molecule inhibitors of the NFAT:AP-1 interaction.

References

Avni O, Lee D, Macian F et al 2002 T(H) cell differentiation is accompanied by dynamic changes in histone acetylation of cytokine genes. Nat Immunol 3:643–651

Bachmaier K, Krawczyk C, Kozieradzki I et al 2000 Negative regulation of lymphocyte activation and autoimmunity by the molecular adaptor Cbl-b. Nature 403:211–216

Boussiotis VA, Freeman GJ, Berezovskaya A, Barber DL, Nadler LM 1997 Maintenance of human T cell anergy: blocking of IL-2 gene transcription by activated Rap1. Science 278:124–128

Chen L, Glover JN, Hogan PG, Rao A, Harrison SC 1998 Structure of the DNA-binding domains from NFAT, Fos and Jun bound specifically to DNA. Nature 392:42–48

Chiang YJ, Kole HK, Brown K et al 2000 Cbl-b regulates the CD28 dependence of T-cell activation. Nature 403:216–220

Crabtree GR 1999 Generic signals and specific outcomes: signaling through Ca^{2+}, calcineurin, and NF-AT. Cell 96:611–614

Crabtree GR, Olson EN 2002 NFAT signaling: choreographing the social lives of cells. Cell 109:S67–79

Dustin ML 2002 Regulation of T cell migration through formation of immunological synapses: the stop signal hypothesis. Adv Exp Med Biol 512:191–201

Dustin ML, Bromley SK, Kan Z, Peterson DA, Unanue ER 1997 Antigen receptor engagement delivers a stop signal to migrating T lymphocytes. Proc Natl Acad Sci USA 94:3909–3913.

Fang D, Elly C, Gao B et al 2002 Dysregulation of T lymphocyte function in itchy mice: a role for Itch in TH2 differentiation. Nat Immunol 3:281–287

Feske S, Giltnane J, Dolmetsch R, Staudt LM, Rao A 2001 Gene regulation mediated by calcium signals in T lymphocytes. Nat Immunol 2:316–324

Fields PE, Gajewski TF, Fitch FW 1996 Blocked Ras activation in anergic CD4+ T cells. Science 271:1276–1278

Giffin MJ, Stroud JC, Bates DL et al 2003 Structure of NFAT1 bound as a dimer to the HIV-1 LTR kappa B element. Nat Struct Biol 10:800–806

Grakoui A, Bromley SK, Sumen C et al 1999 The immunological synapse: a molecular machine controlling T cell activation. Science 285:221–227

Heissmeyer V, Rao A 2004 E3 ligases in T cell anergy — turning immune responses into tolerance. Sci STKE 2004:PE29

Heissmeyer V, Macian F, Im SH et al 2004 Calcineurin imposes T cell unresponsiveness through targeted proteolysis of signaling proteins. Nat Immunol 5:255–265

Hershko A, Ciechanover A 1998 The ubiquitin system. Annu Rev Biochem 67:425–479

Hicke L 2001 A new ticket for entry into budding vesicles-ubiquitin. Cell 106:527–530

Hogan PG, Chen L, Nardone J, Rao A 2003 Transcriptional regulation by calcium, calcineurin, and NFAT. Genes Dev 17:2205–2232

Huppa JB, Gleimer M, Sumen C, Davis MM 2003 Continuous T cell receptor signaling required for synapse maintenance and full effector potential. Nat Immunol 4:749–755

Jin L, Sliz P, Chen L et al 2003 An asymmetric NFAT1 dimer on a pseudo-palindromic kappa B-like DNA site. Nat Struct Biol 10:807–811

Kamradt T, Mitchison NA 2001 Tolerance and autoimmunity. N Engl J Med 344:655–664

Katzmann DJ, Odorizzi G, Emr SD 2002 Receptor downregulation and multivesicular-body sorting. Nat Rev Mol Cell Biol 3:893–905

Kruisbeek AM, Amsen D 1996 Mechanisms underlying T-cell tolerance. Curr Opin Immunol 8:233–244

Lesage S, Goodnow CC 2001 Organ-specific autoimmune disease: a deficiency of tolerogenic stimulation. J Exp Med 194:F31–36

Li W, Whaley CD, Mondino A, Mueller DL 1996 Blocked signal transduction to the ERK and JNK protein kinases in anergic CD4+ T cells. Science 271:1272–1276

Macian F, Garcia-Rodriguez C, Rao A 2000 Gene expression elicited by NFAT in the presence or absence of cooperative recruitment of Fos and Jun. EMBO J 19:4783–4795

Macian F, Lopez-Rodriguez C, Rao A 2001 Partners in transcription: NFAT and AP-1. Oncogene 20:2476–2489

Macian F, Garcia-Cozar F, Im SH et al 2002 Transcriptional mechanisms underlying lymphocyte tolerance. Cell 109:719–731

Macian F, Im SH, Garcia-Cozar FJ, Rao A 2004 T-cell anergy. Curr Opin Immunol 16:209–216

Monks CR, Freiberg BA, Kupfer H, Sciaky N, Kupfer A 1998 Three-dimensional segregation of supramolecular activation clusters in T cells. Nature 395:82–86

Monticelli S, Solymar DC, Rao A 2004 Role of NFAT proteins in IL13 gene transcription in mast cells. J Biol Chem 279:36210–36218

Nalefski EA, Falke JJ 1996 The C2 domain calcium-binding motif: structural and functional diversity. Protein Sci 5:2375–2390

Negulescu PA, Krasieva TB, Khan A, Kerschbaum HH, Cahalan MD 1996 Polarity of T cell shape, motility, and sensitivity to antigen. Immunity 4:421–430

Okamura H, Aramburu J, Garcia-Rodriguez C et al 2000 Concerted dephosphorylation of the transcription factor NFAT1 induces a conformational switch that regulates transcriptional activity. Mol Cell 6:539–550

Perry WL, Hustad CM, Swing DA et al 1998 The itchy locus encodes a novel ubiquitin protein ligase that is disrupted in a18H mice. Nat Genet 18:143–146

Rao A, Luo C, Hogan PG 1997 Transcription factors of the NFAT family: regulation and function. Annu Rev Immunol 15:707–747

Schwartz RH 2003 T cell anergy. Annu Rev Immunol 21:305–334

Seto ES, Bellen HJ, Lloyd TE 2002 When cell biology meets development: endocytic regulation of signaling pathways. Genes Dev 16:1314–1336

Stroud JC, Chen L 2003 Structure of NFAT bound to DNA as a monomer. J Mol Biol 334:1009–1022

Wells AD, Liu QH, Hondowicz B et al 2003 Regulation of T cell activation and tolerance by phospholipase C gamma-1-dependent integrin avidity modulation. J Immunol 170:4127–4133

Yokoi N, Komeda K, Wang HY et al 2002 Cblb is a major susceptibility gene for rat type 1 diabetes mellitus. Nat Genet 31:391–394

DISCUSSION

Hafler: Has anyone examined whether Cbl is effective in signalling to regulatory T cells?

Rao: There are lots of common features, including factors such as CTLA4 in T_{reg} function, and the fact that regulatory T cells impose anergy on their target cells. All I can say is that I am still trying to think of the correct experiments.

Ting: In activated T cells is there a phase where you have NFAT and no Jun/Fos?

Rao: Yes, at the end of the response. I suspect that this whole programme would follow the T cell response.

Rioux: Would your model predict that your programme of negative signalling, if it doesn't work, would be one common pathway to multiple different autoimmune diseases? It would not be specific to any end organ. Would you be able to think of an experiment where you would put in other genes that would direct the specificity of the end-stage disease?

Rao: That's what I would guess. It would be nice to have a common pathway which was then superimposed with different effectors. The organ specificity is likely to be determined by other factors such as the DCs in the organs.

Rioux: On the basis of some of the current knockouts could you predict that by doing double knockouts that you would be able to direct this specificity?

Rao: I am not sure that I know enough about autoimmune disease to be able to answer this.

Goodnow: If you take *CblB*, which is one of your genes, the knockout has a subtle lupus-like phenotype. Yet in the KDP (Komida Diabetes Prone) rat strain the combination of a spontaneous null allele of *CblB* and a particular MHC gives type 1 diabetes. This might be an example.

Abbas: I want to take this one step further. If you accept that we are gradually getting a better handle on the gene programmes associated with activation versus tolerance (and I really believe this), should we, in addition to doing open-ended association mapping studies, be picking candidate genes from these sorts of lists that are appearing?

Wicker: Yes, that is already being done. The ongoing efforts of all these different groups are focusing on these negative signalling molecules where there is polymorphism, because these are prime candidate genes. There is special attention focused on those which have shown effects in animals.

Rioux: We are all doing candidate gene studies because we can't do the genomewide association studies yet. Are we doing the exact same genes? No. But presumably there is a fairly substantial overlap.

Wicker: As soon as someone has published something, in a week everyone has tested that associated SNP.

Wakeland: Was PPN22 originally a candidate gene based on function?

Behrens: Celera Diagnostics picked this up when they were doing their resequencing, and targeted it for testing in rheumatoid arthritis (RA).

Goldstein: There is a difference between just having good candidate genes in your study and trying to have a fairly comprehensive set of genes for a pathway, and trying to test for interactions in that pathway. There is lots of this going on. People are putting good candidates into their studies, but in the areas I am following it is much rarer for someone to try to comprehensively represent a pathway and have some kind of sensible strategy for testing for interactions among polymorphisms in genes in that pathway. We all accept that there will be interactions. If there is a common variant that has a bigger effect independent of genetic background, then it is not going to be a complex trait any more. But our design, even with the sample sizes that we are planning to take on in the future, will not be sufficient to pick up interactions in a genomewide context. We need to be guided in the search and interaction space by the biology. This is a bit more than saying put good candidates into your list.

Abbas: You have said this well. My impression is that the candidate genes are driven frequently by which knockout gives an autoimmune phenotype. What David is saying is that we should look at genes in a pathway and target those as your candidates, and not worry about the knockouts. There is relatively less of this simply because the data aren't in yet about what these pathways are.

Hafler: As we are about to embark on whole genome scans, will this have the power without biological knowledge, or do we have to preconceive what the epistatic and interactive effects are?

Goldstein: Certainly, we will have trouble with power in open-ended searches for interactions.

Kere: If we have one candidate gene at a 30% frequency in the population, a second candidate gene at 20%, and a third at 10%, individuals with all three would represent 0.6% of the general population. If the combination has a sixfold relative risk then we'd expect to see something like 3.6% of our patients to be triple carriers.

Goldstein: It is not only the absolute numbers, but also the statistical space: how many different interactions are you checking for? You don't want only to find what you expect, but we do need to be guided by biology in order to simplify this space as much as possible.

Wicker: Based on the biology of the two genes, we have looked for interaction between *CTLA4* and *PTPN22*. We are thinking of pathways. This is why we looked for associations with IL2R α, β and γ in addition to looking for the *Il2* orthologue in humans. These have been looked for before, but it is necessary to look in a much broader sense: you just can't pick a few SNPs, you have to resequence each gene. It looks like we have some interaction, which you would expect, between these two negative signallers, *CTLA4* and *PTPN22*. But even with 3500 as the number of cases and controls examined, the interaction is not statistically significant; even with a preconceived, biology-based hypothesis it is still not enough, because the allele frequency of the mutant PTPN22 phosphatase is so low.

Rao: I have sat through a day and a half of this and I'm not convinced of its utility. You don't have to do a real experiment; a thought experiment will do. You are going to get alleles in the population that predispose to diseases. It is obvious that if I change the affinity of interaction of Itch with PLCγ by twofold, there is going to be more up-regulation. There are a large number of genes that could come together in the population and give an increase in susceptibility to disease, but what does that tell you ultimately?

Hafler: Let's take MS or diabetes as an example. We don't know which genes are coming together.

Kere: Any family will be different.

Hafler: Take a pathway that is not elevated and therapeutically lower it in patients, and this may increase their risk of an infection. But if we take a pathway that is elevated and causes susceptibility to disease, if we lower this back to baseline we will have the potential to treat patients without exposing them to the risk of immunosuppression.

Abbas: What Anjana Rao proposed at the end of the paper is that you have 20 genes that lead to unregulated NFAT. We are asking whether those 20 genes have a role in autoimmune disease. Her point is just block NFAT and you have achieved the effect anyway. The therapeutic approach is that what is upstream is no longer relevant if you know what the end target is.

Cookson: The whole point of doing genetics is that you don't have to assume that you know the pathway. You just do genetic experiments and you get concrete results.

Seed: This has already been done. We have therapeutic interventions that directly address NFAT activation. They don't work in many autoimmune diseases. Cyclosporine doesn't work in psoriasis and MS or RA.

Rao: By our model, cyclosporine would interfere with the development of anergy.

Goodnow: Cyclosporine is counterproductive. You want a more selective molecule that inhibits only immunogenic pathways and not tolerogenic pathways.

Cookson: What about IL4? There are functional polymorphisms in the promoter of IL4 that show no association with asthma. Anti-IL4 therapy is ineffectual. We could have guessed that and saved a lot of money.

Goldstein: If you are saying there is a tight association between whether there is variation in a gene that is associated with a disease, and whether drugs that target that gene product work, that is not true as a general rule. SCN1A, the α subunit of the Na^+ channel, is a frontline target for antiepileptic drugs. Apparently, however, it has no common variation that associates with common forms of epilepsy (although mutations in it cause rare forms). It is not true that common variation in the gene is a good guide.

Cookson: I am saying that if functional variation is present and it has no effect on the phenotype you are interested in, that is information. That is not the same as what you are saying, which is that if there is no polymorphism it is not a good target.

Goldstein: I would agree that it is more information if there is a common functional variation that is not disease related. But I am not sure it is much better information that the gene is not a good target. We have found that SCN1A has a common functional variant in it that is associated with dosing of anti-epileptic drugs, but it is not associated with epilepsy itself, yet the gene is a good target.

Seed: When you look at network theory and look for stable networks (I think anergy is probably a stable state), often what is seen is a feedback loop that ends up propagating itself. Among those NFAT-regulating genes, do you find anything that feeds back on NFAT? How about NFAT as a downstream effector of itself?

Rao: Some of them shut off the MAPK pathway, whereas others might lead to small increases in basal Ca^{2+} levels, which would maintain NFAT in the nucleus.

Kuchroo: You used the Ca^{2+} pathway, using ionomycin to activate cells and induce anergy. Anergy can be induced by many different mechanisms apart from the Ca^{2+} pathway. If a different method is used to induce anergy, do you still see the same pathway being utilized?

Rao: I haven't tried to look because the literature is a mess. No one agrees on the definition of anergy. The biochemistry points us in a certain direction. What amuses me is that many of the genes that seem to plug into the programme result in autoimmune disease when they are knocked out. This is the *in vivo* validation of the biochemical programme.

Lindgren: It seems to me that the immunologists try to describe how the cascades and signalling pathways are connected to each other. Then they change it experimentally, say, twofold and see what effect that produces. This doesn't mean that this reflects what really happens in the natural, outbred human population. The geneticists are more aiming at trying to find causality of genetic variation in a system, however this is often hard to prove without the immunologist's tools. These two approaches don't have to be in opposition.

Abbas: I agree with you. All the fuss about whether we approach the problem from the genetics angle or basic immunologic angle is unnecessary. CTLA4 and its association with multiple autoimmune diseases is a good example of people going back and forth in both directions. The best examples of where the genetics and basic biology have come together are, not surprisingly, in the relatively rare single gene disorders.

Lindgren: Everyone is trying to reach the same endpoint by different routes. It doesn't mean we have to ask the same questions.

Abbas: There was a specific point to some of this: expression profiling and mining for candidate genes is one approach that is fundamentally different to open-ended linkage analysis and associations. The question is, how do we balance our attempts to do the two? It is not either/or.

Bowcock: I have to defend genetics. Genetics is a reductionist approach: it takes us from a large scale to a smaller one, so we can actually find a variant in a novel gene or region and get novel insights into disease susceptibility.

Abbas: I am not criticizing genetics. I am just saying that there are two alternative approaches. How do we balance them?

Hafler: David Goldstein made the critical point here. Because of gene interactions it is going to be very difficult. With the number of patients we are collecting we may be able to get single hits, but in order to address the issue of interactions we are going to require much larger sample sizes.

Goldstein: I don't think there was any suggestion of dismissing genetics. But the role of genetics shouldn't be overstated, in a sense that there are other routes to therapy. This is clear.

Goodnow: Turn it round the other way, which drugs do we have that have actually come from genetics? The only example I can think of is statins.

Genetic lesions in thymic T cell clonal deletion and thresholds for autoimmunity

Adrian Liston and Christopher C. Goodnow[1]

John Curtin School of Medical Research and The Australian Phenomics Facility, The Australian National University, Canberra, ACT 2601, Australia

Abstract. The cause of common polygenic autoimmune diseases is poorly understood because of genetic and cellular complexity in humans and animals. We have investigated the mechanisms of two genetic causes of organ-specific autoimmunity by tracking the fate of high avidity organ-specific CD4 T cells using a transgenic mouse model. Firstly, we have found that an *Idd*-associated cluster of loci from the NOD strain causes a T cell intrinsic failure to delete during *in vivo* encounter with high-avidity autoantigen, a trait distinguished by the failure to induce the pro-apoptotic gene *Bim*. Secondly, we have found that inactivation of the autoimmune regulator (*Aire*) gene reduces the level of thymic expression of organ-specific genes, in a gene-dose dependent manner. In this paper we describe a model relating efficiency of thymic deletion and susceptibility to autoimmunity. Using this model, subtle quantitative trait loci can have an additive effect on each of the parameters of thymic deletion, and the result of interaction between subtle modifications in the multiple parameters can result in large changes in the susceptibility to autoimmunity.

2005 The genetics of autoimmunity. Wiley, Chichester (Novartis Foundation Symposium 267) p 180–199

Autoimmune diseases, despite being directed against different target antigens and tissues, often cluster together in individuals and families. For example, the relatives of patients with type 1 diabetes (Jaeger et al 2001), rheumatoid arthritis (Prahalad et al 2002, Taneja et al 1993) and multiple sclerosis (Jaeger et al 2001) show a higher susceptibility for autoimmunity, and patients suffering one autoimmune disease, such as type 1 diabetes, have a greater chance of suffering additional autoimmune diseases, such as thyroiditis. This indicates the potential for a broad-spectrum genetic defect in immunological tolerance mechanisms, but the nature of the

---

[1]This paper was presented at the symposium by Christopher C. Goodnow to whom correspondence should be addressed.

cellular or genetic defects has been difficult to elucidate. In the case of susceptibility to organ-specific autoimmunity, defects in peripheral tolerance mechanisms have generally been viewed as likely candidates. In this paper, we discuss two independent lines of research showing that inherited defects in thymic clonal deletion explain autoimmune susceptibility to diabetes and other organ-specific diseases.

Burnet's original concept of clonal deletion as a mechanism to explain actively acquired self-tolerance, applied *à la* Lederberg to T cells bearing antigen receptors (TCRs) with high affinity for self-antigens during their differentiation within the thymus, was the first mechanism to be experimentally established (Kappler et al 1987). Thymocytes rearrange their TCR genes as they differentiate from $CD4^-CD8^-$ double negative (DN) progenitors into immature $CD4^+CD8^+$ double positive (DP) T cells. Each immature DP T cell thus acquires a unique TCR on its surface. T cells whose TCRs bind self antigen and MHC too strongly at this point are triggered to die by TCR signalling of clonal deletion, while cells with TCRs that bind self MHC too weakly fail to receive any TCR signal and die by a separate process of 'neglect'. Only those T cells with TCRs that react weakly with self-MHC transmit a particular type of TCR signal that promotes 'positive selection' into mature $CD4^+8^-$ or $CD4^-8^+$ single positive (SP) T cells that then emigrate to the extrathymic lymphoid tissues of the body.

In the case of tolerance to organ specific antigens, two chief reasons contributed to the view that thymic deletion would be of little significance compared to peripheral tolerance mechanisms. Foremost was the evidence that major protein components of specific organs, such as insulin in the pancreatic islets, or thyroglobulin in the thyroid gland, are present at insignificant quantities in the thymus. Even in the face of growing evidence for promiscuous, trace expression of these and many other organ-specific components in rare cells in the thymic medullary epithelial meshwork (Hanahan 1998, Kyewski et al 2002), it was difficult to see how this could delete more than a small fraction of autoreactive cells before export to the periphery. That view was buttressed by the second reason for disfavouring thymic deletion, namely the ready isolation of T cells and clones in the periphery of autoimmune-prone mice with sufficient autoreactivity to actively transfer disease to lymphopaenic recipients.

The beauty of classical genetic analysis, which starts with a phenotype and proceeds to explain it in cellular and molecular terms, is that it is relatively immune to the conceptual biases that are intrinsic to the elegant but artificed hypothesis-testing experiments in immunology. Here we review our experience analysing the autoimmune phenotypes in a Mendelian autoimmune disorder, autoimmune polyendocrine syndrome 1, and in the NOD mouse. Surprisingly, both genetic approaches indicate that thymic deletion is central to organ-specific tolerance.

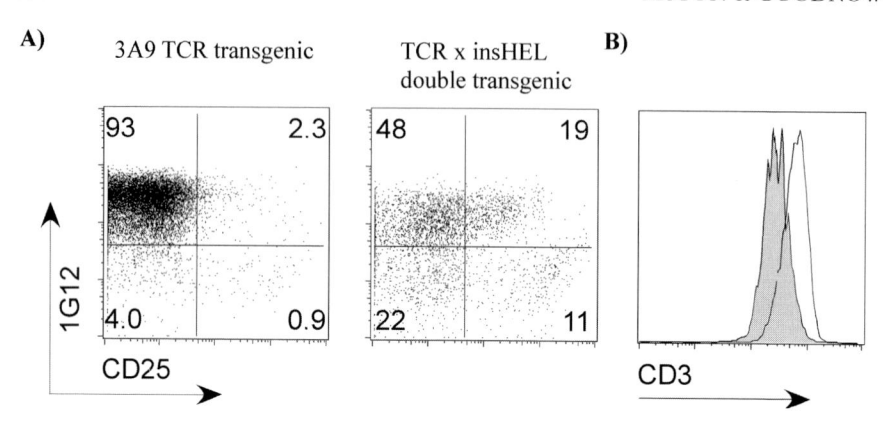

FIG. 1. Development of a regulatory/anergic phenotype in 3A9 TCR transgenic cells in the presence of insHEL. (A) In 3A9 TCR transgenic mice, CD4$^+$ single positive thymocytes are primarily clonotypic 1G12$^+$ and CD25$^-$, while in TCR×insHEL mice, the CD25$^+$ population is enriched. (B) Clonotypic 1G12$^+$ CD4$^+$ single positive thymocytes from TCR×insHEL mice (grey) have decreased levels of CD3 compared to TCR mice (white).

Tracing the cellular effects of autoimmune susceptibility genes

To trace the cellular defects caused by autoimmune susceptibility genes, our studies have used the 3A9 TCR, a high affinity TCR for peptide 46–61 of hen egg lysozyme (HEL) peptide bound to I-A^k (Allen et al 1985). In 3A9 TCR animals crossed with different HEL transgenic mice, thymic clonal deletion results in a graded reduction in the number of HEL-reactive T cells produced in the presence of neo-self HEL depending on the HEL transgene. Titration experiments show that for thymocytes of a fixed avidity, increasing amounts of antigen exposure result in an increase in the level of negative selection, resulting in a dose-response curve. Besides clonal deletion there are additional levels of central tolerance in play, with the enrichment of regulatory cells (Fig. 1A) and the active induction of TCR down-regulation (Fig. 1B) and anergy (Akkaraju et al 1997). Thus the tolerance induced is robust, allowing a certain number of HEL-reactive cells to escape negative selection before clinical autoimmunity is induced. Genetic defects that cause spontaneous autoimmunity in humans or mice would therefore be expected to have one of three cellular consequences when introduced into TCR×HEL animals: (1) there might be no effect, if the gene did not effect one of the tolerance mechanisms operating in these animals, or the effect of the gene was masked by the higher T cell precursor frequency or the nature of the HEL antigen; (2) there might be a disruption of clinical tolerance in the animals, but stemming from other defects not involving the TCR-bearing cells (e.g. target organ defects, B cell or dendritic cell [DC] defects); and (3) the susceptibility gene might selectively disrupt thymic or peripheral deletion, anergy, CD25$^+$ cell enrichment, or TCR down-regulation.

Monogenic lesions in central tolerance

The human monogenic autoimmune disease, autoimmune polyendocrinopathy syndrome type 1 (APS1) represents one of the most striking examples of a generalized failure of tolerance to organ-specific antigens. Clinical manifestations of APS1 include a variety of organ-specific autoimmune diseases, the most common of which are hypoparathyroidism and primary adrenocortical failure, accompanied by chronic mucocutaneous candidiasis (Betterle et al 1998), with many other organs often compromised by autoimmunity including the thyroid and pancreatic islet β cells. APS1 is caused by homozygous mutations in a novel gene *AIRE* (Nagamine et al 1997, The Finnish-German APACED Consortium 1997) whose function in tolerance was obscure. *Aire*-deficient mice also develop multi-organ autoimmune symptoms, (Anderson et al 2002, Ramsey et al 2002) and we therefore asked which if any of the tolerance mechanisms observed in TCR×HEL animals would be disrupted by introducing a truncating *Aire* mutation that mirrors one of the most common human mutations (Ramsey et al 2002).

Aire appears to be a transcription factor, as it localizes in nuclear speckles (Heino et al 1999, 2000), interacts with CBP (transcriptional coactivator CREB-binding protein) (Pitkanen et al 2000), and is able to activate transcription in luciferase assays (Bjorses et al 2000, Pitkanen et al 2000). Expression studies show that it is expressed most highly in rare thymic stromal cells (Ramsey et al 2002, Heino et al 1999, Bjorses et al 1999), although it is also expressed by scattered cells in peripheral lymphoid tissue. Experiments by Anderson et al (2002) found that medullary epithelial cells isolated from *Aire* knockout mice had lost promiscuous expression of insulin mRNA, and simultaneous research from our laboratory showed that the thymus in *Aire* knockout mice had lost the ability to delete 3A9 CD4$^+$ T cells recognizing HEL antigen expressed under control of the insulin promoter (insHEL) (Fig. 2) (Liston et al 2003). The loss of *Aire* abolishes thymic expression of HEL under the insulin promoter, resulting in the maturation and escape from the thymus of large numbers of CD4$^+$1G12$^+$ CD25$^-$ HEL-reactive cells. These cells make up ∼2% of the peripheral lymphoid repertoire in *Aire*-deficient animals, compared with 0.2% in controls, and result in a high incidence and very early onset of autoimmune diabetes (Liston et al 2004a).

Remarkably, a ∼2.5-fold decrease in thymic expression resulting from loss of a single copy of *Aire* allows three times more autoreactive T cells to mature and escape from the thymus (Fig. 2), and the 0.8% contribution this makes to the splenic lymphoid repertoire is sufficient to result in a high frequency of diabetes

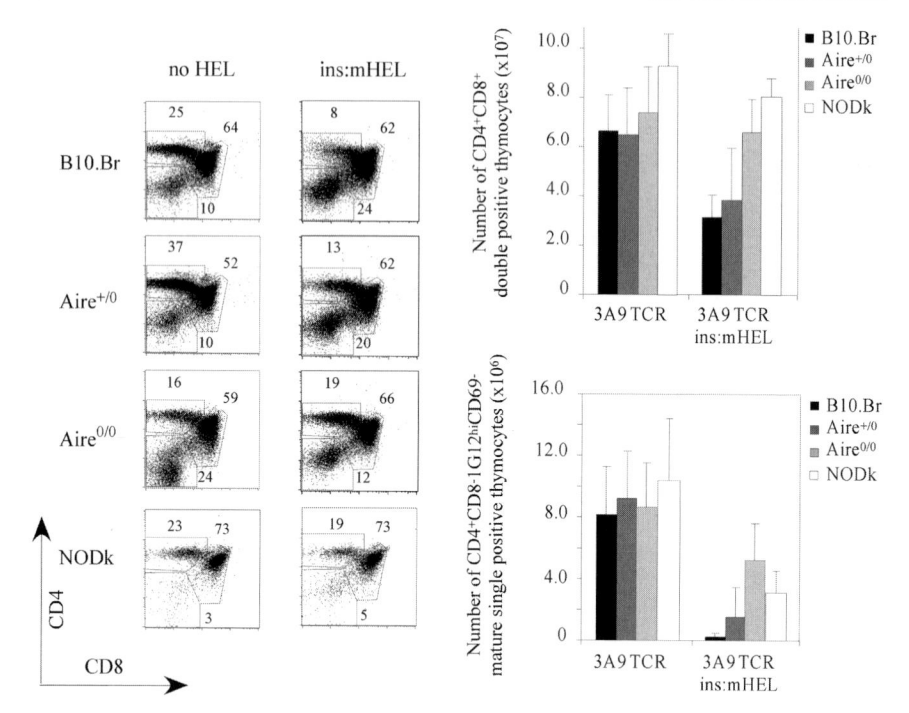

FIG. 2. Defective thymic deletion: a common consequence of *Aire* defects or non-MHC genes from the NOD autoimmune mouse strain. Shown are flow cytometric profiles of thymocytes, and numerical data obtained from these analyses, from 3A9 TCR transgenic mice with or without a HEL transgene controlled by the insulin gene promoter. All mice are H-2k congenic, and differ either in their non-MHC strain background (B10.BR vs. NODk) or in their *Aire* genotypes (B10.BR and NOD are both *Aire*[+/+]).

(Fig. 3). The *Aire* pathway for thymic deletion thus appears to be acutely sensitive to small reductions in function for at least a subset of *Aire*-dependent antigens, rather than being saturated or buffered against small changes. Further analysis of the effect of *Aire* on central tolerance to neo-self HEL under other promoters have identified a subset of promoters that are profoundly *Aire* dependent for triggering thymic deletion (insulin, thyroglobulin), while others are partially dependent (metallothionein) or fully independent (H-2K^b). For those promoters that are *Aire*-dependent, there was a clear gene-dose affect, with loss of a single copy of *Aire* reducing the thymic expression of, and thymic deletion towards, the organ-specific antigen (Liston et al 2004a).

Although APS1 is classified as a strictly recessive disorder with complete penetrance based on the inheritance pattern of the unusual combination of symptoms (Ahonen 1985), there are anecdotal data of mutations in a single copy of *AIRE* being associated with human autoimmunity (Buzi et al 2003, Cetani et al

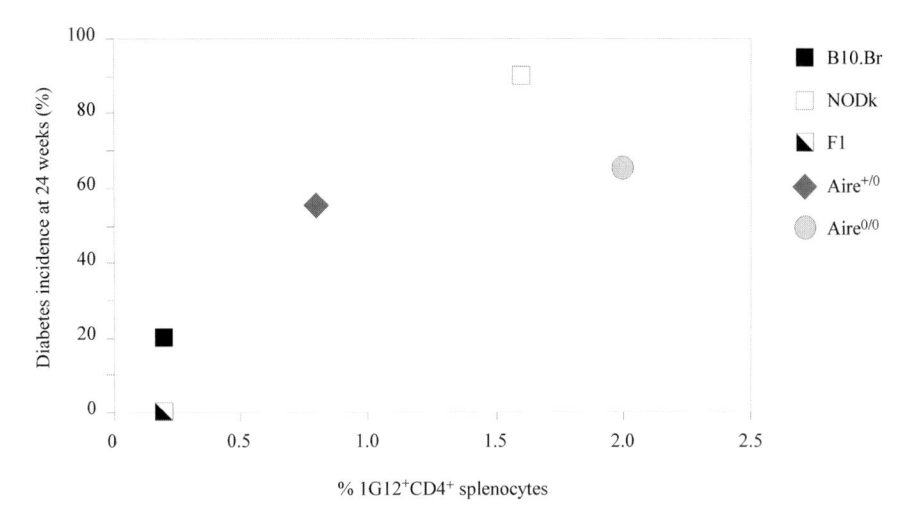

FIG. 3. Scatterplot of the incidence of diabetes at 24 weeks of age, and the percentage of splenic lympocytes that are CD4$^+$1G12$^+$, on TCR×insHEL double transgenic mice of various backgrounds.

2001, Soderbergh et al 2000). The possibility that heterozygous carriers have an increased prevalence of discrete autoimmune diseases has not yet been systematically addressed. The striking dose dependency revealed in *Aire* heterozygous mice as described above suggest such an effect may also occur in human carriers, but likely only revealed in conjunction with other genetic factors weakening the pathway (see general discussion).

Polygenic lesions in central tolerance

Like APS1, the NOD mouse strain also exhibits generalized susceptibility to autoimmune diseases, most notably insulin-dependent diabetes mellitus, but inherited in a highly polygenic fashion. NOD mice exhibit spontaneous type 1 diabetes, sialitis and dacryoadenitis, and are highly susceptible to autoimmune encephalitis, prostatitis, autoimmune haemolytic anaemia or systemic lupus upon exposure to particular exogenous challenges (Wicker et al 1995, Baker et al 1995, Oldenborg et al 2002, Boulard et al 2002, Zaccone et al 2002, Braley-Mullen et al 1999, Rivero et al 1998, Takahashi et al 1997, Ridgway et al 1996, Baxter et al 1994). Over 20 loci have been linked to diabetes development in the NOD mouse (*Idd* loci), some of which appear to specifically cause susceptibility to diabetes (e.g. *Idd1*), while others are associated with enhanced susceptibility to a range of autoimmune diseases (e.g. *Idd3*, *Idd5*). The specific mechanism of susceptibility contribution of most of these loci remains to be elucidated. However it is likely that a subset of *Idd* loci result in an inherited propensity towards autoimmunity generally, with the specific target antigens and tissues varying depending upon additional loci and specific environmental factors (Wicker et al 1989, Bias et al 1986, Lesage & Goodnow 2001).

Given the focus on peripheral defects in NOD mice, it was a surprise to find that the chief effect of non-MHC NOD genes was a profound defect in thymic clonal deletion that parallels the homozygous *Aire* defect described above (Fig. 2). *In vitro* studies by Kishimoto & Sprent showed that semi-mature thymocytes, intermediate between the immature CD4$^+$8$^+$ DP cells and CD4$^+$8$^-$ SP cells, are relatively resistant to cell death when their TCRs are cross-linked in tissue culture with different doses of anti-TCR antibody. This defect was unique to strains with non-MHC NOD genes, and appeared unique to the semi-mature stage of differentiation as there was no difference in TCR-induced death of immature DP cells *in vitro* (Kishimoto & Sprent 2001). In parallel *in vivo* studies using the 3A9 TCR system, we found an almost complete failure of thymic deletion in TCR×insHEL mice backcrossed to the NOD.H-2^k background (Fig. 2) and results in diabetes onset (Fig. 3; Lesage et al 2002). By backcrossing other HEL transgenes to the NODk background, we find that the *in vivo* deletion defect is not limited to semi-mature T cells but applies equally for deletion occurring at all stages of DP-SP thymocyte maturation, for CD25$^+$ and CD25$^-$ subsets, and is observed with varying dose and anatomical source of self antigens (Liston et al 2004b). Unlike the *Aire* defect, the NOD defect is not due to any change in expression in the thymus, but acts cell autonomously within the autoreactive thymocytes themselves. The comparative analysis of deletion in mice with different HEL transgenes shows that the deletion response of NOD thymocytes is not absolutely crippled, but rather the thymic antigen dose-response is shifted by approximately tenfold compared to T cells with B10 alleles. Thus the NOD thymocytes have an intrinsic resistance to negative selection, resulting in a shift of the antigen dose-response curve to the right (Fig. 4A). For antigens expressed at concentrations close to the threshold of autoimmunity, this shift can result in a decrease in clonal deletion to the point where autoimmunity occurs, while for antigens expressed at much higher levels, the defect in clonal deletion that occurs can be of no physiological consequence (Fig. 4A).

We analysed the inheritance pattern of the thymic deletion defect by measuring the frequency of autoreactive mature T cells in 149 backcross B10.BR > NODk N2 animals that were TCR×insHEL double transgenic females. Mapping of the 'non-deleter' trait identified six loci contributing in an apparently additive manner — four NOD loci conferring susceptibility to defective thymic deletion in homozygotes, and interestingly two B6 loci conferring susceptibility to defective thymic deletion in B6/NOD heterozygotes (Liston et al 2004b). Strikingly, all four

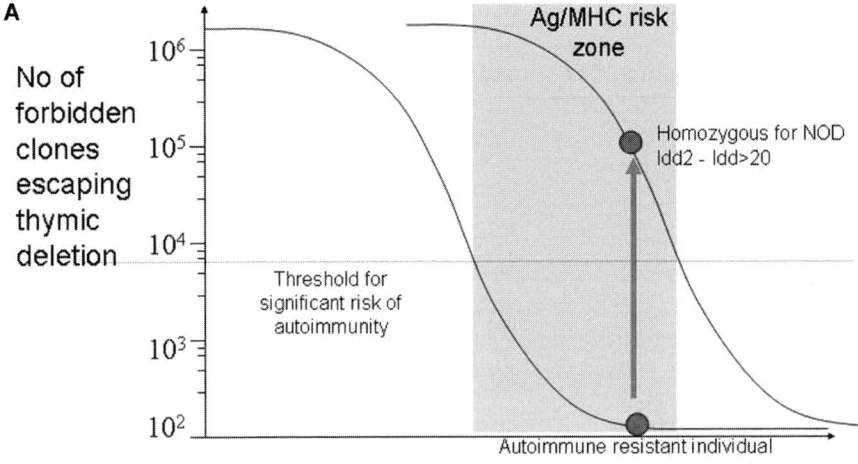

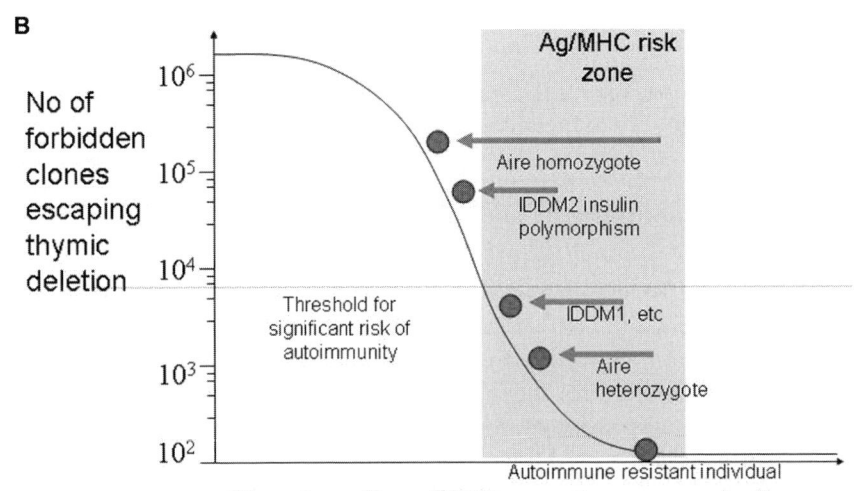

GENETIC LESIONS IN THYMIC CLONAL DELETION   187

A

No of forbidden clones escaping thymic deletion

10^6
10^5 — Homozygous for NOD Idd2 - Idd>20
10^4
Threshold for significant risk of autoimmunity
10^3
10^2
Autoimmune resistant individual

Ag/MHC risk zone

Thymic antigen/MHC complex concentration

B

No of forbidden clones escaping thymic deletion

10^6
10^5 — Aire homozygote
IDDM2 insulin polymorphism
10^4
Threshold for significant risk of autoimmunity — IDDM1, etc
10^3 — Aire heterozygote
10^2
Autoimmune resistant individual

Ag/MHC risk zone

Thymic antigen/MHC complex concentration

FIG. 4. Schematic illustrating the relationship between the display of tissue antigens in the thymus and the frequency of high-avidity T cells escaping the thymus, and how this relationship is altered by different autoimmune susceptibility genes. Variants in *Aire*, autoantigen genes, or MHC can elevate the frequency of forbidden clones by diminishing the display of tissue antigens in the thymus, whereas variants in the apoptotic machinery of thymocytes diminish the effect of a given degree of display. The effects of these variants will be greatest for antigen/MHC combinations that are most limiting normally and thus lie in a 'risk zone' where quantitative effects can elevate the frequency of forbidden clones above a threshold for autoimmune susceptibility.

of the NOD susceptibility loci colocalize with regions previously identified as diabetes susceptibility loci, and the two B6 susceptibility loci colocalize with B6 diabetes susceptibility loci noted previously (Ghosh et al 1993). This colocalization of defective thymic deletion to *Idd* loci reinforce the earlier prediction that a subset of *Idd* loci control general susceptibility to autoimmunity by allowing forbidden T cell clones to escape the thymus.

Molecular analysis of thymic deletion in TCRinsHEL transgenic B10 or NOD animals, by oligonucleotide microarray profiling of mRNA expression in highly purified *ex vivo* subsets of T cell in the early stages of positive or negative selection, or prior to selection, revealed a striking set of apoptosis inducing genes that are selectively induced during negative selection in B10 and poorly induced in NOD. In particular, the pro-apoptotic Bcl2 family inhibitor, *Bim*, was strongly induced in autoreactive $CD4^+IG12^+$ thymocytes in B10 mice at the mRNA and protein level, yet was not detectably induced in the NOD counterparts (Liston et al 2004b). Given the essential role for *Bim* as a mediator of thymic clonal deletion (Villunger et al 2004, Bouillet et al 2002) and the clear evidence that even loss of a single copy of *Bim* causes a marked defect in thymocyte apoptosis and greatly increased incidence of autoimmunity, we conclude that defective thymic deletion and generalized autoimmunity in NOD arises by multiple *Idd* genes acting additively to diminish *Bim* induction in response to TCR engagement by high avidity autoantigen.

Thresholds for autoimmunity and additive effects of genes acting at multiple points in thymic deletion

The robust nature of immunological tolerance buffers the presence of a low number of forbidden T cell clones with high autoantigen avidity in the peripheral circulation. A small number of autoreactive cells can be tolerated. However, if this number rises above a given threshold of buffering capacity, the chance of autoimmunity increases. Whether this is a bipolar distribution or a linear progression, the changes can be modelled using a set 'autoimmune threshold', above which the chance of autoimmunity will drastically increase. Experimentally, this allowable threshold of autoreactive cells in the TCR×insHEL mouse is in the range of 0.2–0.8% of splenic lymphocytes (or rather, lower than 0.2–0.8% of splenic lymphocytes, as this figure includes HEL-reactive regulatory and anergic cells), as genetic backgrounds that allow a higher proportion of HEL-reactive cells to escape have a high incidence of diabetes, while strains with a lower proportion of HEL-reactive cells have a low incidence of diabetes (Fig. 3). The specific threshold for autoimmunity will vary from antigen to antigen, based on intrinsic properties to the antigen and the expressing organ, and extrinsic properties of mechanisms of immune tolerance, however it is likely that for any given antigen, a certain threshold of autoreactive cells can be tolerated without autoimmunity occurring.

The analysis of *Aire* mutants highlights a pathway for thymic display of peripheral antigens that can be influenced by genes acting in concert at multiple points (Fig. 4B). Loss of a single copy of *Aire* reduces thymic expression of *Aire*-dependent autoantigen genes by half. A common natural polymorphism in the insulin gene promoter (*Iddm2*) causes a comparable two- to threefold decrease in thymic insulin gene expression (Vafiadis et al 1997) which is strongly linked to diabetes susceptibility (Vafiadis et al 1997, Pugliese et al 1997). Likewise, heterozygous loss of the Myelin P0 protein is associated with increasing T cell responses and autoimmunity to this autoantigen (Miyamoto et al 2003). It is thus reasonable to predict that *Aire* heterozygosity is likely to be a strong autoimmune susceptibility factor if its effects are compounded by the *Iddm2* susceptibility allele (Fig. 4B). If insulin peptides are less efficiently presented by diabetes-associated *Iddm1* MHC alleles (Corper et al 2000, Ogino et al 2000, Stratmann et al 2000), one can readily see how multiple small effects could additively diminish thymic display of specific tissue antigens, allowing the frequency of forbidden clones with high avidity for these antigens to rise above the threshold for autoimmune disease to develop (Fig. 4B).

The NOD mouse analysis illustrates how defects in the same pathway can also arise downstream of thymic autoantigen display, acting within forbidden thymocyte clones to decrease their apoptotic response (Fig. 4A). Resistance to thymic deletion could come about through global decreases in TCR signalling, such as point mutations in ZAP70 (Sakaguchi et al 2003), reduced induction of apoptosis from reduced *Bim* levels (Bouillet et al 2002), or the polygenic NOD trait which results in a functional 'knock-down' of *Bim* (Lesage et al 2002). With a decrease in apoptotic response to antigen, the dose response curve of thymocytes results in a shift to the right, such as has been defined for the NOD mouse.

Based on our findings with the 3A9 TCR, for a given TCR avidity there is a relatively narrow range of thymic concentrations of peripheral autoantigen — a 'risk zone' — where small changes in the efficiency of thymic display or apoptotic response translate into an increase in circulating autoreactive cells (Fig. 4). Antigens expressed at levels above this point may be less likely to become targets of autoimmunity, even with a partial defect in antigen display or apoptosis. Whereas *Aire* defects and apoptotic defects are likely to elevate the risk of autoimmunity for a range of antigens within this risk zone, other defects in the pathway such as allelic variants of MHC or of autoantigen genes such as insulin, will elevate the risk of autoimmunity only for specific target antigens and tissues.

Increasing resistance to autoimmunity

The converse to the above studies in genetic defects in negative selection is the potential augmentation of resistance to autoimmunity. It is reasonable to predict that a relatively modest increase in *AIRE* activity, induced in a therapeutic fashion, could, in addition to protecting *AIRE* null patients from APS1, markedly lower the incidence of type 1 diabetes and other organ-specific autoimmune diseases in individuals with wild-type *AIRE*. Likewise, enhanced susceptibility to negative selection (the reverse of the NOD trait) could heighten resistance to autoimmunity across a broad range of antigens, although the potential effects on repertoire restriction are unknown. For both of these reasons, it will be important for future work to define the other components responsible for thymic tolerance.

References

Ahonen P 1985 Autoimmune polyendocrinopathy — candidosis — ectodermal dystrophy (APECED): autosomal recessive inheritance. Clin Genet 27:535–542

Akkaraju S, Ho WY, Leong D et al 1997 A range of CD4 T cell tolerance: partial inactivation to organ-specific antigen allows nondestructive thyroiditis or insulitis. Immunity 7: 255–271

Allen PM, Matsueda GR, Haber E, Unanue ER 1985 Specificity of the T cell receptor: two different determinants are generated by the same peptide and the I-Ak molecule. J Immunol 135:368–373

Anderson MS, Venanzi ES, Klein L et al 2002 Projection of an immunological self-shadow within the thymus by the aire protein. Science 298:1395–1401

Baker D, Rosenwasser OA, O'Neill JK, Turk JL 1995 Genetic analysis of experimental allergic encephalomyelitis in mice. J Immunol 155:4046–4051

Baxter AG, Horsfall AC, Healey D et al 1994 Mycobacteria precipitate an SLE-like syndrome in diabetes-prone NOD mice. Immunology 83:227–231

Betterle C, Greggio NA, Volpato M 1998 Clinical review 93: autoimmune polyglandular syndrome type 1. J Clin Endocrinol Metab 83:1049–1055

Bias WB, Reveille JD, Beaty TH, Meyers DA, Arnett FC 1986 Evidence that autoimmunity in man is a Mendelian dominant trait. Am J Hum Genet 39:584–602

Bjorses P, Pelto-Huikko M, Kaukonen J et al 1999 Localization of the APECED protein in distinct nuclear structures. Hum Mol Genet 8:259–266

Bjorses P, Halonen M, Palvimo JJ et al 2000 Mutations in the AIRE gene: effects on subcellular location and transactivation function of the autoimmune polyendocrinopathy-candidiasis-ectodermal dystrophy protein. Am J Hum Genet 66:378–392

Bouillet P, Purton JF, Godfrey DI et al 2002 BH3-only Bcl-2 family member Bim is required for apoptosis of autoreactive thymocytes. Nature 415:922–926

Boulard O, Fluteau G, Eloy L et al 2002 Genetic analysis of autoimmune sialadenitis in nonobese diabetic mice: a major susceptibility region on chromosome 1. J Immunol 168: 4192–4201

Braley-Mullen H, Sharp GC, Medling B, Tang H 1999 Spontaneous autoimmune thyroiditis in NOD.H-2h4 mice. J Autoimmun 12:157–165

Buzi F, Badolato R, Mazza C et al 2003 Autoimmune polyendocrinopathy-candidiasis-ectodermal dystrophy syndrome: time to review diagnostic criteria? J Clin Endocrinol Metab 88:3146–3148

Cetani F, Barbesino G, Borsari S et al 2001 A novel mutation of the autoimmune regulator gene in an Italian kindred with autoimmune polyendocrinopathy-candidiasis-ectodermal dystrophy, acting in a dominant fashion and strongly cosegregating with hypothyroid autoimmune thyroiditis. J Clin Endocrinol Metab 86:4747–4752

Corper AL, Stratmann T, Apostolopoulos V et al 2000 A structural framework for deciphering the link between I-Ag7 and autoimmune diabetes. Science 288:505–511

Ghosh S, Palmer SM, Rodrigues NR et al 1993 Polygenic control of autoimmune diabetes in nonobese diabetic mice. Nat Genet 4:404–409

The Finnish-German APACED Consortium TF-GA 1997 An autoimmune disease, APECED, caused by mutations in a novel gene featuring two PHD-type zinc-finger domains. Nat Genet 17:399–403

Hanahan D 1998 Peripheral-antigen-expressing cells in thymic medulla: factors in self-tolerance and autoimmunity. Curr Opin Immunol 10:656–662

Heino M, Peterson P, Kudoh J et al 1999 Autoimmune regulator is expressed in the cells regulating immune tolerance in thymus medulla. Biochem Biophys Res Commun 257:821–825

Heino M, Peterson P, Sillanpaa N et al 2000 RNA and protein expression of the murine autoimmune regulator gene (Aire) in normal, RelB-deficient and in NOD mouse. Eur J Immunol 30:1884–1893

Jaeger C, Hatziagelaki E, Petzoldt R, Bretzel RG 2001 Comparative analysis of organ-specific autoantibodies and celiac disease-associated antibodies in type 1 diabetic patients, their first-degree relatives, and healthy control subjects. Diabetes Care 24:27–32

Kappler JW, Roehm N, Marrack P 1987 T cell tolerance by clonal elimination in the thymus. Cell 49:273–280

Kishimoto H, Sprent J 2001 A defect in central tolerance in NOD mice. Nat Immunol 2:1025–1031

Kyewski B, Derbinski J, Gotter J, Klein L 2002 Promiscuous gene expression and central T-cell tolerance: more than meets the eye. Trends Immunol 23:364–371

Lesage S, Goodnow CC 2001 Organ-specific autoimmune disease: a deficiency of tolerogenic stimulation. J Exp Med 194:F31–6

Lesage S, Hartley SB, Akkaraju S et al 2002 Failure to censor forbidden clone of CD4 T cells in autoimmune diabetes. J Exp Med 196:1175–1188

Liston A, Lesage S, Wilson J, Peltonen L, Goodnow CC 2003 Aire regulates negative selection of organ-specific T cells. Nat Immunol 4:350–354

Liston A, Gray DH, Lesage S et al 2004a Gene dosage—limiting role of Aire in thymic expression, clonal deletion, and organ-specific autoimmunity. J Exp Med 200:1015–1026

Liston A, Lesage S, Gray DH et al 2004b Generalized resistance to thymic deletion in the NOD mouse; a polygenic trait characterized by defective induction of Bim. Immunity 21:817–830

Miyamoto K, Miyake S, Schachner M, Yamamura T 2003 Heterozygous null mutation of myelin P0 protein enhances susceptibility to autoimmune neuritis targeting P0 peptide. Eur J Immunol 33:656–665

Nagamine K, Peterson P, Scott HS et al 1997 Positional cloning of the APECED gene. Nat Genet 17:393–398

Ogino T, Sato K, Miyokawa N, Kimura S, Katagiri M 2000 Importance of GAD65 peptides and I-Ag7 in the development of insulitis in nonobese diabetic mice. Immunogenetics 51:538–545

Oldenborg PA, Gresham HD, Chen Y, Izui S, Lindberg FP 2002 Lethal autoimmune hemolytic anemia in CD47-deficient nonobese diabetic (NOD) mice. Blood 99:3500–3504

Pitkanen J, Doucas V, Sternsdorf T et al 2000 The autoimmune regulator protein has transcriptional transactivating properties and interacts with the common coactivator CREB-binding protein. J Biol Chem 275:16802–16809

Prahalad S, Shear ES, Thompson SD, Giannini EH, Glass DN 2002 Increased prevalence of familial autoimmunity in simplex and multiplex families with juvenile rheumatoid arthritis. Arthritis Rheum 46:1851–1856

Pugliese A, Zeller M, Fernandez A, Jr et al 1997 The insulin gene is transcribed in the human thymus and transcription levels correlated with allelic variation at the INS VNTR-IDDM2 susceptibility locus for type 1 diabetes. Nat Genet 15:293–297

Ramsey C, Winqvist O, Puhakka L et al 2002 Aire deficient mice develop multiple features of APECED phenotype and show altered immune response. Hum Mol Genet 11:397–409

Ridgway WM, Fasso M, Lanctot A, Garvey C, Fathman CG 1996 Breaking self-tolerance in nonobese diabetic mice. J Exp Med 183:1657–1662

Rivero VE, Cailleau C, Depiante-Depaoli M, Riera CM, Carnaud C 1998 Non-obese diabetic (NOD) mice are genetically susceptible to experimental autoimmune prostatitis (EAP). J Autoimmun 11:603–610

Sakaguchi N, Takahashi T, Hata H et al 2003 Altered thymic T-cell selection due to a mutation of the ZAP-70 gene causes autoimmune arthritis in mice. Nature 426:454–460

Soderbergh A, Rorsman F, Halonen M et al 2000 Autoantibodies against aromatic L-amino acid decarboxylase identifies a subgroup of patients with Addison's disease. J Clin Endocrinol Metab 85:460–463

Stratmann T, Apostolopoulos V, Mallet-Designe V et al 2000 The I-Ag7 MHC class II molecule linked to murine diabetes is a promiscuous peptide binder. J Immunol 165:3214–3225

Takahashi M, Ishimaru N, Yanagi K et al 1997 High incidence of autoimmune dacryoadenitis in male non-obese diabetic (NOD) mice depending on sex steroid. Clin Exp Immunol 109:555–561

Taneja V, Singh RR, Malaviya AN, Anand C, Mehra NK 1993 Occurrence of autoimmune diseases and relationship of autoantibody expression with HLA phenotypes in multicase rheumatoid arthritis families. Scand J Rheumatol 22:152–157

Vafiadis P, Bennett ST, Todd JA et al 1997 Insulin expression in human thymus is modulated by INS VNTR alleles at the IDDM2 locus. Nat Genet 15:289–292

Villunger A, Marsden VS, Zhan Y et al 2004 Negative selection of semimature CD4(+)8(-) HSA+ thymocytes requires the BH3-only protein Bim but is independent of death receptor signaling. Proc Natl Acad Sci USA 101:7052–7057

Wicker LS, Miller BJ, Fischer PA, Pressey A, Peterson LB 1989 Genetic control of diabetes and insulitis in the nonobese diabetic mouse. Pedigree analysis of a diabetic H-2nod/b heterozygote. J Immunol 142:781–784

Wicker LS, Todd JA, Peterson LB 1995 Genetic control of autoimmune diabetes in the NOD mouse. Annu Rev Immunol 13:179–200

Zaccone P, Fehervari Z, Blanchard L et al 2002 Autoimmune thyroid disease induced by thyroglobulin and lipopolysaccharide is inhibited by soluble TNF receptor type I. Eur J Immunol 32:1021–1028

DISCUSSION

Hafler: An interesting way of testing some of these hypotheses in complex human disease would be to assess the frequency of autoreactive T cells and their relationship to thymic expression of the antigen. It would be tough to get subject's approval to remove thymuses, so what is the surrogate marker to do this with? Can we take peripheral blood lymphocytes or epidermal cells?

Wicker: Pugliese has published that he also observes antigen presenting cells in peripheral lymphoid organs that are that are producing self proteins normally found only in specific tissues, such as insulin (Pugliese et al 2001).

Goodnow: Polychronakos has published an interesting paper in which he took mice with a beautiful allelic series of pro-insulin deficiencies (Chentoufi & Polychronakos 2002). He sees a linear relationship with the spontaneous proliferation when he puts either insulin C peptide or proinsulin into cultures. I don't understand how he does those experiments, because in an unprimed mouse, to get an antigen-specific proliferative response in culture is almost a miracle.

Kuchroo: If the frequency is high enough then you can get the response. For example, if you put PLP peptide on the lymph node cells from a naïve SJL mouse, you get background proliferation. This correlates with the lack of expression of PLP in the thymus. If you reintroduce it, then the endogenous frequency goes down (Anderson et al 2000).

Goodnow: Is this without priming?

Kuchroo: Yes.

Hafler: Maybe the experiment to do would be to get newborn thymus from surgery and examine for expression of self-antigens in relationship to self-antigen reactivity.

Abbas: Before you ask whether these genes that we are picking up influence thymic expression of antigen, the first experiment would be to ask what the number of autoreactive T cells is in a person. This may be because of failure of thymic selection, or it may be because of peripheral activation. In human autoimmune disease, except for some of the things that you and the MS community have done, in all the other diseases we just don't know if there is an increased frequency of autoreactive T cells in the circulation. Some of this is feasible because you have done it with MS and DR2-myelin basic peptide tetramers. The same principle should be applicable to similar situations.

Goodnow: Technically it is hard. I spent a period of time in Gus Nossal's lab trying to do single cell measurements in the pretransgenic area. It is bashing your head against a wall.

Hafler: The first thing we need is a surrogate measure of thymic expression of self-antigen. For example, peripheral blood T cells express the goli form of myelin basic protein. If we had a surrogate marker in peripheral blood we could then examine these factors.

Abbas: So you are not just looking for a marker for antigen expression in the thymus, you are also looking for a marker for cells that have failed negative selection in the thymus. That is going to be very tough.

Kuchroo: One of the outcomes of thymic expression of self antigen is obviously deletion. The other is the induction of the $CD4^+CD25^+$ cells. In the data from Christoph Benoist's lab, when they made the Aire knockout mouse there was no defect in the $CD4^+CD25^+$ cells. The knockout they made was different from your knockout. Is there a defect in the induction of the $CD4^+CD25^+$ cells in the Aire knockout mouse?

Goodnow: Lena Peltonen's group made this knockout. It has essentially a stop codon almost in the same place as the most common of the APS1 mutants. There is some question as to whether it is completely null, or whether the small N-terminal fragment still does something. Anyway, it mirrors the most common APS1 human mutation. We see normal numbers of $CD25^+$ cells. In these negative-selecting mice the proportion of forbidden clones that are not deleted that are $CD25^+$ becomes very high. This is abolished in our knockout. If you look at the percentage of $CD4^+$ cells that are T_{reg}s you can get excited about what you might assume is a defect in T_{reg} production. But this is purely because the $CD25^+$ cells are very refractory to thymic deletion. They are essentially left over when you delete the other guys. Their absolute numbers actually go down slightly. We just don't have any evidence that there is a T_{reg} problem. Diane Mathis' group have recently done an experiment where they make a mouse with two thymuses: a wild type thymus that should be able to make T_{reg}s and an *Aire*-deficient thymus. Autoimmunity is dominant in this condition. This argues that the primary role is to get rid of cells rather than to make T_{reg} cells.

Kuchroo: Which of the NOD loci did you pick up in your mapping?

Goodnow: The strongest loci are a chromosome 15 locus that showed up in the original insulitis/diabetes screen and an EAE locus, and a locus on chromosome 7 that has been shown to be an important NOD diabetes susceptibility locus by a congenic approach but is missed in genome scans presumably because a NOD resistance locus is present more proximally on chromosome 7. The weaker loci are ones that sit on *Idd5* and also where *Idd13* has been mapped which includes the *Bim* gene itself. Then there are two loci with quite strong chi squares where the B10 is contributing a resistance to thymic deletion, paradoxically. Interestingly, those two loci match up with two loci that were in John and Linda's original mapping of diabetes and insulitis. One of them had a high chi square, *Idd8*, where the B10 was contributing to a susceptibility locus, and another one had suggestive link-up that matched. These seemed to match with our two. Again, this is one of those situations where the resistance strain does seem to have some susceptibility alleles. This is interesting because in our original TCR islet HEL double transgenic mice we get 20% progressing to diabetes on the B10 background and 90% on the NOD, and in the F1 it is completely suppressed.

Cookson: Would you like to comment on the tissues that are involved in the human AIRE knockout? It is not all peripheral tissues: there is something relatively specific about it. Also in humans there are particular clusterings of autoimmune disease. For example, the thyro-gastric cluster, with pernicious anaemia and thyroiditis. Do you have any feeling for why there are these differences?

Goodnow: That is a great question. The short answer is that I don't. The diagnosis for APS1 is at least two of Addisons, parathyroid and candidiasis. Diabetes and thyroiditis are only 15% of cases. Then there are cutaneous manifestations. One speculation for candidiasis is that it is autoimmunity against Paneth cells.

Hafler: Thinking of this in terms of FoxP3, you see the same thing with multiple endocrine and enzymic processes disrupted. This raises an important question. We have just found a decrease in regulatory T cells in the peripheral blood of MS patients, yet in the FoxP3 knockout there is no CNS disease. At first this bothered me a lot. But when one has a knockout one is looking at a very different type of phenotype than might be the case with a more subtle defect.

Abbas: Let me give you another hypothesis. It is curious that many of these mutants are showing up with autoimmune diseases affecting endocrine tissues. One hypothesis, which relates to Bill Cookson's comment about a requirement for a second signal, is that the frequency of cellular necrosis is higher in endocrine tissues than in any other. If necrotic death activates second signals, you are constantly generating second signals within endocrine organs. So they are the ones that are the most poised to be involved by failure of regulation. The minute you allow forbidden clones to increase or regulatory cells to decrease, this is the place where autoimmune reactions develop. It is an interesting hypothesis that is obviously difficult to prove.

Hafler: The point is that the defect in FoxP3 or AIRE doesn't mean that this won't be relevant for other autoimmune diseases.

Kuchroo: In humans, the AIRE defect on different backgrounds gives different phenotypes. Even though there is this mutation, there may be other genes coming in and directing the autoimmunity or potentiating it.

Seed: This is a speculation. Possibly, these same cells that are present in thymic epithelium might be located elsewhere in the body. They might be stem cells: they might be progenitors of differentiated thymic epithelium, which because of AIRE perhaps has a generalized TATA box activation. One thought is that you might be able to find or generate these cells in other locations, so you wouldn't have to search for them in the thymus. Identifying the characteristics that define these cell types would be helpful. I have a comment on the endocrine hypothesis. There are two other phenomena associated with endocrine-type lineage cells. That is, they have a strongly focused transcriptional and translational apparatus that is engaged in producing a small number of secretory proteins. They are unusually focused compared with generalized epithelium. And they are mostly directly exposed to the circulation. This also probably helps in terms of identification of the antigen in the first place.

Abbas: It is not only endocrine cells. If you look at the AIRE knockout paper it may be neuroendocrine cells in the gastric epithelium. It is the retinal pigment epithelium that becomes the target of autoantibodies. There are a few tissues.

Goodnow: In APS1 there is 17% autoimmune hepatitis.

Behrens: It looks to me in the thymic epithelium that AIRE is *trans*-activating stochastically. For instance, why are you only seeing the thyroglobulin antigen induced in just a couple of cells? What is known about the specificity of particular proteins up-regulated by AIRE? The fact that those who have looked for specific autoantigens in purified populations of these thymic epithelial cells really only see a limited spectrum of autoantigens makes me wonder whether there are there other AIRE homologues or AIRE-like transcription factors that haven't been looked at.

Goodnow: As I understand it there are no other genes in the genome that have the same configurations of motifs. There are other proteins with SAND domains and some of these other domains that look like they might have a similar role, but not much is known about them. In terms of what is going on, one idea is that it is making all the genes turn on randomly in rare cells, and a bit like haemopoietic stem cells they are promiscuously trying all genetic programmes. Then there is another idea suggested by Andy Farr in Seattle. When he sections thymus he finds rare patches of cysts. Some of them look at the electron microscopy level like a little thyroid follicle, and others like ciliated epithelium. One scenario is that there is a controlled version of a teratocarcinoma making a little bit of each part of the body, and it really is an immunological homunculus. One experiment that could test this would be to ask whether the insulin expression in the thymus is still dependent on the insulin-activating transcription factors such as Pdx1.

Behrens: Besides the mutants that cause the full blown disease, is there any known variation of this protein in human populations?

Goodnow: Not that I know of.

Wicker: There is variation, but it is not associated with type 1 diabetes.

Goodnow: There are lots of different variants that are now being reported, some of which are being found in what appear to be heterozygotes. Are they dominant negatives or is there an unascertained second permutation on the other allele? Or are they really heterozygotes?

Wicker: Again, a lot of those are too rare to test for disease association. There is no common variation discernable in the structure of the potentially mutant alleles.

Vyse: When you did your experiments with your HEL TCR transgenic, have you just got one transgenic line in which you can do these experiments, or do you have variants with potentially different affinities to HEL? If the latter is the case, you could carry out the same experiments with these and look for variation at the receptor level to see how it influences things, both in the AIRE and NOD mouse.

Goodnow: We don't, but Anne O'Garra made another TCR transgenic to HEL that sees HEL in the context of I-A^b. This is an epitope that has always been described as inefficiently presented or subdominant. When you cross that to the same Ins HEL transgene there is no deletion in the thymus. It is hard to say whether it is a low affinity TCR or just a peptide that is less efficiently presented. It comes out of the thymus fine. They don't develop spontaneous autoimmune diabetes. It is essentially an ignorant T cell that comes out and doesn't pose much danger on its own. If you push things you can make that T cell diabetogenic. There has always been this argument against the idea that thymic tolerance had anything to do with organ-specific autoimmunity. You can find all these clones such as BDC2.5 and autoreactive T cells circulating in the blood and this can mediate disease under various circumstances. The assumption was that thymic deletion wasn't important. Now my way of looking at this is that there are peaks of very high anergic T cells which would pose a great danger of being prime movers of an autoimmune response, and then there are lower avidity T cells that pose a risk but are less likely to be prime movers, except under certain circumstances such as T$_{reg}$ deficiency.

Hafler: Do they provide a potential benefit? Are they there to regulate responses to injury in some fashion?

Goodnow: No, I think it is just holes in the repertoire. This is a bad thing. The primary function of the immune system is to get rid of viruses and bacteria. If you get a bit of autoimmunity as a result of being a bit generous with what you let out of the thymus it is probably going to have a weaker selection pressure than getting knocked off by *Mycobacterium tuberculosis*.

Abbas: I want to suggest an issue of strategy. I think it is fair to say that these transgenic systems have taught us more about pathways of tolerance than any other type of experimental system. The question is, if you have identified genes from genome scans and want to test their role in autoimmunity, why not go straight into a transgenic system?

Kuchroo: It is being done. We have been crossing the BDC2.5 onto the *Idd9* congenics, looking at how it affects the T cell responses.

Abbas: I think it is extremely powerful and people should keep these in mind.

Hafler: Michael Karin took a particular NOD2 haplotype from a human and put it into a mouse. He saw more inflammatory disease in the gut. How would you interpret this? Should we just knock out genes or should we be able to take the haplotypes or gene regions and put these into experimental models to see what they do?

Abbas: I am taking it one step further, and saying instead of an experimental model being just a mouse, redesign your experimental models to look for particular pathways.

Rao: You should have picked up agenesis phenotypes, which could be detected by magnetic resonance imaging (MRI) scans. Have you seen these?

Goodnow: We didn't screen for them, but I am sure that you would get whatever you screened for on the basis of the T cell scan.

Rao: You have emphasized that you have got mostly mutations in the protein coding genes, rather than the non-coding transcripts. Is that because mutations in non-coding transcripts are less sensitive to the kinds of mutations that ENU induces?

Goodnow: ENU does have a high preference for mutating A or T bases over C and Gs. They are not particularly enriched in terms of these non-coding regions. If a non-coding element can tolerate a base change more than a coding element, why are they as conserved as exons at the nucleotide level?

Foote: Could you set up a sensitised screen to get some of these more subtle phenotypes?

Goodnow: You'd have to do a 10-generation iterative selection strategy.

Wijmenga: Can't you just sequence a bunch of them to see whether you have the mutant?

Goodnow: That is the other possibility.

Wakeland: In a recent journal I was reading a synopsis of a meeting at Cold Spring Harbor Laboratory at which Ed Rubin reported deleting over a megabase of DNA (http://www.newscientist.com/article.ns?id=dn5063) that contained a huge series of these highly conserved elements in a mouse. He reported that this resulted in no apparent phenotype or impact on viability. This result argues against the idea that these highly conserved sequences will always have a significant impact on function.

Vyse: You are going to get multiple hits with your ENU screen. Perhaps the phenotypes that you start out with that are dependent on multiple smaller QTL-type problems drop out in your breeding scheme and you ignore them. You are deliberately selecting for the more penetrant effects.

Goodnow: We had two instances of mice where these individuals looked like they must be mutant but where we didn't see it breed true. There were only two drop-outs. For neither do we have good evidence that they were mutant to start with, because they were single individuals in a family. In every case where we had at least two clear, independent phenotypes they bred through as a monogenic disorder. So we don't have this kind of ascertainment bias, but there is this big ascertainment bias that for us to even call it 'interesting' it had to be two standard deviations from normal.

Wakeland: By focusing on highly penetrant phenotypes, you are excluding a lot of mutations, many of which might be similar to the types of natural polymorphism involved in disease susceptibility.

Goodnow: Absolutely.

References

Anderson AC, Nicholson LB, Legge KL, Turchin V, Zaghouani H, Kuchroo VK 2000 High frequency of autoreactive myelin proteolipid protein-specific T cells in the periphery of naive mice: mechanisms of selection of the self-reactive repertoire. J Exp Med 191:761–770

Chentoufi AA, Polychronakos C 2002 Insulin expression levels in the thymus modulate insulin-specific autoreactive T-cell tolerance: the mechanism by which the IDDM2 locus may predispose to diabetes. Diabetes 51:1383–1390

Pugliese A, Brown D, Garza D et al 2001 Self-antigen-presenting cells expressing diabetes-associated autoantigens exist in both thymus and peripheral lymphoid organs. J Clin Invest 107:555–564

An autoimmune disease-associated CTLA4 splice variant lacking the B7 binding domain signals negatively in T cells

Lalitha Vijayakrishnan, Jacqueline M. Slavik, Zsolt Illés, Dan Rainbow, Laurence B. Peterson, Arlene S. Sharpe, Linda S. Wicker and Vijay K. Kuchroo[1]

Center for Neurologic Diseases, Department of Neurology, Brigham and Women's Hospital and Harvard Medical School, Boston, MA 02115, USA

Abstract. Cytotoxic T lymphocyte-associated antigen 4 (CTLA4) plays a critical role in down-regulating T cell responses. A number of autoimmune diseases have shown genetic linkage to the *CTLA4* locus. We have cloned and expressed an alternatively spliced form of CTLA4 that has genetic linkage with type 1 diabetes in NOD mice. This splice variant of CTLA4, named ligand-independent CTLA4 (liCTLA4), lacks exon 2 including the MYPPPY motif essential for binding to the costimulatory ligands B7-1 and B7-2. liCTLA4 is expressed as a protein in primary T cells and strongly inhibits T cell responses by binding and dephosphorylating the TcRζ chain. Expression of liCTLA4, but not full length CTLA4 (flCTLA4), was higher in memory/regulatory T cells from diabetes resistant NOD congenic mice compared to susceptible NOD mice. Transgenic expression of liCTLA4 in autoimmune prone *Ctla4*$^{-/-}$ mice inhibited spontaneous T cell activation and prevented early lethality in the *Ctla4*$^{-/-}$ mice. Thus, increased expression and negative signalling delivered by the liCTLA4 may play a critical role in regulating the development of T cell-mediated autoimmune diseases.

2005 The genetics of autoimmunity. Wiley, Chichester (Novartis Foundation Symposium 267) p 200–218

Type 1 diabetes is an autoimmune disease that shows familial aggregation and appears to be genetically determined. The Non-obese diabetic (NOD) mouse serves as a good model for human disease, because the disease appears spontaneously and bears pathogenetic features remarkably similar to human type 1 diabetes. Diabetes susceptibility in NOD mice has been subjected to genetic

---

[1]This paper was presented at the symposium by Vijay K. Kuchroo to whom correspondence should be addressed.

analysis and at least 18 genetic loci have been identified that contribute to susceptibility (Costa et al 2000). Some of the same genetic loci have also been identified in other autoimmune diseases (Becker et al 1998) raising the possibility that there may be a set of common 'autoimmune genes' that confer susceptibility to multiple autoimmune diseases. Identification of such genes may help us identify a common pathway that is dysregulated and results in the development of autoimmunity. It was also found that susceptibility loci that have been identified in autoimmune diseases in mice also overlap with other human autoimmune diseases and one such locus is present on chromosome 1 in mice and chromosome 2q33 in humans (Hill et al 2000). This chromosomal segment harbours an immunologically important family of costimulatory receptors.

By congenic mapping it was established that this locus, defined as *Idd5.1*, contains costimulatory molecules CD28, CTLA4 and ICOS. Introgression of the costimulatory genes of *Cd28*, *Ctla4* and *Icos* from the diabetes-resistant B10 strain, could confer resistance to diabetes (Lamhamedi-Cherradi et al 2001, Hill et al 2000). In humans, autoimmune diseases such as multiple sclerosis (Harbo et al 1999, Ebers et al 1996), insulin-dependent diabetes mellitus (IDDM) (Fajardy et al 2002, Cosentino et al 2002, Abe et al 2001, Redondo et al 2001), Graves' disease (Kotsa et al 1997, Kinjo et al 2002, Kouki et al 2000, Tomer & Davies 1997) Hashimoto's thyroiditis (Nithiyananthan et al 2002), lupus (Hudson et al 2002) and rheumatoid arthritis (Grennan 2002) have been shown to be associated with the locus. In each case the genetic cause for disease has been mainly attributed to single nucleotide polymorphisms (SNPs) in *Ctla4* ($-319>T$, $+49A>G$, $+1822C>T$ and [AT] n-3′UTR). However, a causal polymorphism resulting in functional variants has not been defined. A soluble isoform of CTLA4 (sCTLA4) generated by alternate splicing and deletion of exon 3 has previously been described in both mouse and humans, and its level in human plasma was found to be elevated among a population of patients with autoimmune thyroid disease (Grennan 2002). The expression of this soluble form of CTLA4 relative to the wild-type form, and its function in terms of T cell activation/inhibition has not been defined.

CD28 and CTLA4 costimulatory molecules in T cells

CD28 is expressed on the surface of unactivated T cells and provides a positive costimulatory signal for the activation of T cells. CTLA4, on the other hand, is up-regulated on the cell surface following T cell activation (Zhang et al 1997, Linsley et al 1996, Alegre et al 1996). CTLA4 shares 31% amino acid identity with CD28 with only limited conservation between the cytoplasmic domains. There is 100% conservation between the cytoplasmic domains of murine and human CTLA4, suggesting a conserved signalling function. In contrast to CD28,

CTLA4 induces a negative signal into T cells (Krummel & Allison 1995). This has been most clearly demonstrated by CTLA4-deficient mice, which develop a severe lymphoproliferative disorder and die at a young age due to multi-organ autoimmune disease (Tivol et al 1995, Bergman et al 2001, Chambers et al 1997). Both CD28 and CTLA4 have to the same ligands B7-1 and B7-2, which are expressed on the surface of antigen-presenting cells (APCs).

Molecular mechanisms which mediate CTLA4 function in T cells

Considering the pivotal role for CTLA4 in T cell regulation, many groups have studied the molecular mechanism by which CTLA4 mediates negative regulation. Major functions attributed to CTLA4 have been its ability to deliver cell cycle checkpoints in a transition from the G1 to S phase (Alegre et al 2001, Walunas et al 1994, Greenwald et al 2002) and inhibition of interleukin (IL)2 secretion (Krummel & Allison 1996). These attributes have made it a major player in the maintenance of peripheral tolerance (Perez et al 1997, Walunas & Bluestone 1998, Allison et al 1998, Frauwirth et al 2000, Fecteau et al 2001, Greenwald et al 2001). Much of the protein remains trapped in clathrin-coated pits of early endosomes (Zhang et al 1997) but once expressed on the cell surface, its extracellular domain, by virtue of being a higher affinity ligand for B7 molecules on APCs, redirects B7 away from CD28 interaction. At the same time the intracellular domain concentrates major phosphates like PP2A (Chuang et al 2000, Baroja et al 2002) and SHP2 (Schneider et al 1995, Lee et al 1998) within the immunological synapse where they interact with the TCRζ chain (Lee et al 1998). Therefore, a combination of negative signals via its cytoplasmic domain, together with sequestration of B7 molecules by the extracellular domain of CTLA4 at the synapse, mediates negative regulation of T cells (Carreno et al 2000). A direct interaction of CTLA4 with the phosphorylated form of CD3ζ within the glycolipid-enriched microdomains associated with the T cell signalling complex was observed. In this setting, CTLA4 regulated the accumulation/retention of TCRζ in the signalling complex, as the lipid raft fractions from CTLA4 knockout (KO) T cells contained significantly higher amounts of the TCR components when compared with wild-type littermates. In contrast, coligation of CTLA4 with the TCR during T cell activation selectively decreased the amount of TCRζ that accumulated in the rafts. These results suggest that CTLA4 functions to regulate T cell signalling by controlling TCR accumulation and/or retention within this critical component of the immunological synapse.

While it is clear that CTLA4 plays a pivotal role in the regulation of autoimmune disease, but its association with genetic susceptibility has remained a mystery. No strong polymorphisms have been identified that can account for the genetic susceptibility. However, recently alternately spliced forms for CTLA4 have been associated with the genetic susceptibility to autoimmune diseases in humans and mice. In human autoimmune diseases, association with the soluble form of CTLA4 (sCTLA4) and in mice with the liCTLA4 has been reported (Ueda et al 2003).

While amplifying CTLA4 from the activated spleen cells of C57Bl/6 mice by reverse transcriptase (RT)-PCR reaction we identified three different bands of CTLA4: (1) full-length form of *Ctla4*, (*flCtla4*); (2) soluble *Ctla4*, (*sCtla4*); and (3) novel *Ctla4* splice variant of approximately 300 bp (Fig. 1). On sequencing, it was found that the novel splice variant lacked exon 2 and the major IgV domain essential for interaction with B7 molecules. It was hence named ligand-independent *Ctla4* or *liCtla4*. Using cDNA from C57Bl/6 spleen cells activated with anti-CD3 and a specific 5' primer at the junction between exon 1 and exon 3 and a 3' primer in a region around the stop codon of *Ctla4*, we were able to specifically amplify only the splice variant, yielding a PCR product corresponding to the expected size of the variant *Ctla4* (Fig. 1A, Lane 4 and 5). We thus confirmed that the variant form does exist in the cell and encodes for a message distinct from that encoded by the wild-type *Ctla4*. The *liCtla4* is expressed as a protein, as transfection of the cDNA of *liCtla4* cloned within the multiple cloning site of pCMV-MYC in HEK293 cells yielded a protein species of approximately 8 kDa, detected on a reducing gel with antibodies directed to the MYC tag as compared to a 36 kDa full-length protein of CTLA4 (Fig. 1C). Furthermore, we were able to detect the novel splice variant liCTLA4 in activated T cells along with the flCTLA4 by using an antibody directed to the cytoplasmic motif of CTLA4 (Fig. 1D) which can recognize both the flCTLA4 and liCTLA4 since the coding amino acids are the same for both forms of CTLA4. The full-length form has three predicted N-linked glycosylation sites; the novel form has none. To identify whether the liCTLA4 was also expressed in normal T cells we undertook Western blotting analysis with an antibody directed to the tail of CTLA4. Thus in the Western blot for the detection of CTLA4 iosforms in T cells, we found flCTLA4 expressed as doublet band showing highly glycosylated flCTLA4 migrating at $\sim$ 36 kDa. liCTLA4 was found to be expressed in T cells as an 8 kDa protein conforming to the predicted size of liCTLA4. liCTLA4 lacked exon 2 of the flCTLA4 and had a deletion of a major portion of the extracellular domain of CTLA4 including the critical MYPPPY sequence essential for interaction with B7 molecules (Fig. 1D).

We established function of liCTLA4 by cloning these molecules in a retroviral vector pGCIRES (Fig. 2) and expressing it in the T cells. The pGCIRES vector (an MMLV-based vector) has been engineered to contain a multiple cloning site for incorporation of genes expressing the test protein and a downstream selectable marker, GFP. The GFP encoded by the retroviral vector was used as surrogate marker for protein expression of both the isoforms of CTLA4 (Costa et al 2000).

T cells from triple knockout (TKO) mice lacking B7.1/B7.2 and CTLA4 and double knockout mice which lack B7.1 and B7.2 were infected with retrovirus expressing either CTLA4, liCTLA4 or empty vector control. Infected populations of cells were monitored for GFP expression by flow cytometry to normalize for expression levels of either protein as shown in Fig. 2A and then sorted for GFP expression by flowcytometry. Figure 2B shows a Western blot analysis for the expression CTLA4 or liCTLA4 protein in the lysates of sorted populations of GFP-positive cells. The sorted T cells were then activated with

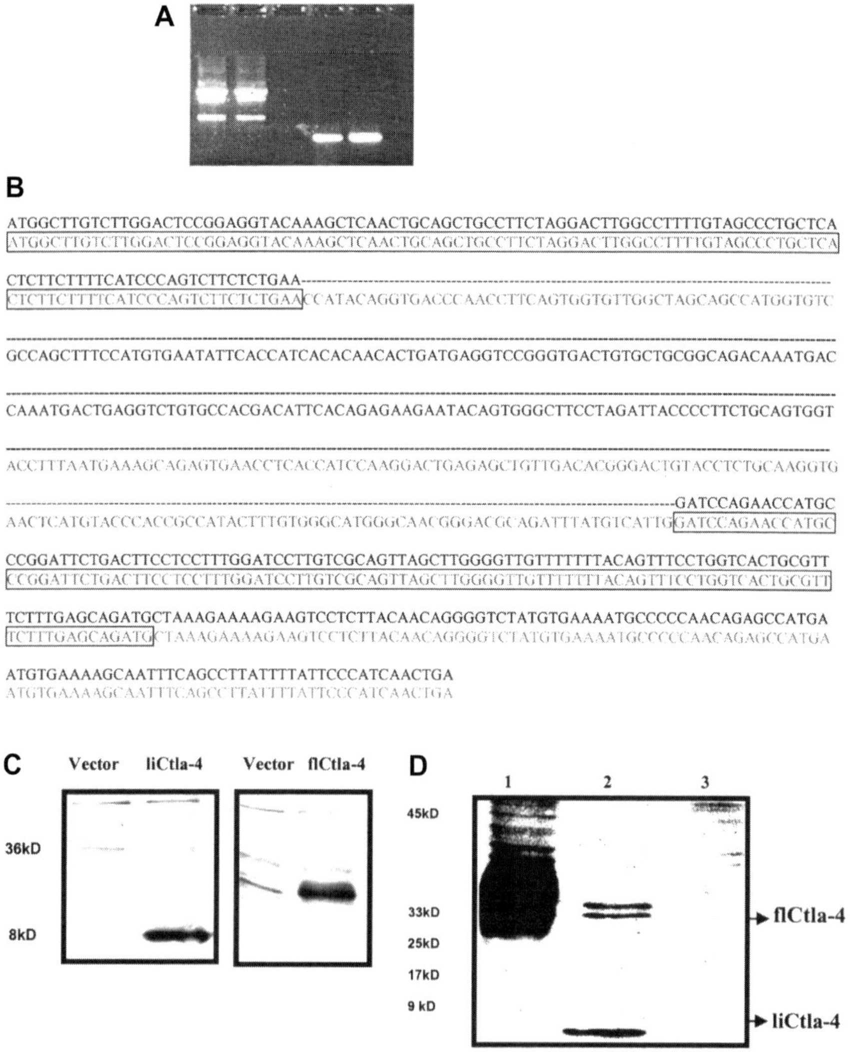

A

B

ATGGCTTGTCTTGGACTCCGGAGGTACAAAGCTCAACTGCAGCTGCCTTCTAGGACTTGGCCTTTTGTAGCCCTGCTCA
ATGGCTTGTCTTGGACTCCGGAGGTACAAAGCTCAACTGCAGCTGCCTTCTAGGACTTGGCCTTTTGTAGCCCTGCTCA

CTCTTCTTTTCATCCCAGTCTTCTCTGAA---
CTCTTCTTTTCATCCCAGTCTTCTCTGAA CATACAGGTGACCCAACCTTCAGTGGTGTTGGCTAGCAGCCATGGTGTC

GCCAGCTTTCCATGTGAATATTCACCATCACACAACACTGATGAGGTCCGGGTGACTGTGCTGCGGCAGACAAATGAC

CAAATGACTGAGGTCTGTGCCACGACATTCACAGAGAAGAATACAGTGGGCTTCCTAGATTACCCCTTCTGCAGTGGT

ACCTTTAATGAAAGCAGAGTGAACCTCACCATCCAAGGACTGAGAGCTGTTGACACGGGACTGTACCTCTGCAAGGTG

---GATCCAGAACCATGC
AACTCATGTACCCACCGCCATACTTTGTGGGCATGGGCAACGGGACGCAGATTTATGTCATTGGATCCAGAACCATGC

CCGGATTCTGACTTCCTCCTTTGGATCCTTGTCGCAGTTAGCTTGGGGTTGTTTTTTTACAGTTTCCTGGTCACTGCGTT
CCGGATTCTGACTTCCTCCTTTGGATCCTTGTCGCAGTTAGCTTGGGGTTGTTTTTTTACAGTTTCCTGGTCACTGCGTT

TCTTTGAGCAGATGCTAAAGAAAAGAAGTCCTCTTACAACAGGGGTCTATGTGAAAATGCCCCCAACAGAGCCATGA
TCTTTGAGCAGATGCTAAAGAAAAGAAGTCCTCTTACAACAGGGGTCTATGTGAAAATGCCCCCAACAGAGCCATGA

ATGTGAAAAGCAATTTCAGCCTTATTTTATTCCCATCAACTGA
ATGTGAAAAGCAATTTCAGCCTTATTTTATTCCCATCAACTGA

C Vector liCtla-4   Vector flCtla-4   **D**

36kD

8kD

45kD
33kD
25kD
17kD
9 kD

→ flCtla-4
→ liCtla-4

varying concentrations of soluble anti-CD3 in the presence of antigen-presenting cells from normal Balb/c mice. We found that liCTLA4, which lacks extracellular IgV domain required for interaction with B7 molecules, seemed to be as capable of inhibiting T cell responses as the full length molecule, both in terms of proliferation and interferon (IFN)γ secretion. (Fig. 2C,D). Thus the novel isoform of CTLA4 identified by us is functional in T cells. However, the mechanism by which it mediates negative effects without binding to B7 molecules is not clearly understood.

It has been demonstrated that flCTLA4 associates with the TCRζ chain within the immunological synapse. This association recruits negative regulators of T cell activation, like the phosphatase SHP2, into the synapse. To determine whether the liCTLA4 associates with the TCRζ and recruits SHP2, lysates from purified normal CD3$^+$ T cells from naïve and anti-CD3 plus anti-CD28 activated T cells were subjected to imunoprecipitation followed by Western blotting with a CTLA4 tail-specific antibody. These Western blotting analyses suggested that the flCTLA4 and liCTLA4 heterodimerize in both resting and (to a lesser extent) in activated T cells. However, even after immunoprecipitation with the anti-flCTLA4 specific antibody (4F10), in the lysates there was a pool of liCTLA4 that existed independent of flCTLA4. Additionally, flCTLA4 immunoprecipitates which also contained associated liCTLA4 could associate with the TCRζ and SHP2 in both resting and activated T cells. In contrast, though liCTLA4 was able to associate with the TCRζ chain in activated T cells it did not associate with SHP2 in either resting or activated T cells. So it is likely, that unlike flCTLA4, the inhibitory effect of liCTLA4 may not require SHP2 recruitment.

Our data demonstrate both flCTLA4 and liCTLA4 associate with the TCRζ but the association of liCTLA4 with TCRζ was activation dependent. Although

---

FIG. 1. Identification, cloning and expression of a novel splice variant of murine *Ctla4*. (A) RT-PCR amplification of *Ctla4* from cDNA of C57/Bl6 spleen cells. Lane 1, unactivated; 2, activated; 3, water control. Lanes 4–6, RT-PCR amplification of *liCtla4* using a junctional primer at exon1/exon3 and reverse primer in exon 4 of *liCtla4* from cDNA of C57/Bl6 spleen cells. Lane 4, unactivated; 5, activated; 6, water control. The forward exon 1/exon 3 primer was TCTCGAAGATCCAG and reverse primer in exon 4 was TCCTTCTTCTTCATAAACGGC. (B) Comparative nucleotide sequence of *liCtla4* (black font, upper line) and *flCtla4* (grey font, lower line). Exons are indicated by: boxed letters, first two lines, Exon1; grey font lines 2, 5 and 6, Exon2; boxed letters lines 6–8, Exon3; and grey font lines 8 and 9, Exon4. (C) Expression of *Ctla4* isoforms in HEK293 cells. *liCtla4* was cloned into expression vector pCMV-MYC and *flCtla4* was cloned into expression vector pCMV-HA and expressed in HEK293 cells. Western blot analysis of HEK293 cell lysates immunoblotted with anti-MYC antibody (left panel) or anti-CTLA4 (right panel). (D) Detection of CTLA4 isoforms in T cells. Lysates from: Lane 1, positive control, recombinant cDNA of flCtla-4 expressed in HEK293 cells; lane 2, spleen cells from C57/Bl6 mice; lane 3, spleen cells from *Ctla4*$^{-/-}$ mice.

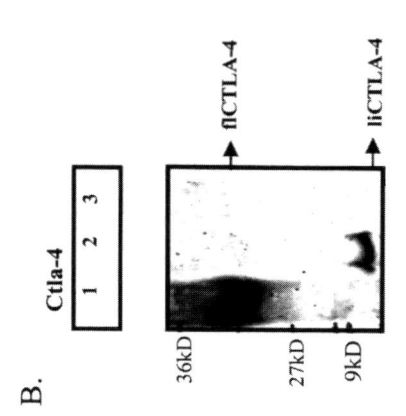

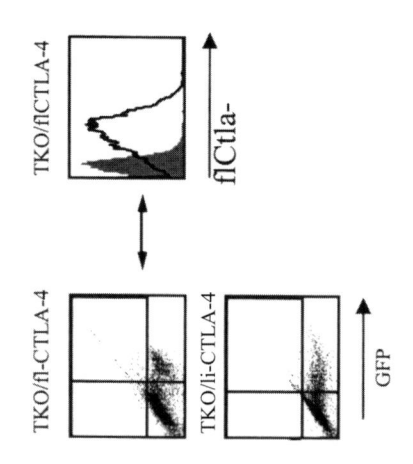

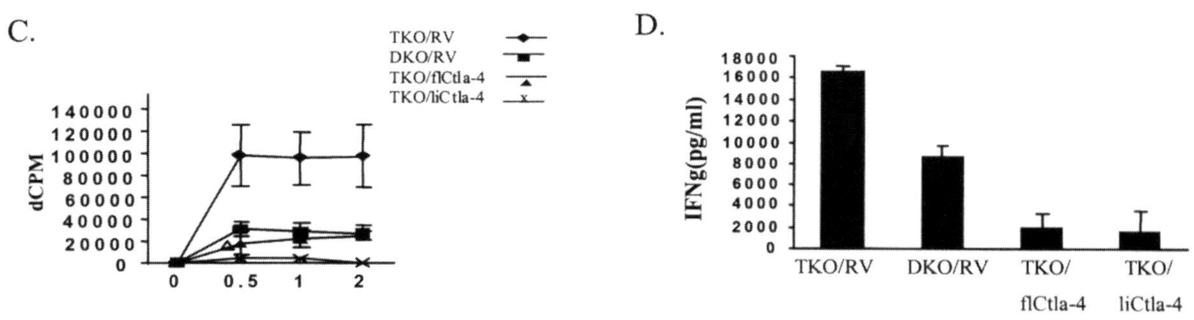

FIG. 2. Functional analysis of flCtla-4 and liCtla-4 in T cells. Activated CD3+ T cells from triple knockout mice (TKO) that lack CTLA4, B7-1 and B7-2 and double knockout (DKO) mice which lack B7-1 and B7-2 were infected with retrovirus pGCIRES expressing either the *flCtla4*, *liCtla4* or empty vector (RV). Infected cells were stimulated with antigen presenting cells from normal Balb/c mice in the presence of varying concentrations of anti-CD3. (A) FACS analysis of retrovirus infected TKO T cells showing comparable levels of GFP expression in the TKO T cells infected with *flCtla4* and *liCtla4*. (B) Western Blot analysis of cell lysates prepared from retrovirus infected GFP+ TKO T cells for the expression of flCTLA4 and liCTLA4. CTLA4 isoforms were detected by an anti-CTLA4 antibody designed to recognize its cytoplasmic domain. Lane 1, flCTLA4; lane 2, liCTLA4; and lane 3, empty vector, RV. (C) Inhibition of T cell proliferative responses to varying anti-CD3 concentrations. D. Inhibition of IFNγ secretion by flCTLA4 and liCTLA4 in TKO T cells infected with retrovirus expressing flCTLA4 or liCTLA4A. Cells were activated with anti-CD3 at 1 μg/ml. Data represent pooled values from two independent experiments. Error bars indicate standard error of mean.

flCTLA4 associates with SHP2, liCTLA4 does not. However, it was not clear whether the ability of flCTLA4 to associate with the TCRζ and SHP2 requires associated liCTLA4. To address this we utilized $Ctla4^{-/-}$ T cells in which flCTLA4 and liCTLA4 were independently expressed by retroviral infection. Lysates were prepared from resting or activated TKO T cells infected with liCTLA4 or flCTLA4. CTLA4 immunoprecipitates (using a C19 anti-CTLA4 antibody which recognizes both forms of CTLA4) were blotted independently with the anti-TCRζ chain antibody and SHP2 antibody to examine CTLA4/TCRζ association in this system. The association of both liCTLA4 and flCTLA4 with the TCRζ was activation dependent. However, unlike our observation in normal T cells when either liCTLA4 or flCTLA4 was expressed independently in $Ctla4^{-/-}$ T cells, both molecules failed to interact with SHP2 in either resting or activated T cells suggesting that the inhibitory signalling complex formed by the association between the flCTLA4, TCRζ and SHP2 seen in normal T cells requires the presence of liCTLA4.

It has been shown previously that the interaction of TCRζ and CTLA4 mediates TCRζ dephosphorylation. To analyse the consequences of flCTLA4 and liCTLA4 on the TCRζ chain, we examined the phosphorylation status of TCRζ in $Ctla4^{-/-}$ T cells infected with vector alone, liCTLA4 or flCTLA4. In resting TKO T cells infected with vector alone, liCTLA4 or flCTLA4 phosphorylation of the TCRζ was not observed. But upon CD3 cross-linking of TKO T cells infected with the vector alone, maximal phosphorylation of the TCRζ chain was achieved, indicated by the appearance of a phosphotyrosine band of p22. Infection of $Ctla4^{-/-}$ T cells with flCTLA4 decreased the extent of TCRζ tyrosine phosphorylation, such that the bands corresponding to TCRζ now were of a lower molecular mass (p15, p18). Strikingly, in $Ctla4^{-/-}$ T cells infected with liCTLA4, no tyrosine phosphorylation of the TCRζ chain was observed. These data demonstrate that both flCTLA4 and liCTLA4 can mediate dephosphorylation of the TCRζ chain even in the absence of SHP2 recruitment, suggesting that alternative negative signalling phosphatases may associate with the TCRζ/CTLA4 complex. Secondly, the total ablation of TCRζ phosphorylation in liCTLA4 infected $Ctla4^{-/-}$ T cells suggests that even in the absence of B7 ligation, liCTLA4 is more potent than flCTLA4 in preventing phosphorylation of TCRζ chain. It should be noted that our conclusions are drawn from an overexpression system where the expression of both molecules is calculated and compared based on GFP expression. Nevertheless, based on this data one could conclude that the liCTLA4 is a potent inhibitory molecule with an ability to regulate proximal T cell signalling events as demonstrated by its ability to dephosphorylate the TCRζ in activated T cells.

We next examined the expression of flCTLA4 and liCTLA4 in the prototypic diabetes susceptible NOD and resistant B6/H2g7 mice. For comparison we also

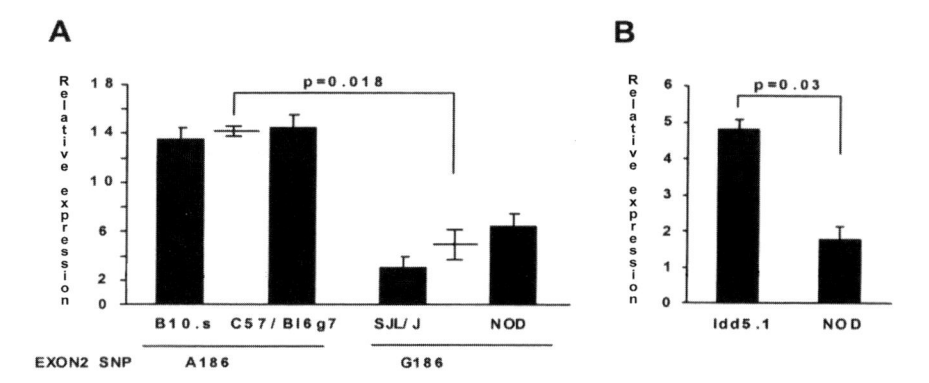

FIG. 3. Expression of *flCtla4* and *liCtla4* in CD4+CD45RB[low] cells of autoimmune resistant and susceptible mouse strains. (A) mRNA expression of *flCtla4* and *liCtla4* in CD4+ T cells of different mouse strains. (B) mRNA expression of *flCtla4* and *liCtla4* in T cells of NOD and *Idd5.1* congenic mice. mRNA was obtained from T cells of autoimmune susceptible (SJL/J, NOD) and resistant strains (B10.S, C57/Bl6g7) and *Idd5.1* congenic and wild-type NOD mice. Expression of *liCtla4* was examined by real-time RT-PCR. The values represent $2^{-\Delta\Delta Ct}$ ratio of the individual samples relative to expression levels of GAPDH. A point mutation within exon 2 of *Ctla4* that varied between SJL/NOD (G186) and B10.S/B6 (A186) within exon2 of *flCtla4* is also shown. Mean data obtained from two separate experiments are indicated.

tested another pair of mouse strains that are susceptible/resistant to another autoimmune disease, experimental autoimmune encephalomyelitis (EAE). We also compared the expression of liCTLA4 in EAE-susceptible SJL and -resistant B10.S by the real-time TAQMAN PCR. The expression levels of *flCtla4* and *liCtla4* differed between the prototypic diabetes and EAE-susceptible strains (SJL and NOD) and resistant (B6/Iag7 and B10.S) strains of mice. We found a consistently higher (four-to-sixfold) expression in the mRNA levels of *liCtla4* in the CD45RB[low] CD4+ (memory/regulatory) T cells of the autoimmune resistant strains than in the CD4+ T cells of the autoimmune susceptible strains (Fig. 3A,B). However, how the variant liCTLA4 form is expressed following activation with regard to the flCTLA4 is not clear. It is possible that the flCTLA4 and liCTLA4 are regulated and expressed differently in T cells following activation.

Construction of *liCtla4* transgenic mice

To determine whether enhanced expression levels of *liCtla4* altered the phenotype of T cells in terms of activation, differentiation and effector functions, we created mice transgenic for the *liCtla4*. The *liCtla4* constructs were generated on the CD2 promoter and injected into the oocytes of NOD and B6 mice. We have bred the liCTLA4 transgenic mice onto the $Ctla4^{-/-}$ background and tested the effect of transgenic expression of *liCtla4* in curing early lethality and CTLA4-disease in the $Ctla4^{-/-}$ mice×*liCtla4* transgenic mice. Preliminary data suggest that constitutive expression of *liCtla4* does protect $liCtla4^{-/-}$ mice from early lethality. The mechanism by which liCTLA4 protects $Ctla4^{-/-}$ mice from multi-organ autoimmune disease will be discussed.

Our data provide strong evidence for an inhibitory role of a novel isoform of CTLA4 (called liCTLA4), which in mice is genetically linked to autoimmunity in that it is overexpressed in the resistant strains of mice. The liCTLA4 attenuates T cell responses even though it lacks an extracellular domain required for interaction with B7 molecules. However, its expression kinetics and mechanism of negative regulation seem to be distinct from that of flCTLA4. Genetic evidence in human autoimmune disease suggests that protection from diabetes is also not due to a structural polymorphism in the coding sequence of CTLA4 gene but instead is correlated with the expression level of an alternatively spliced form of CTLA4 (sCTLA4). The causative variant associated with diabetes susceptibility is mapped to a non-coding 6.1 kb 3′ region of CTLA4, which determines lower levels of the sCTLA4 transcript (Ueda et al 2003). These data suggest that genetic modulation of the expression of alternatively spliced forms of CTLA4 contributes to the genetic control of autoimmunity in both mice and humans.

References

Abe T, Yamaguchi Y, Takino H et al 2001 CTLA-4 gene polymorphism contributes to the mode of onset of diabetes with antiglutamic acid decarboxylase antibody in Japanese patients: genetic analysis of diabetic patients with antiglutamic acid decarboxylase antibody. Diabet Med 18:786

Alegre ML, Noel PJ, Eisfelder BJ et al 1996 Regulation of surface and intracellular expression of CTLA4 on mouse T cells. J Immunol 157:4762–4770

Alegre ML, Frauwirth KA, Thompson CB 2001 T-cell regulation by CD28 and CTLA-4. Nat Rev Immunol 1:220–228

Allison JP, Chambers C, Hurwitz A et al 1998 A role for CTLA-4-mediated inhibitory signals in peripheral T cell tolerance? In: Immunological tolerance (Novartis Found Symp 215). Wiley, Chichester, p 92–102

Baroja ML, Vijayakrishnan L, Bettelli E et al 2002 Inhibition of CTLA-4 function by the regulatory subunit of serine/threonine phosphatase 2A. J Immunol 168:5070–5078

Becker KG, Simon RM, Bailey-Wilson JE et al 1998 Clustering of non-major histocompatibility complex susceptibility candidate loci in human autoimmune diseases. Proc Natl Acad Sci USA 95:9979–9984

Bergman ML, Cilio CM, Penha-Goncalves C et al 2001 CTLA-4-/- mice display T cell-apoptosis resistance resembling that ascribed to autoimmune-prone non-obese diabetic (NOD) mice. J Autoimmun 16:105–113

Carreno BM, Bennett F, Chau TA et al 2000 CTLA-4 (CD152) can inhibit T cell activation by two different mechanisms depending on its level of cell surface expression. J Immunol 165:1352–1356

Chambers CA, Sullivan TJ, Allison JP 1997 Lymphoproliferation in CTLA-4-deficient mice is mediated by costimulation-dependent activation of CD4+ T cells. Immunity 7:885–895

Chuang E, Fisher TS, Morgan RW et al 2000 The CD28 and CTLA-4 receptors associate with the serine/threonine phosphatase PP2A. Immunity 13:313–322

Cosentino A, Gambelunghe G, Tortoioli C, Falorni A 2002 CTLA-4 gene polymorphism contributes to the genetic risk for latent autoimmune diabetes in adults. Ann N Y Acad Sci 958:337–340

Costa GL, Benson JM, Seroogy CM et al 2000 Targeting rare populations of murine antigen-specific T lymphocytes by retroviral transduction for potential application in gene therapy for autoimmune disease. J Immunol 164:3581–3590

Ebers GC, Kukay K, Bulman DE et al 1996 A full genome search in multiple sclerosis. Nat Genet 13:472–476

Fajardy I, Vambergue A, Stuckens C et al 2002 CTLA-4 49 A/G dimorphism and type 1 diabetes susceptibility: a French case-control study and segregation analysis. Evidence of a maternal effect. Eur J Immunogenet 29:251–257

Fecteau S, Basadonna GP, Freitas A et al 2001 CTLA-4 up-regulation plays a role in tolerance mediated by CD45. Nat Immunol 2:58–63

Frauwirth KA, Alegre ML, Thompson CB 2000 Induction of T cell anergy in the absence of CTLA-4/B7 interaction. J Immunol 164:2987–2993

Greenwald RJ, Boussiotis VA, Lorsbach RB, Abbas AK, Sharpe AH 2001 CTLA-4 regulates induction of anergy in vivo. Immunity 14:145–155

Greenwald RJ, Oosterwegel MA, van der Woude D et al 2002 CTLA-4 regulates cell cycle progression during a primary immune response. Eur J Immunol 32:366–373

Grennan DM 2002 Re: An association between the CTLA4 exon 1 polymorphism and early rheumatoid arthritis with autoimmune endocrinopathies, by Vaidya et al. Rheumatology (Oxford) 41:1213 (author reply 1213)

Harbo HF, Celius EG, Vartdal F, Spurkland A 1999 CTLA4 promoter and exon 1 dimorphisms in multiple sclerosis. Tissue Antigens 53:106–110

Hill NJ, Lyons PA, Armitage N et al 2000 NOD Idd5 locus controls insulitis and diabetes and overlaps the orthologous CTLA4/IDDM12 and NRAMP1 loci in humans. Diabetes 49:1744–1747

Hudson LL, Rocca K, Song YW, Pandey JP 2002 CTLA-4 gene polymorphisms in systemic lupus erythematosus: a highly significant association with a determinant in the promoter region. Hum Genet 111:452–425

Kinjo Y, Takasu N, Komiya I et al 2002 Remission of Graves' hyperthyroidism and A/G polymorphism at position 49 in exon 1 of cytotoxic T lymphocyte-associated molecule-4 gene. J Clin Endocrinol Metab 87:2593–2596

Kotsa K, Watson PF, Weetman AP 1997 A CTLA-4 gene polymorphism is associated with both Graves disease and autoimmune hypothyroidism. Clin Endocrinol (Oxf) 46:551–554

Kouki T, Sawai Y, Gardine CA et al 2000 CTLA-4 gene polymorphism at position 49 in exon 1 reduces the inhibitory function of CTLA-4 and contributes to the pathogenesis of Graves' disease. J Immunol 165:6606–6611

Krummel M, Allison J 1995 CD28 and CTLA4 have opposing effects on the response of T cells to stimulation. J Exp Med 182:459–466

Krummel MF, Allison JP 1996 CTLA-4 engagement inhibits IL-2 accumulation and cell cycle progression upon activation of resting T cells. J Exp Med 183:2533–2540

Lamhamedi-Cherradi SE, Boulard O, Gonzalez C et al 2001 Further mapping of the Idd5.1 locus for autoimmune diabetes in NOD mice. Diabetes 50:2874–2878

Lee KM, Chuang E, Griffin M et al 1998 Molecular basis of T cell inactivation by CTLA-4. Science 282:2263–2266

Linsley P, Bradshaw J, Greene J et al 1996 Intracellular trafficking of CTLA4 and focal localization towards sites of TcR engagement. Immunity 4:535–543

Nithiyananthan R, Heward JM, Allahabadia A, Franklyn JA, Gough SC 2002 Polymorphism of the CTLA-4 gene is associated with autoimmune hypothyroidism in the United Kingdom. Thyroid 12:3–6

Perez V, Vanparijis L, Biuckians A et al 1997 Induction of peripheral T cell tolerance in vivo requires CTLA-4 engagement. Immunity 6:411–417

Redondo MJ, Fain PR, Eisenbarth GS 2001 Genetics of type 1A diabetes. Recent Prog Horm Res 56:69–89

Schneider H, Prasad KV, Shoelson SE, Rudd CE 1995 CTLA-4 binding to the lipid kinase phosphatidylinositol 3-kinase in T cells. J Exp Med 181:351–355

Tivol E, Borriello F, Schweitzer A et al 1995 Loss of CTLA-4 leads to massive lymphoproliferation and fatal multiorgan destruction, revealing a critical negative regulatory role of CTLA-4. Immunity 3:541–547

Tomer Y, Davies TF 1997 The genetic susceptibility to Graves' disease. Baillieres Clin Endocrinol Metab 11:431–450

Ueda H, Howson JM, Esposito L et al 2003 Association of the T-cell regulatory gene CTLA4 with susceptibility to autoimmune disease. Nature 30:30

Walunas TL, Bluestone JA 1998 CTLA-4 regulates tolerance induction and T cell differentiation in vivo. J Immunol 160:3855–3860

Walunas TL, Lenschow DJ, Bakker CY et al 1994 CTLA-4 can function as a negative regulator of T cell activation. Immunity 1:405–413

Zhang B, Yamamura T, Kondo T, Fujiwara M, Tabira T 1997 Regulation of experimental autoimmune encephalomyelitis by natural killer (NK) cells. J Exp Med 186:1677–1687

DISCUSSION

Abbas: I have a question for both you and Linda Wicker. I thought that the splice variant was associated with diabetes. Is this true?

Wicker: If you have more of the splice variant you are protected from disease.

Rao: Can you see a problem with splicing?

Wicker: There is a synonymous SNP in exon 2 of *Ctla4* that alters the efficiency of an exon splicing silencer motif. The SNP present in the protective allele allows the protein complex that binds via the motif to interact with higher affinity thereby causing the exon to be excluded from the mature message.

Abbas: How common do you think disease associated splice variants will prove to be?

Cookson: Very common.

Kuchroo: If you look at the *Tim3* splice variant you find a big difference in Balb/c versus B6. This may partly affect the Th1/Th2 balance.

Wakeland: There are splice variants in the CD150 family that are characteristic of the two different CD150 haplotypes in inbred strains. We believe that these are strong candidates for causing autoimmunity.

Cookson: CD1 has splice variants.

Kere: Regulation of splice variation may be a major mechanism for complex disease.

Behrens: There are also some recent data showing that if you look across all autoantibodies in humans and mice, there is an over-representation of antibodies against proteins that are known to undergo splicing.

Rao: Is the expression level of this truncated thing much higher than you'd expect if you completely eliminated the contribution from the ligand-binding domain? If your molecule has two functions and you have eliminated one of them, is the transgenic mouse overexpressing this form that has only one function?

Kuchroo: It does express the form at higher levels, but in a wild-type mouse it is together with the full-length form. In the knockout mouse we are looking at the function in the absence of the full-length form. The best experiment is when we can knock down only one of the forms by RNAi. Christophe Benoist and Diane Mathis have started to make a construct to knock-down only the liCTLA4. We can then start asking whether in the absence of the ligand independent form, the full length form still has all the functions.

Abbas: There has been this thought that CTLA4 functions as a negative signalling molecule and as a competitive inhibitor. Obviously the ligand-independent version is missing the competition for function. It is striking that the negative signalling seems to be enough.

Foote: Have you made the reciprocal transgene that just expresses the full length form?

Kuchroo: It has been made.

Foote: Has it been made in the same construct?

Kuchroo: We haven't done this.

Rao: One thing about the tailless variant is that it is much less susceptible to degradation.

Abbas: Craig Thompson's lab have also made a tailless variant. The problem is that CTLA4 is a strange beast. 95% of it is inside the cell and it rapidly cycles to the plasma membrane. The tailless variant loses its normal trafficking properties and is constitutively expressed at very high levels on the cell surface.

Wakeland: Do these all rescue the knockout?

Wicker: Craig Thompson showed that the tailless trangene rescued the *Ctla4* knockout partially. It wasn't completely rescued.

Kuchroo: One other thing is that because of trafficking, this seems to get into the synapse complex quickly. You can see a lot of it with the zeta chain very quickly.

Seed: It is often the case that the surface molecules that don't have N-linked glycans won't make it out of the endoplasmic reticulum unless they are co-transported. It might be interesting to look at what is carrying the extracellular domain to the surface. It might be association but it might also be that something else ferries it to the cell surface.

Kuchroo: Some of the biochemistry suggests that it moves as a complex. We haven't teased this apart.

Goodnow: You mentioned that *Ctla4* knockout mice have multi-organ autoimmune disease. How clear is it that they actually have an autoimmune disease?

Kuchroo: I gave you the party line. No one has shown that those cells that infiltrate into the skeletal or cardiac muscles are actually autoreactive. No one has shown the specificity of those cells.

Goodnow: Do they have autoantibodies?

Abbas: No, they do not have anti-DNA antibodies. The problem is that they are dying by the time you wean them, so they might not have had enough time to make antibodies. The *Ctla4* knockout mice have cell infiltrates in the heart, muscle and every organ, and die of a myocarditis. All of us have seen this for years, but people ask, is it autoimmune? This raises the problem that if you are looking at infiltrative diseases, how do we know they are autoimmune? The one thing we can say is that if we cross the *Ctla4* knockout mouse onto a true germ-free background they still get disease.

Hafler: For MS and diabetes, do we really know that they are infiltrating diseases?

Abbas: It has been an absolute nightmare trying to figure out the peptide specificity of the infiltrating T cells. This is a general issue in all autoimmune diseases. Why do we care? I am not sure how critical the question is.

Goodnow: I would say it is highly critical if we are talking about mapping pathways. When T cells are activated they do extravasate across all sorts of vessels in the tissues. This kind of pathology in the *Ctla4* knockout could be explained by spontaneous polyclonal activation. This is a very different mechanistic pathway from autoimmunity.

Abbas: Something has got to engage the antigen receptor.

Goodnow: They can't get out of the thymus if they don't recognize MHC, so we know that they are always having their antigen receptors engaged.

Hafler: But the level it takes to activate the cell may be low, and there is incredible degeneracy of the TCR.

Kuchroo: If we take the data from the EAE model, the activated T cells will go all over the place. But in order to keep them homed to the target tissue, they need some sort of specificity for binding and activation in the target organ, or the T cells just go in and come back out again.

Abbas: Dale Umetsu's work fits in nicely with what Vijay Kuchroo presented about the *Tim* genes; Dale's lab was the one that identified *Tim* genes as susceptibility genes for asthma. He is going to present some of his results now.

Umetsu: My background is in immunology, not genetics. We have been studying the immunology for asthma and allergy for many years. These diseases have increased in prevalence quite dramatically over recent decades. We thought we would learn a great deal about regulation of asthma taking a genetic approach, and identifying an asthma susceptibility gene. However, we knew that finding such a gene in humans would be a formidable task, so we decided to use a mouse model of asthma. We have been studying BALB/c mice, which produce high levels of IL4 and develop severe airway hyperreactivity (AHR) when these mice are immunized with antigen. We have also been using DBA/2 mice, which produce low levels of IL4 and have normal airway reactivity when these mice are immunized in the same way.

Identification of an asthma susceptibility gene even in laboratory mouse strains, however, is a formidable task, and therefore we thought we would further simplify this problem by using congenic mice. We screened a panel of BALB/c congenic mice containing DBA/2 chromosomal segments and found one strain that stood out. It had the BALB/c background except for a chromosome 11 segment inherited from DBA/2. This chromosome 11 segment turned out to be syntenic to human 5q23-35, a region which has been repeatedly linked with asthma. Most importantly, this chromosome 11 segment converted the BALB/c mouse from one that produced low levels of IL4 and had normal airway reactivity to one with higher levels of IL4 and AHR. We used linkage analysis and genotyped 3000 N2 mice crossed between BALB/c and positionally cloned a new gene family which we call Tims. *Tim3*, the third member of this family encodes a protein that regulates the development of immune diseases, and Vijay Kuchroo has shown that this is preferentially expressed on Th1 cells. We found in mice that *Tim1* regulates the development of asthma and allergy. Furthermore, *Tim1* is preferentially expressed on Th2 cells. Therefore these studies indicated that the Tims were particularly involved in regulating adaptive immunity and the function of CD4+ T cells.

Now, what about the human TIMs; are they involved in the regulation human disease? We know that the Tims are located on chromosome 5q33.2, which has been repeatedly linked with asthma and autoimmune diseases in humans. We sequenced the coding region of *TIM1* in 40 individuals and found significant polymorphisms, including a 6 amino acid insertion/deletion polymorphism. It also turns out that the human *TIM1* is the receptor for the hepatitis A virus (HAV). In humans infection with HAV has been associated with protection against the development of asthma and allergy. But because HAV is not a respiratory virus and is transmitted through faecal–oral routes, most people have assumed that infection with HAV is a merely a marker of poor hygiene, and it is poor hygiene rather than HAV that protects against asthma and allergy.

We examined the relationship between HAV, asthma and the 6 amino acid insertion polymorphism in *TIM1*. We found that in HAV seropositive individuals, having one or two copies of this insertion polymorphism is associated with a significant reduction in atopy. In contrast, in HAV seronegative people there is no association of this polymorphism with the development of atopy. These studies therefore indicate that *TIM1* is a significant atopy susceptibility gene, but only in HAV seropositive individuals. Secondly, these studies suggest that HAV can directly prevent the development of atopy by binding to its receptor, TIM1, and changing the development of T cells, reducing Th2 development and thus atopy. We believe that the HAV binds very efficiently to the long form of TIM1 (and the 6 amino acid polymorphism) and infects T cells. This results in less Th2 development resulting in less atopy and asthma. In contrast, HAV binds less efficiently to the short form of TIM1, resulting in less efficient infection and leading to greater Th2 cell development. Most importantly, these studies provide a molecular mechanism for the hygiene hypothesis. The incidence of infections such as HAV is significantly decreased in industrialized countries. For HAV, it has been reduced from nearly 100% 20 years ago to about 20% in the USA. This protective mechanism due to HAV binding to TIM1 is therefore much less common today than 20 years ago, which could explain why the prevalence of asthma and allergy have increased so dramatically over the past two decades.

To summarize, we have used linkage analysis in a murine model of asthma to identify the *Tim* genes. We also showed that *TIM1* is an important atopy susceptibility gene in humans, but only in HAV seropositive individuals. Therefore *TIM1* integrates environmental factors with genetic factors in explaining some of the observations in human asthma and allergy.

Abbas: Do hepatitis A seropositive individuals have virus floating around? I would imagine they are the ones who don't have virus. You are arguing that the virus is directly ligating TIM1 and changing T cell patterns, so this is important.

Umetsu: Hepatitis A virus infection tends to be a self-limited one, although there are individuals who have more severe and longer courses. 20 years ago infection with HAV used to be very common, so re-exposure might have been very common. It is possible that re-exposure might enhance the effects of hepatitis A virus in some of those individuals. Clearly, the infection is now much rarer today.

Behrens: Would one exposure to hepatitis A change your Th2 repertoire for a long period?

Umetsu: We don't know, but that what the epidemiology of HAV infection suggests. We are now trying to do some virology and immunological studies to see exactly what hepatitis A does to T cells, and how it might have long term effects on the immune system.

Behrens: Do you see any autoantibodies against the TIMs in these hepatitis infected individuals? I am just wondering how a short-term viral infection could have a long-lasting effect on susceptibility. Perhaps it is inducing some response.

Umetsu: That is a possibility. It is clear that hepatitis A virus is associated with protection against atopy, and we are starting to define the molecular explanation.

Cookson: Just a comment on the epidemiology. The population you examined for the polymorphisms was mixed racially and ethnically. Usually that is a problem for these kinds of studies.

Umetsu: This is a cross-sectional study. We actually broke down all the groups into specific ethnic backgrounds. The frequency of the polymorphism changes a little, but the significance remained in all the groups when we broke it down.

Abbas: Have you done the direct experiments of adding viral particles to T cells and seeing if it changes the cytokine balance?

Umetsu: We are doing this now.

Rao: Epidemiologically, is seropositivity more prevalent if you have the insertion?

Abbas: It's a chicken and egg scenario.

Umetsu: We have looked at this. The percentage of individuals who are seropositive for hepatitis is the same in both groups independent of the insertion. We don't think the frequency of infection is different, but we think the result of infection is quite different in the two groups.

Hafler: There is the flip side of what a virus might do: we know that a viral infection can change the T cell repertoire in subsequent T cell responses, via active viral infection. Without persistence, this could have a major effect on what happens later. This is another mechanism that should be figured out.

Abbas: For all of us who worry about the relationship between infection and autoimmunity, it really is a puzzle that in many of these diseases infections seem to protect while in others they precipitate disease. No one has a clue about the mechanisms. In the transgenic models many of us use, we tend to downplay the significance of infection.

Goodnow: We have lots of clues, it is answers we are short of.

Cookson: Just because you can't see the infections that precipitate disease, it doesn't mean that they aren't there. The patterns of infections have changed. The same thing was seen with clustering of leukaemia cases. Eventually, a particular infection was traced. I imagine that a precipitating infection for type I diabetes might be found. Doesn't multiple sclerosis look like a chronic infection?

Hafler: What has clearly been shown by a number of epidemiological studies is that exacerbations of MS are preceded by upper respiratory infections.

Abbas: The transgenic mouse model that Joan Goverman described was very interesting. This was an MBP-specific TCR transgenic where about half the mice were getting an EAE type of disease. When the lab moved from California to Washington State the disease went away. They had to re-derive all their mice into a pathogen-free colony, and now when they infect the mice half of them would get the disease again. Enterobacter infections will trigger autoimmunity. It is equally clear that in type 1 diabetes in the NOD mouse, infection cures them.

Wicker: Only some infections, not all.

Bowcock: We need to clarify the difference between infections for protection and susceptibility.

Abbas: That is the point. Even within Th1-mediated classic autoimmune disease we can see both effects.

Hafler: I am not sure that you can compare what goes on in NOD and EAE transgenics with human diseases.

Umetsu: Respiratory viral infections can acutely exacerbate asthma in individuals with known asthma. However, the relationship with infection and the development of asthma is unclear. I have a question for the autoimmune people. The prevalence of autoimmune diseases has also gone up considerably, in association with a general drop in infection rates. Is there a hypothesis that there are infections that can protect against the development of autoimmune disease?

Goodnow: Do you see an association between the *Tim* polymorphism and hepatitis A virus in type 1 diabetes which is also rocketing?

Umetsu: That is possible, but it hasn't been looked at.

Rioux: Has anyone done binding studies to show that there is a difference between the insertion and the normal?

Umetsu: A virologist we are working with, Gerardo Kaplan, has looked at the interactions with versions of *Tim1* with or without a mucin domain. The mucin domain seems to be critical for the uncoating of the virus. In the short form the mucin domain is reduced in length by 20%. We think the short form is much less effective in uncoating of the virus. We are looking at this now.

Rioux: Whenever we take our data set and split into two different groups, the one thing we have to worry about is that randomly choosing subgroups wouldn't give you an equally interesting difference between subsets. In other words, if you just randomly select the same number of subsets, would this remain a significant observation?

Umetsu: I rely on our statistician, Neil Risch, who was happy with this analysis. Clearly, it needs to be replicated in other populations. We are doing this.

Rioux: Vijay, when you look at the transgenic expression of the ligand-independent CTLA4 and correct for diabetes, what happens if you look at all the mice? Is there a spectrum of the quantitative trait?

Kuchroo: They all express ligand-independent CTLA4 and it is a puzzle why only 50% are protected. This is a gene that is controlled pretty well, so it must be a threshold of T cell activation. What we are trying to do is to see how the repertoire is evolving in these mice.

Rioux: How do you quantitatively or qualitatively say that they have protection or not?

Kuchroo: The only thing we have to go on is the clinical phenotype: they are sick or not sick. We undertake urinalysis to see sugar levels in urine and we plan to support this with histology.

Large-scale screens for cDNAs with *in vivo* activity

Adrian Ting, Stefan Lichtenthaler, Ramnik Xavier, Soon-Young Na, Shahrooz Rabizadeh, Tara Holmes and Brian Seed[1]

Harvard Medical School, Massachusetts General Hospital, 55 Fruit Street, Molecular Biology, Wellman 911, Boston, MA 02114, USA

> *Abstract.* The pace of biological investigation has been greatly accelerated by technologies that permit comprehensive inventory of gene expression under diverse conditions. We have been developing and using approaches to understand gene function that are based on functional assessments of gene activity, using automated expression cloning followed by gene knockdown using shRNA or by gene knockout. Some recent developments in expression screens and methods to expedite the formation of targeted mutations in mice are discussed. A resource for large scale quantitative profiling of mRNA abundance is also described.
>
> *2005 The genetics of autoimmunity. Wiley, Chichester (Novartis Foundation Symposium 267) p 219–230*

Expression cloning, the isolation of cDNAs, genomic DNAs, or RNAs having or directing the synthesis of a biological activity of interest, has been practised for over 20 years with considerable success (Jolly et al 1983, Aruffo & Seed 1987). However, for the most part it has been practised with a single object or desired activity in mind. Only recently has expression cloning come to be applied to the systematic itemization of large collections of cDNAs that may have related activities *in vivo* (Chanda et al 2003, Huang et al 2004). Many of the strategies and rationales for historical expression cloning practices have had to be modified to accommodate larger scale programmes. For example, when the target of interest is a particular biological activity for which it can be reasonably anticipated that there are no more than a few candidate cDNAs, the objective of the screen is usually to identify any one member of the target group, possibly to be followed by enumeration of the remaining members by homology or database mining. In

---

[1]This paper was presented at the symposium by Brian Seed to whom correspondence should be addressed.

such cases it is usually sufficient to find one cDNA, and hence physical selection methods, such as sorting, panning, or metabolic selections, which typically result in the isolation of one or at most a small number of independent isolates, are appropriate. However, physical selections frequently result in a winnowing or narrowing of the candidate DNA pools that selectively favours the most robust clones or the clones with the most potent activity. In comprehensive screens, a large number of weaker clones with less potent activity are of interest and need to be retained and analysed. In this setting physical selection methods can be detrimental, and non-destructive methods, such as sib-selection or screening, are preferable. Such methods are sometimes called pool subdivision screens, and have the attractive property that they allow the collection of all clones that have the capacity to exceed some sensitivity threshold, typically determined by the size of the pool and the signal to noise properties of the assay. Sib-selection screens are more laborious than physical or metabolic selections, however, as the creation of the master collection of pools and the subsequent hit deconvolution usually require very large numbers of DNA preparations. As a result, sib-selection screens are ideal candidates for laboratory automation. Automation poses hurdles of its own. The equipment is frequently expensive and the methodologies required by robotic procedures do not always conform well to familiar lab techniques. It is not uncommon to find that processes that work well when performed manually do not work at all, or work very poorly, when placed in an automation setting. In this contribution we describe our initial experiences with conducting expression cloning screens for cDNAs having a desired activity, initially by manual methods, and subsequently by automated methods.

Among the first projects initiated in this programme was a screen for cDNAs that induce the expression of a transcriptional reporter dependent on activation of NF-κB. The reporter was constructed from a multimerized NF-κB binding site placed upstream from a strong synthetic basal promoter (TATA element). The initial readout was expression of codon-optimized green fluorescent protein (GFP) (Haas et al 1996), and both transient and stably transfected reporter lines were used. In these studies cDNA libraries that had been prepared by a method that gives a high yield of full-length clones were employed. Two types of libraries were chosen, from activated human T cells and from human brain tissues. The former was chosen for its proximity to the biological system of interest, T cell activation, and the latter was chosen because of the diversity of the mRNA known to be expressed in the tissue source. Pools of clones were assembled by plating approximately 500 colonies per 10 cm bacterial plate, and the DNA prepared by harvesting the cells from each plate and performing standard non-automated purifications. Pools were transfected into cells in culture using the calcium phosphate coprecipitation method, and the transfected cultures were inspected manually for the presence or absence of GFP expression. Pools that seemed to contain rare cells expressing GFP were selected for subdivision. The pooled DNA was transformed into *Escherichia coli* and a fivefold coverage of the initial pool size was replated, in pools that were five- to 10-fold smaller than the initial pool. Fivefold coverage should result in the loss of any one clone at a frequency of less than 1%. The subclone pools were worked up in the same way, followed by another round of division and then a final round in which individual clones were analysed. The hit density in the activated T cell library was approximately twofold lower than in the brain library, but higher than anticipated: approximately one in 3000 brain library clones had activity. Several known inducers of NF-κB were detected in this screen, validating the approach and building confidence in the general approach. Figure 1 illustrates the appearance of pools in the successive steps toward isolation of a cDNA clone encoding BCMA, an atypical member of the tumour necrosis factor (TNF) receptor superfamily.

To reduce the labour involved, as many of the steps as possible were automated. The libraries were picked robotically with a Genetix Q-Bot into 384 well plates and grown individually. The resulting cultures were pooled robotically into groupings of 96 wells each, in two dimensions. Initial pooling attempts were made by using pin transfer heads, but these were found to have high variability and were susceptible to carry-over cross-contamination. Although pin transfer was attractive because of its low cost, it was ultimately abandoned in favour of a liquid handling device that was programmed to rinse the pipette tips by aspiration of bleach followed by water and ethanol. Carryover was negligible under these conditions and the cost was supportable because individual tips could be reused extensively.

The two dimensions in which the pools were formed were called the 'plate to well' and the 'well to well' dimensions, conforming to their origin in the pooling scheme. In the 'plate to well' dimension, a fraction of each of 96 of the 384 well cultures was removed and expelled into a single well. This was done with a single 96 head pipetting tool mounted on a robotic liquid handling platform (Beckman Coulter Biomek FX). In the 'well to well' dimension, a fraction of each of the wells in the same relative location on 96 successive plates was removed, and expelled into a single well. Thus in the 'well to well' pool, each of the, for example, 'A3' wells would have come from well A3 of 96 consecutive plates, whereas in the 'plate to well' pool, each well would contain one-quarter of an entire 384 well plate. An assemblage of $96 \times 96 = 9216$ clones are then screened in 192 transfections, comprising 96 well to well pools, and 96 plate to well pools. If there were to be a single hit in the 96 well to well pools and a single hit in the 96 plate to well pools, the locations of those hits would identify the plate and well of the active cDNA uniquely among the 9216 clones sampled. In practice,

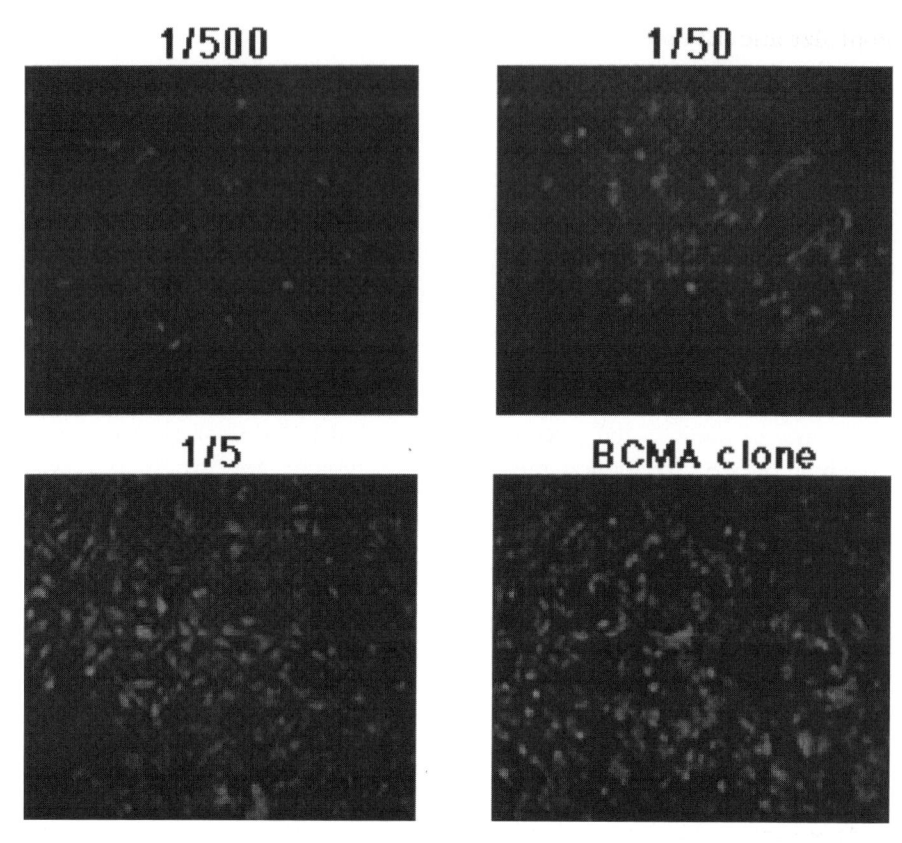

FIG. 1. Isolation of a cDNA clone encoding BCMA. Shown are representative images of fluorescence micrographs of pools containing BCMA at the indicated approximate dilutions.

screenings generate multiple hits per 96×96 pool, and from 9216 clones, historical rates predicted three hits per NF-κB screen. To accommodate the variability (and to some extent, imprecision) of determination of activity, the five most active wells were chosen from each dimension, and the 25 possible intersections of the well to well and plate to well pools were individually assayed for activity. Because it was found that several of the initially identified cDNA clones that activated NF-κB also induced apoptosis, and that apoptosis tended to decrease the signal due to GFP, we prepared cell lines stably transfected with Bcl-X$_L$ (Boise et al 1993) and CrmA, two anti-apoptotic proteins that act on the mitochondrial release and caspase activation steps, respectively, of the apoptotic cascade.

Pool size and hit density

In an ordered pool deconvolution strategy to interrogate x^2 clones requires $2x$ transfections of pools of x clones followed by y^2 transfections of the possible locations of the y hits in the pool. Thus if the pool is too large, most of the work will lie in the individual deconvolution transfections. Ignoring the possibility that a positive row or column can harbour two hits (a reasonable approximation when the hit density is low), the total number of transfections is $2x + y^2$, and the frequency of positive clones is $f=y/x^2$. We would like to minimize the transfection frequency, which is the total number of transfections divided by the total number of clones. This is

$$(2x+y^2)/x^2 = 2/x + f^2x^2$$

Minimizing this function means setting the first derivative with respect to x to 0, or

$$-2/x^2 + 2f^2x = 0$$

which implies

$$f^2/x^3 = 1$$

a surprisingly simple result that indicates the optimal pool size (column or row length) is $x=f^{-2/3}$. For a hit frequency of 1/5000, x should be ~292, for example, whereas for a hit frequency of 1/1000, x should be 100.

At present our hit densities in a variety of screens, including assays for secreted proteins, transcription factor activation, and apoptosis, have been relatively high, perhaps surprisingly so, on the order of 1/1000 to 1/2500 clones. Based on these figures, a pool size of 96 is appropriate.

A simple example can help illustrate the contributing factors above. Suppose the hit density is 1/1000, but the pool size is 400. Then to screen 400×400=160 000 clones requires only 800 primary transfections, from which 160 positives emerge. However there are 160×160 possible intersections, leading to an additional 25 600 transfections to sort out the true positives, for a total of 26 400 transfections to enumerate all of the positive clones. If the same 160 000 clones are broken into 16 subpools of 100×100, screening will require 3200 primary transfections with an average hit density of 10 positives each. The 10 positives translate to 100 intersections for each of the 16 subpools, or another 1600 transfections, for a total of 4800 transfections to define all the positive clones. Hence if the hit density is 1/1000, the required number of transfections to exhaustively enumerate all hits in a 400×400 matrix is over five times greater than the number of transfections to enumerate all hits in the same number of clones at a pool size of 100.

Once the candidate intersections of positive rows and columns have been identified, the filter mats are pulled and a small circle of each of the desired spotted dried lysates is punched out. The circle is rinsed in water and eluted by allowing it to stand in a small volume of Tris/EDTA. The resulting eluate typically provides between 10–100 colonies upon transformation into chemically competent bacteria of modest competency. Individual colonies are inoculated into 96 deep well blocks and grown in a high-density oxygenated shaker for DNA preparation. The individual DNA preparations are tested for activity and sequenced.

Selected results for some preliminary screens of approximately one million clones each are shown below. In picking projects we typically amass clones in modules of $384 \times 384 = 147\ 456$ clones, and 7 modules are collected (1 032 192 clones) per library. The preliminary screens described below have been carried out on clones picked from a human brain library, which has a high diversity relative to other libraries we have evaluated. We have recently completed primary screens for genes that induce NF-κB and serum response element (SRE) transcriptional activity in the complete set of a million clones and are analysing the individual transfectants.

Screening by microscopy allowed clones that have a predominantly intracellular action to be distinguished from those that show a predominantly extracellular action. In the former case, a fraction of the cells appear positive, whereas in the latter, a nearly uniform induction is seen. This is because the non-transfected cells can respond nearly as efficiently as the transfected cells when the cDNA encodes a secreted agent, such as a pro-inflammatory cytokine. Figure 2 illustrates this with a representative image of a primary screen field from a hit plate containing cDNA encoding a secreted protein, compared to a hit plate containing a cDNA encoding an intracellular mediator.

However, visual inspection screens can be time consuming and more challenging to automate compared to screens based on more easily automated quantitative measurements, such as ELISA or enzymatic reporter activity. Reporters based on the *Photinus* luciferase (de Wet et al 1985) were found to be sensitive and relatively fit for automation. Some of the variability inherent in making luciferase determinations from cellular lysates was reduced by performing the assays in triplicate and ranking the activity numerically for each plate. The numerical rank orders were added for the triplicate plates and the wells with the lowest score were chosen for deconvolution. The non-parametric rank order test was more robust than a number of other parametric measures that proved to be vulnerable to differences in counting efficiency, reaction composition and other variables that produced significant plate-to-plate variation. Transient cotransfection of the reporter construct and the library pools worked well in this setting. In some screens a normalization for transfection

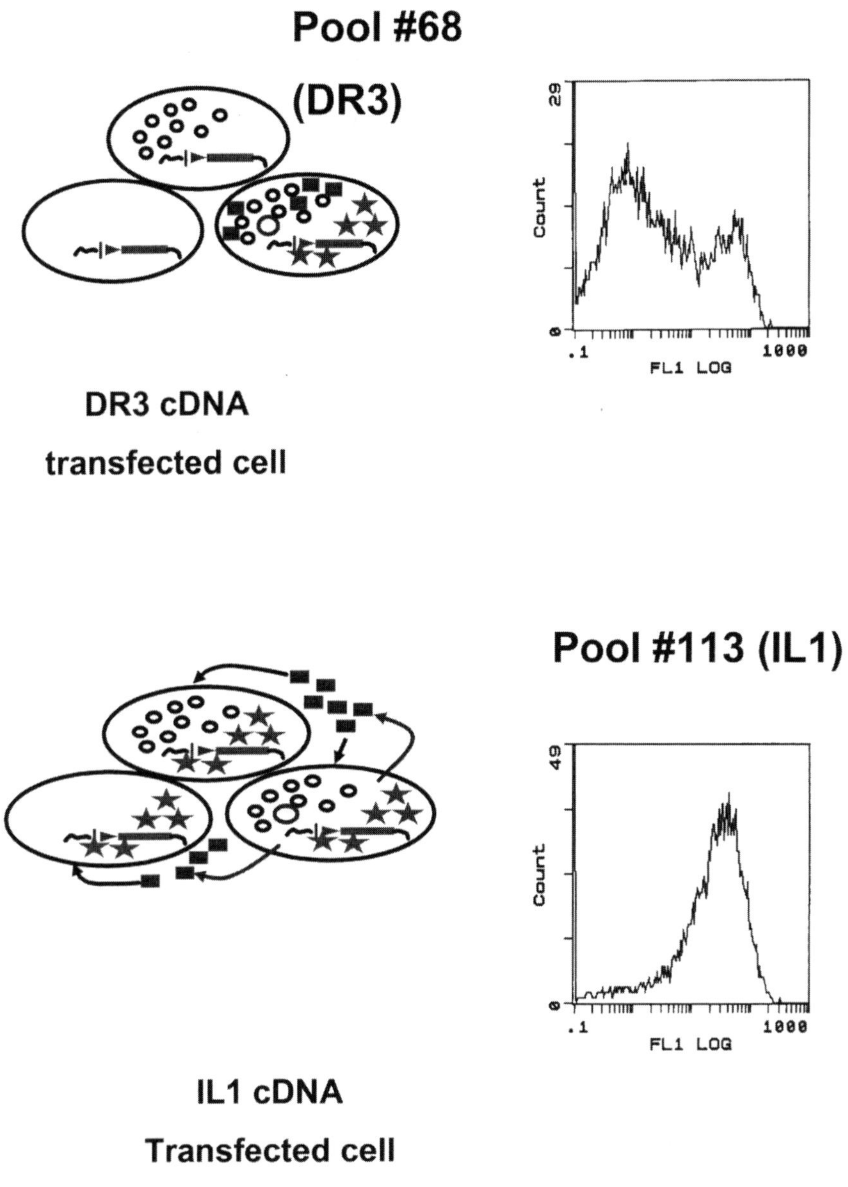

FIG. 2. Visual identification of a secreted effector compared to an intracellular mediator.

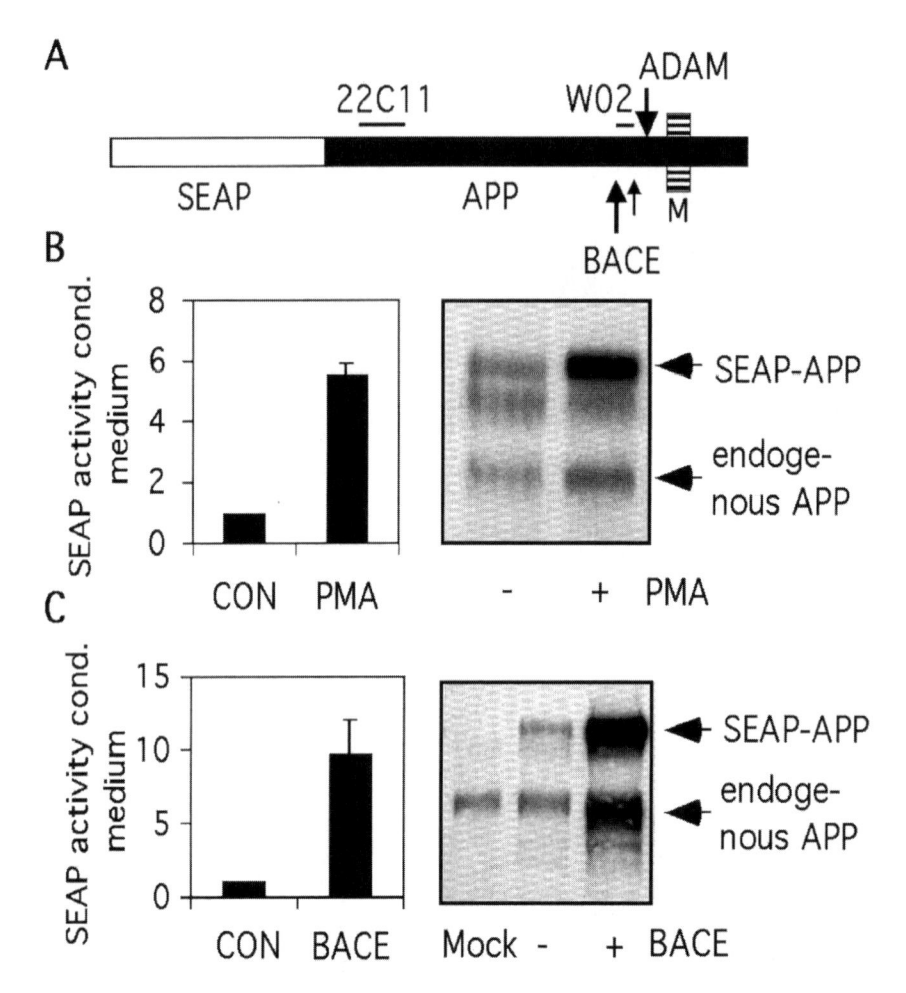

FIG. 3. Alkaline phosphatase reporter assay for the ectodomain shedding of the amyloid precursor protein (APP). (A) Schematic drawing of the SEAP-APP fusion protein. The ectodomain of secretory alkaline phosphatase (SEAP) was fused to the N-terminus of full-length APP695 lacking its signal peptide. The horizontal bar indicates the epitope recognized by the monoclonal antibody 22C11. Arrows indicate the proteolytic cleavage sites of ADAM-metalloproteases and BACE within the APP ectodomain. BACE has a major and a minor (small arrow) cleavage site. M: membrane. (B, C) 293 cells stably expressing SEAP-APP were treated with (B) the phorbol ester PMA (1 μM) or (C) transfected with a BACE-encoding plasmid or control vector. PMA and the overexpression of BACE stimulate the secretion of SEAP-APP as measured by Western blotting using antibody 22C11 (right panels) or by the increased alkaline phosphatase activity in the conditioned medium relative to the control cells (left panels). The phosphatase activity represents the mean of two independent experiments. Mock: vector transfected control cells only secrete the endogenous APP but no SEAP-APP.

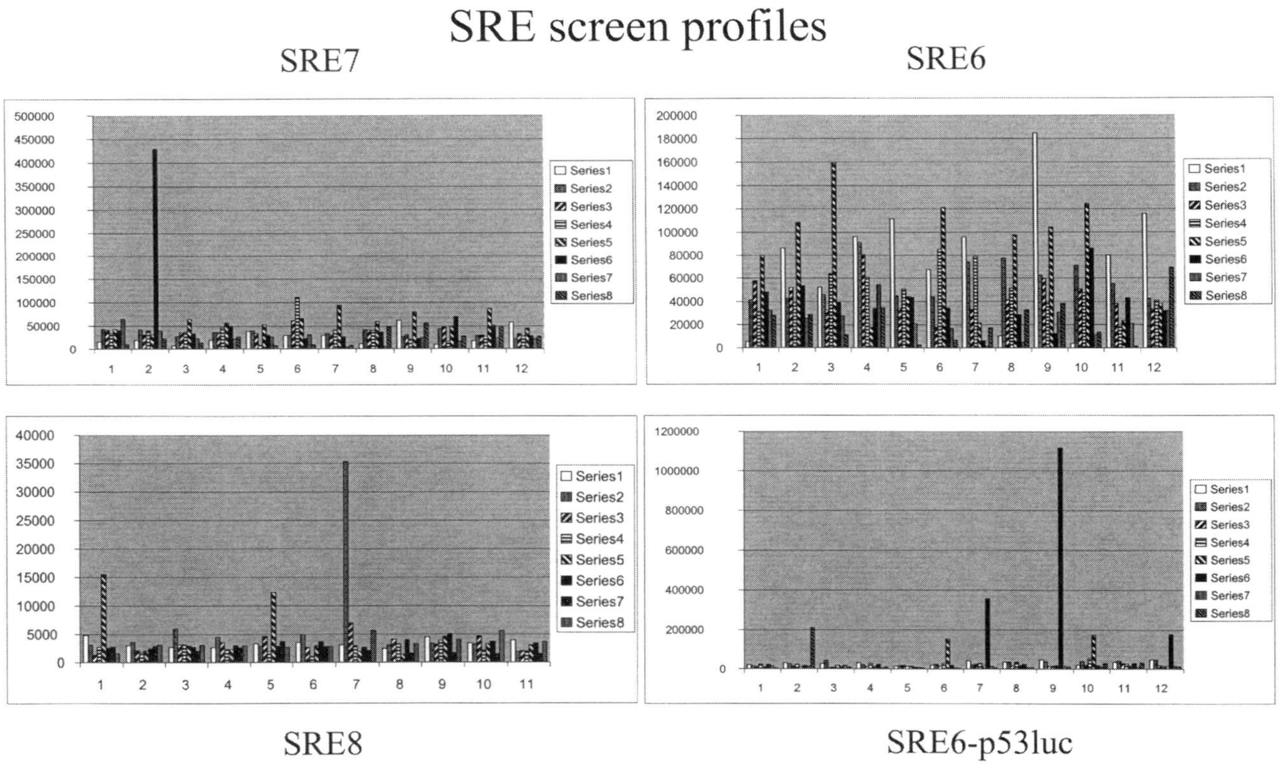

LARGE-SCALE SCREENS 227

FIG. 4. Contrast of SRE and p53 screen profiles in primary screen. Top, screen for activators of the serum response element. Bottom, screen for activators of p53 transcriptional activity.

efficiency using the *Renilla* luciferase was used. Because the substrate requirements are different — *Photinus* luciferase requiring luciferin and ATP (de Wet et al 1985) and *Renilla* luciferase requiring coelenterazine (Matthews et al 1977) — it is possible to conduct both assays sequentially using the same sample. However, variation in the activity of the latter led to greater variability, and because of the increased expense this approach was not made standard.

Several screens have been carried out for localization or functional activity that does not depend on a transcriptional activation. For example, a screen to identify cDNAs that have the capacity to increase the release of the extracellular domains of integral membrane proteins was undertaken, using a model engineered transmembrane protein. The model protein consisted of the catalytic domain of alkaline phosphatase joined to the extracellular, transmembrane and intracellular domains of the amyloid precursor protein, APP (Fig. 3). This protein showed little basal release into the medium (quantified by alkaline phosphatase activity), and release could be augmented by exposure of the cells to mediators known to facilitate ectodomain shedding, or to cDNAs known to have this property. Among the clones in an initial screen of a brain library were two independent isolates of *BACE1*, previously shown to encode a β-secretase responsible for the formation of the amyloid β fragment (Sinha et al 1999, Vassar et al 1999, Hussain et al 1999), as well as one clone encoding APLP1, an amyloid precursor like protein. The discovery of the former validated the screen and the identification of the latter suggested there may be regulatory circuits that heighten ectodomain shedding in the presence of excess substrate. In addition to these cDNAs a number of novel cDNAs were found, as well as a few whose activity had been previously demonstrated to lead to ectodomain release, such as MEKK1 (Liao et al 2004) and PKA (Kumar et al 1999).

Among the transcriptional assays considerable variation was found in the behaviour of reporters and the signal-to-noise levels of the pool transfections. The NF-κB screen, for example, gave large numbers of hits which resulted in a continuum of activities in the primary screening wells, making discrimination of the top five wells sometimes challenging. A screen for activators of serum response element (SRE) dependent transcription was consistently cleaner, with a relatively few high amplitude responses observed in primary screens (Fig. 4). Hit deconvolution was more straightforward with this screen, which was validated by the discovery of several known activators of the serum response.

In summary, automated expression screens promise to reveal activity of cDNAs or genomic DNAs in a variety of useful contexts. The application of robotics and laboratory automation principles is essential to make full use of this powerful technology. Adaptation to automation is not always straightforward and requires time and careful attention to all steps. However, the result can be a dramatic improvement in efficiency.

References

Aruffo A, Seed B 1987 Molecular cloning of a CD28 cDNA by a high-efficiency COS cell expression system. Proc Natl Acad Sci USA 84:8573–8577

Boise LH, Gonzalez-Garcia M, Postema CE et al 1993 bcl-x, a bcl-2-related gene that functions as a dominant regulator of apoptotic cell death. Cell 74:597–608

Chanda SK, White S, Orth AP et al 2003 Genome-scale functional profiling of the mammalian AP-1 signaling pathway. Proc Natl Acad Sci USA 100:12153–12158

de Wet JR, Wood KV, Helinski DR, DeLuca M 1985 Cloning of firefly luciferase cDNA and the expression of active luciferase in *Escherichia coli*. Proc Natl Acad Sci USA 82:7870–7873

Haas J, Park EC, Seed B 1996 Codon usage limitation in the expression of HIV-1 envelope glycoprotein. Curr Biol 6:315–324

Huang Q, Raya A, DeJesus P et al 2004 Identification of p53 regulators by genome-wide functional analysis. Proc Natl Acad Sci USA 101:3456–3461

Hussain I, Powell D, Howlett DR et al 1999 Identification of a novel aspartic protease (Asp 2) as beta-secretase. Mol Cell Neurosci 14:419–427

Jolly DJ, Okayama H, Berg P et al 1983 Isolation and characterization of a full-length expressible cDNA for human hypoxanthine phosphoribosyl transferase. Proc Natl Acad Sci USA 80:477–481

Kumar A, La Rosa FG, Hovland AR et al 1999 Adenosine 3′,5′-cyclic monophosphate increases processing of amyloid precursor protein (APP) to beta-amyloid in neuroblastoma cells without changing APP levels or expression of APP mRNA. Neurochem Res 24:1209–1215

Liao YF, Wang BJ, Cheng HT, Kuo LH, Wolfe MS 2004 Tumor necrosis factor-alpha, interleukin-1beta, and interferon-gamma stimulate gamma-secretase-mediated cleavage of amyloid precursor protein through a JNK-dependent MAPK pathway. J Biol Chem 279:49523–49532

Matthews JC, Hori K, Cormier MJ 1977 Substrate and substrate analogue binding properties of *Renilla* luciferase. Biochemistry 16:5217–5220

Sinha S, Anderson JP, Barbour R et al 1999 Purification and cloning of amyloid precursor protein beta-secretase from human brain. Nature 402:537–540

Vassar R, Bennett BD, Babu-Khan S et al 1999 Beta-secretase cleavage of Alzheimer's amyloid precursor protein by the transmembrane aspartic protease BACE. Science 286:735–741

DISCUSSION

Rao: There are obviously advantages and disadvantages to your overexpression strategy. I am assuming your library is pretty much full length. One would imagine you could put in a kinase by overexpression and it wouldn't work. First, you would need full length kinase, and second you would need the effector which activates it. Have you thought of a knockdown or RNAi-type screen?

Seed: Yes, we have an effector and we are working on that.

Rao: The alternative technology is to use the same kind of RNAi screen in *Drosophila*, find the *Drosophila* proteins, and then go after the mammalian homologues.

Seed: The pathways don't always match up all that well.

Rao: I agree. Some are conserved, though.

Seed: I suppose as a way of collecting candidate genes it is robust, easy and cheap.

Abbas: If we can get a read-out for a tolerance signal, is it conceivable that we can take cDNAs from patients with autoimmunity versus controls, and then do this kind of screening using that readout to ask who is deficient in tolerance signals? We could identify individual genes using this sort of biological screen.

Seed: I think we would probably be a little more catholic in our approach. The idea that the cDNA is likely to be overexpressed is itself a hypothesis. By taking an unbiased look at all possible cDNAs that could impinge on a pathway we may be in a better position. There are examples where we have syndromes or cell types that have unique expression of cDNAs, but we would like to get around this.

Rao: What you would need to do in that case is to find a biochemical marker for tolerance in one or other cell type, and then put cells of that nature through the screen.

Abbas: As complements to genomic mapping that idea is an interesting one. I think we may not know enough about the pathways and the markers to distinguish between tolerance and non-tolerance, though.

Goodnow: I noticed in some of your transfections you were including CremA and Bcl-XL expressing cells. Do you do that all the time?

Seed: Yes. The reason for this is that it has increased our hit rate. This is probably because there are a reasonable number of apoptotic genes out there. Particularly in an NF-κB screen where we started many of these inducers have dual action.

Goodnow: If you are trying to make retroviruses, is it worth including those things when you are packaging in 293 cells?

Seed: That's what we do. We typically use the Bcl-XL CrmA cells as our platform.

Genomic mining of new genes and pathways in innate and adaptive immunity

Jenny Ting

Department of Microbiology–Immunology, Lineberger Comprehensive Cancer Center, University of North Carolina at Chapel Hill, Chapel Hill, NC 27599, USA

> *Abstract.* Plant disease resistant (R) genes constitute a large family that mediates host response to bacteria, viruses and fungi. Large mammalian proteins containing a nucleotide binding domain (NBD) and C-terminal leucine-rich repeats (LRRs) are similar in structure to the TLR/NBD/LRR subfamily of R proteins and have been suggested as a link between innate and acquired immunity. Because of our long term interest in one of these, the class II transactivator (CIITA), and recent reports linking mutations in two new NBD/LRR proteins (Nod2/CARD 15 and CIAS 1/cryopyrin) to various autoimmune and inflammatory disorders, we have performed a comprehensive search of the human genome and found a multigene family which we termed the CATERPILLAR (CARD, Transcription Enhancer, R[purine]-binding, Pyrin, Lots of Leucine Regions)family. The N-termini of these genes are varied although the majority have a pyrin domain and few have a CARD domain. The genomic organization of these genes demonstrates a high degree of conservation with the NBD encoded as a single large exon and the LRRs encoded in two basic arrangements. Detailed analysis and new functional data regarding a number of the CATERPILLAR proteins will be described, including CIITA, cryopyrin and Monarch 1.
>
> *2005 The genetics of autoimmunity. Wiley, Chichester (Novartis Foundation Symposium 267) p 231–241*

Plant disease resistance genes

Disease resistance in plants is mediated by a large family of R genes encoding R proteins (Fig. 1). These proteins consist of different conserved structural domains. The largest group of R proteins contains a nucleotide binding domain (NBD)/C-terminal leucine-rich repeats (LRRs) structure and constitutes the major immune defence network. The N-terminal domain of this subclass of R proteins can be of different domains, the most common is a TLR-IL1R (TIR) domain found in insect/mammalian Toll-like receptors (TLRs) and the interleukin (IL)1 receptor. Others have a coiled-coil structure including leucine zippers. R genes are crucial for immune defence against bacteria, virus, fungus, nematodes, insects, oomycetes and even synthetic products such as insecticides (Nimchuk et al 2003). As a reflection of their importance, they comprise 1% of the *Arabidopsis* genome and to date 125+ R genes have been found in this genome (Meyers et al 1999). The rice genome has an even larger number of R proteins, estimated to be 600+ R genes. R proteins mediate the recognition of pathogen-derived molecules, which are encoded by the A*vr* (avirulence) genes, although direct recognition has not been demonstrated for most R proteins, and even in rare cases where recognition is demonstrated, *in vivo* evidence is lacking. The avirulence designation arises from the observation that R proteins can neutralize the effects of pathogen, rendering the pathogen avirulent. In this scenario, the *Avr* gene product elicits a protective defence response in the host that expresses the appropriate R gene product, leading to a hypersensitive response (HR) that includes programmed cell death of the infected cells, and a limiting of pathogen spread.

Identification of mammalian R-like proteins: CIITA and the CATERPILLER family

The identification of the CATERPILLER (CARD, Transcription Enhancer, R[purine]-binding, Pyrin, Lots of Leucine Repeats) gene family (Harton et al 2002) was initiated because of our longstanding interest in the class II transactivator (CIITA) (Ting & Trowsdale 2002). CIITA is a founding member of a new family of NTPases that consists of NAIP, CIITA, HET-E and TP1 (Koonin & Aravind 2000). The NACHT motif consists of seven signature motifs, including the ATP/GTPase-specific P-loop, the Walker A and B motifs Mg^{2+}-binding site and five more specific motifs. Structure–function analyses of CIITA have revealed the presence of both conventional domains expected of transcription activators, such as the acidic domain at the N-terminus (residues 1–125) that is required for transactivation function, and unorthodox sequences, such as a mid-section of the protein defined as a GTP-binding domain (residues 337–702), which exhibits weak GTP-binding activity (Chin et al 1997, Harton et al 2002) *in vitro* and *in vivo* (Fig. 2). One of the functions of this domain is in protein oligomerization. We suggest that the multimerization of CIITA may be similar to the induced proximity of Apaf1 to enhance interactions with other proteins in the complex. CIITA also contains a C-terminal leucine rich region (LRR) which affects nuclear translocation and the self-association process.

When CIITA was first described, no other mammalian gene with a similar structure was found. When the NOD1 (nucleotide oligomerization domain) and NOD2 proteins were discovered, it was first noted that CARD/NOD proteins shared structural homology with CIITA in the presence of the NBD/LRR (Nickerson et al 2001). Simultaneously, our laboratory was also searching for other genes that may share a similar domain structure as CIITA. Using the NBD

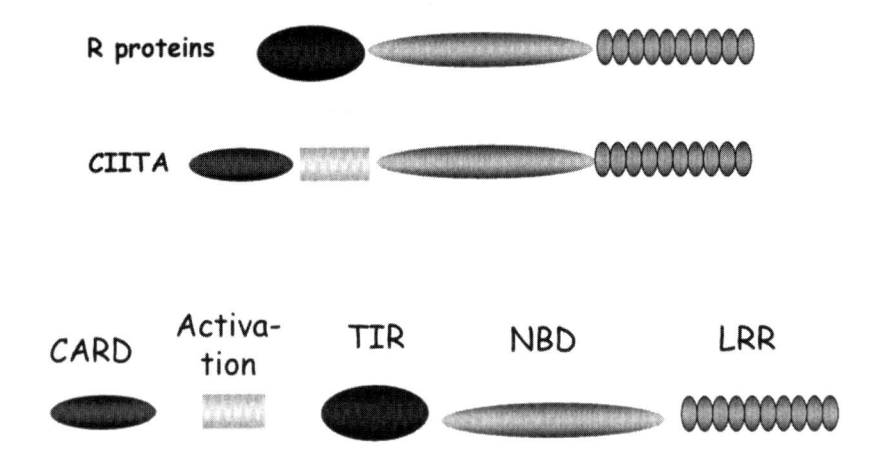

FIG. 1. CIITA and homology to plant R proteins. CIITA bears strong homology to the large family of TIR–NBD–LRR subclass of R proteins found in plants. These proteins are believed to mediate the recognition of products from pathogens, although direct recognition does not take place with regards to most R proteins. CARD, caspase activating and recruiting domain; NBD, nucleotide binding domain; LRR, leucine rich repeats.

and LRR as search criteria, we have found at least 22 known and novel family members (Harton et al 2002). Subsequently others have found a similar family and called these the NOD family (Inohara & Nunez 2003). Another group has delineated the pyrin–NBD-LRR subclass as the NALP protein (Tschopp et al 2003). A few of the genes have also been named PAAD (Pawlowski et al 2001).

Upon surveying these proteins, we found that the CATERPILLER proteins are linked to a limited number of distinct N-terminal domains. CIITA has an authentic acidic transactivation domain found in many strong transcriptional activators. A few of the CATERPILLER proteins have a CARD domain. Most have a pyrin domain, defined as having structural similarity to the PYRIN protein. Mutations in the *PYRIN* gene are genetically associated with susceptibility to familial Mediterranean fever (MEFV), a type of hereditary periodic inflammatory disorder (Ben-Chetrit et al 2002). Most recently, a mutation of this gene in mice produced exaggerated responses to LPS, suggesting that it is a negative regulator of inflammatory responses (Chae et al 2003). This raises the intriguing possibility that other family members may be critical in the control of inflammatory and immune responses.

The association of CATERPILLER genes with immune disorders

One of the most intriguing features of these CATERPILLER genes is their association with a number of inherited immunological disorders (Fig. 3). CIITA

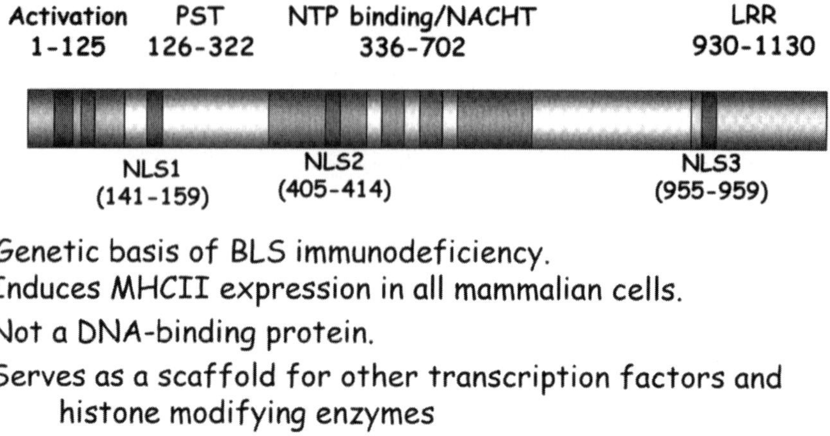

Activation	PST	NTP binding/NACHT		LRR
1-125	126-322	336-702		930-1130

NLS1	NLS2	NLS3
(141-159)	(405-414)	(955-959)

Genetic basis of BLS immunodeficiency.
- Induces MHCII expression in all mammalian cells.
- Not a DNA-binding protein.
- Serves as a scaffold for other transcription factors and histone modifying enzymes

FIG. 2. CIITA the master regulator of MHCII. CIITA has a number of important domains, including a conventional acid activation domain found in most transcriptional activators, several nuclear localization sequences (NLS) and a proline–serine–threonine rich region. However it also contains the signature nucleotide binding domain (also known as NACHT, see text) and leucine rich repeats.

is the master regulator of MHC-II genes (Boss 1999, Steimle et al 1993, Reith & Mach 2001, Ting & Trowsdale 2002). Genetic lesions in this gene result in the immunodeficiency Type II bare lymphocyte syndrome (BLS) (Group A). Mice or humans lacking CIITA have greatly reduced (>99%) *MHC-II* expression. Mutations in *NOD2/CARD15* have been implicated in susceptibility to the inflammatory bowel disease, Crohn's and a granulomatous disorder known as Blau syndrome (Beutler 2001, Hugot et al 2001, Miceli-Richard et al 2001, Ogura et al 2001). Most recently, mutations in the *CIAS* (cold-induced autoinflammatory syndrome) gene, which encodes *CIAS*/cryopyrin/*PYPAF1*, have been found to predispose patients to a variety of autoinflammatory disorders (Dode et al 2002, Feldmann et al 2002, Hoffman et al 2001).

In addition to their linkage to immune disorders, CIITA, NOD2 and CIAS also share a restricted expression pattern in cells of the immune system. CIITA is expressed by monocytes/macrophages, dendritic cells and lymphocytes, while NOD2 and CIAS are primarily expressed by monocytes (Ogura et al 2001, Manji et al 2002). These studies all support the strong possibility that other CATERPILLER gene family members may be important players both in the maintenance of normal immune responses and the onset of inflammatory disorders. More recently, the NOD1 protein has been found to mediate the recognition of a peptidoglycan derived primarily from Gram-negative bacteria

GENOMIC MINING

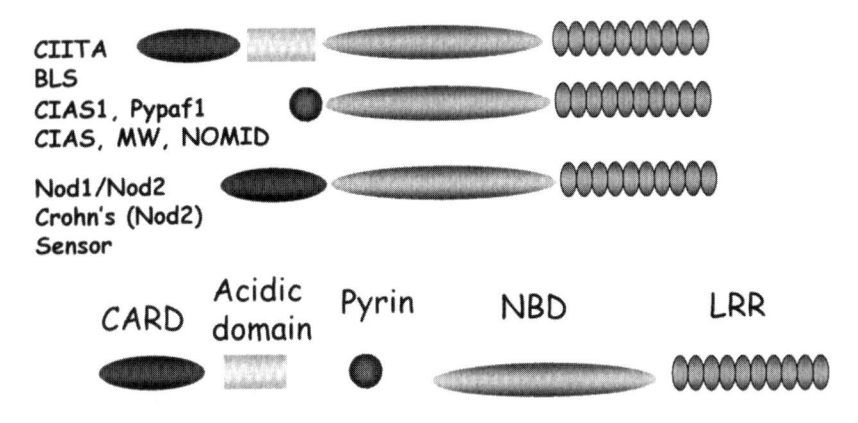

FIG. 3. CATERPILLER family members and disease association. A cartoon depicting the different domain structure present in three CATERPILLER family members. Each is associated with an immunological disorder. BLS, bare lymphocyte syndrome; CIAS, cold induced autoinflammatory syndrome; MW, Muckle–Wells disease; NOMID, neonatal onset of multisystem inflammatory disease (also known as CINCA, chronic infantile neurologic, cutaneous, articular syndrome). The NOD2 protein is also found to be a sensor of bacterial-derived muramyl dipeptide.

(Girardin et al 2003, Chamaillard et al 2003), while NOD2 mediates the recognition of muramyl dipeptide (Girardin et al 2003, Inohara et al 2003). These findings support the provocative but seminal idea that this family of proteins serves as intracellular sensors of bacterial products.

The CATERPILLER gene, *Monarch 1/PYPAF7*

The CATERPILLER gene, *Monarch 1/PYPAF7*, is primarily expressed by cells of innate immunity, namely, granulocytes and monocytes (Williams et al 2003). The gene sequence for *Monarch 1* was deposited into the NCBI database by us and by Millenium Pharmaceuticals under the name *PYPAF7* (Wang et al 2002). Monarch 1/PYPAF7 has the typical pyrin, NBD and LRR configuration. Unpublished data indicate that *Monarch 1* mRNA level is rapidly reduced by agonists of TLR2 and TLR4 1 h post-stimulation, while cells transfected with *Monarch 1* show reduced activation of AP-1 and NF-κB. These experiments indicate that Monarch 1 may constitute a negative regulatory factor of the TLR pathway, and its presence can prevent inflammatory responses from occurring. However the function of Monarch 1 or other pyrin family members may be dependent on the existence of other modifiers. For example, the Millennium group has found that NF-κB activity is greatly induced when Monarch 1 is co-expressed with another pyrin-containing protein called ASC (apoptosis-associated speck-like protein containing a CARD) (Wang et al 2002). Another recent analysis indicates that the role of ASC in modulating NF-κB activation is dependent on the cellular context (Stehlik et al 2002). While the coexpression of ASC with CIAS increases NF-κB activity, ASC alone has an inhibitory influence on NF-κB activation by various proinflammatory stimuli, including tumour necrosis factor (TNF)α, IL1β and lipopolysaccharide (LPS). These studies forecast a complex array of interactions among the CATERPILLER protein family with ASC and other yet-to-be-identified partners.

The CATERPILLER gene, *CIAS/cryopyrin*

The *CIAS* or *cryopyrin* gene encodes a protein with an N-terminal pyrin domain, followed by a mid-NBD and a C-terminal LRR sequence. Mutations in *CIAS* have been genetically associated with several autoinflammatory diseases, such as Muckle–Wells syndrome (MWS), familial cold autoinflammatory syndrome (FCAS), and chronic infantile neurological cutaneous and articular syndromes (CINCA)/neonatal-onset multisystem inflammatory disease (NOMID) (Hoffman et al 2001, Feldmann et al 2002, Aksentijevich et al 2002). Most of these mutations are concentrated in the NBD region. Initial characterization of the relevance of CIAS has focused on its role in TLR signalling pathways and host innate immune defence mechanisms. CIAS is expressed primarily in cells of myeloid lineage (Wang et al 2002). Data from our laboratory show that several agonists of the TLR pathway induce CIAS expression (O'Connor et al 2003). Initial biochemical characterizations of CIAS function have been performed by transfecting expression plasmids into non-myeloid cells. These studies indicate a negative regulatory role on NF-κB activity and therefore a role in the control of inflammatory responses. This is reminiscent of the recently described IRAK-M molecule, which is a negative regulator of the endotoxin response and is also induced by TLR agonists (Kobayashi et al 2002). The negative regulatory role of CIAS is consistent with the presence of overzealous inflammation in autoimmune diseases where it is mutated. Two recent analyses of variant forms of CIAS1 found in autoinflammtory diseases provide evidence that the disease-associated form of CIAS1 spontaneously activates proinflammatory responses (Dowds et al 2004, Agostini et al 2004). One found that variant forms of CIAS caused enhanced NF-κB activation and IL1 production while another showed that monocytes from a CIAS patient produce more IL1β in response to LPS.

CATERPILLER proteins and the generation of diversity

Several domains of the CATERPILLER proteins have been proposed to be important for pathogen recognition, self oligomerization and association with other proteins, including other CATERPILLER proteins (Damiano et al 2004). Heterodimer formation among the various CATERPILLER proteins may provide a powerful way to exponentially increase the recognition repertoire of this protein. In addition, many of the genes coding for these proteins undergo differential splicing particularly in the LRR domain, to create a large number of variant proteins. These may also have different recognition and signalling properties. Finally, since these genes reside predominantly in the subtelomeric region of the chromosome, it is possible that they undergo increased recombination and may be more susceptible to mutagenesis, thus increasing the chance of allelic differences.

In summary, a large number of mammalian genes and proteins that may be the evolutionary equivalents of plant disease resistance genes have now been discovered and found to have an increasing role in inflammatory disorders ranging from periodic fever to inflammatory bowel disease to immunodeficiency. It is likely that these proteins will not only control innate immunity, but also affect adaptive immunity in a direct or indirect way, and rival TLRs in their importance.

Acknowledgements

I thank past and present members of my laboratory who have been instrumental in conducting the work described here. Without their enthusiasm, creativity, dedication and insight, this work would not be possible. The work is supported by NIH grants.

References

Agostini L, Martinon F, Burns K et al 2004 NALP3 forms an IL-1beta-processing inflammasome with increased activity in Muckle–Wells autoinflammatory disorder. Immunity 20:319–325

Aksentijevich I, Nowak M, Mallah M et al 2002 *De novo* CIAS1 mutations, cytokine activation, and evidence for genetic heterogeneity in patients with neonatal-onset multisystem inflammatory disease (NOMID): a new member of the expanding family of pyrin-associated autoinflammatory diseases. Arthritis Rheum 46:3340–3348

Ben-Chetrit E, Cohen R, Chajek-Shaul T 2002 Familial Mediterranean fever and Behçet's disease–are they associated? J Rheumatol 29:530–534

Beutler B 2001 Autoimmunity and apoptosis: the Crohn's connection. Immunity 15:5–14

Boss JM 1999 A common set of factors control the expression of the MHC class II, invariant chain, and HLA-DM genes. Microbes Infect 1:847–853

Chae JJ, Komarow HD, Cheng J et al 2003 Targeted disruption of pyrin, the FMF protein, causes heightened sensitivity to endotoxin and a defect in macrophage apoptosis. Mol Cell 11:591–604

Chamaillard M, Hashimoto M, Horie Y et al 2003 An essential role for NOD1 in host recognition of bacterial peptidoglycan containing diaminopimelic acid. Nat Immunol 4:702–707

Chin KC, Li G, Ting JP 1997 Activation and transdominant suppression of MHC class II and HLA-DMB promoters by a series of C-terminal class II transactivator deletion mutants. J Immunol 159:2789–2794

Damiano JS, Oliveira V, Welsh K, Reed JC 2004 Heterotypic interactions among NACHT domains: implications for regulation of innate immune responses. Biochem J 381:213–219

Dode C, Le Du N, Cuisset L et al 2002 New mutations of CIAS1 that are responsible for Muckle–Wells syndrome and familial cold urticaria: a novel mutation underlies both syndromes. Am J Hum Genet 70:1498–1506

Dowds TA, Masumoto J, Zhu L, Inohara N, Nunez G 2004 Cryopyrin-induced interleukin 1beta secretion in monocytic cells: enhanced activity of disease-associated mutants and requirement for ASC. J Biol Chem 279:21924–21928

Feldmann J, Prieur AM, Quartier P et al 2002 Chronic infantile neurological cutaneous and articular syndrome is caused by mutations in CIAS1, a gene highly expressed in polymorphonuclear cells and chondrocytes. Am J Hum Genet 71:198–203

Girardin SE, Travassos LH, Herve M et al 2003 Peptidoglycan molecular requirements allowing detection by Nod1 and Nod2. J Biol Chem 278:41702–41708

Harton JA, Linhoff MW, Zhang J, Ting JP 2002 Cutting edge: CATERPILLER: a large family of mammalian genes containing CARD, pyrin, nucleotide-binding, and leucine-rich repeat domains. J Immunol 169:4088–4093

Hoffman HM, Mueller JL, Broide DH, Wanderer AA, Kolodner RD 2001 Mutation of a new gene encoding a putative pyrin-like protein causes familial cold autoinflammatory syndrome and Muckle–Wells syndrome. Nat Genet 29:301–305

Hugot JP, Chamaillard M, Zouali H et al 2001 Association of NOD2 leucine-rich repeat variants with susceptibility to Crohn's disease. Nature 411:599–603

Inohara N, Nunez G 2003 NODs: intracellular proteins involved in inflammation and apoptosis. Nat Rev Immunol 3:371–382

Inohara N, Ogura Y, Fontalba A et al 2003 Host recognition of bacterial muramyl dipeptide mediated through NOD2. Implications for Crohn's disease. J Biol Chem 278:5509–5512

Kobayashi K, Hernandez LD, Galan JE et al 2002 IRAK-M is a negative regulator of Toll-like receptor signaling. Cell 110:191–202

Koonin EV, Aravind L 2000 The NACHT family—a new group of predicted NTPases implicated in apoptosis and MHC transcription activation. Trends Biochem Sci 25:223–224

Manji GA, Wang L, Geddes BJ et al 2002 PYPAF1, a PYRIN-containing Apaf1-like protein that assembles with ASC and regulates activation of NF-kappa B. J Biol Chem 277:11570–11575

Meyers BC, Dickerman AW, Michelmore RW et al 1999 Plant disease resistance genes encode members of an ancient and diverse protein family within the nucleotide-binding superfamily. Plant J 20:317–332

Miceli-Richard C, Lesage S, Rybojad M et al 2001 CARD15 mutations in Blau syndrome. Nat Genet 29:19–20

Nickerson K, Sisk TJ, Inohara N et al 2001 Dendritic cell-specific MHC class II transactivator contains a caspase recruitment domain that confers potent transactivation activity. J Biol Chem 276:19089–19093

Nimchuk Z, Eulgem T, Holt BF, 3rd, Dangl JL 2003 Recognition and response in the plant immune system. Annu Rev Genet 37:579–609

O'Connor W Jr, Harton JA, Zhu X, Linhoff MW, Ting JP 2003 Cutting edge: CIAS1/Cryopyrin/PYPAF1/NALP3/CATERPILLER 1.1 Is an inducible inflammatory mediator with NF-kappaB suppressive properties. J Immunol 171:6329–6333

Ogura Y, Bonen DK, Inohara N et al 2001 A frameshift mutation in NOD2 associated with susceptibility to Crohn's disease. Nature 411:603–606

Pawlowski K, Pio F, Chu Z, Reed JC, Godzik A 2001 PAAD—a new protein domain associated with apoptosis, cancer and autoimmune diseases. Trends Biochem Sci 26:85–87

Reith W, Mach B 2001 The bare lymphocyte syndrome and the regulation of MHC expression. Annu Rev Immunol 19:331–373

Stehlik C, Fiorentino L, Dorfleutner A et al 2002 The PAAD/PYRIN-family protein ASC is a dual regulator of a conserved step in nuclear factor kappaB activation pathways. J Exp Med 196:1605–1615

Steimle V, Otten LA, Zufferey M, Mach B 1993 Complementation cloning of an MHC class II transactivator mutated in hereditary MHC class II deficiency (or bare lymphocyte syndrome). Cell 75:135–146

Ting JP, Trowsdale J 2002 Genetic control of MHC class II expression. Cell 109:S21–33

Tschopp J, Martinon F, Burns K 2003 NALPs: a novel protein family involved in inflammation. Nat Rev Mol Cell Biol 4:95–104

Wang L, Manji GA, Grenier JM et al 2002 PYPAF7, a novel PYRIN-containing Apaf1-like protein that regulates activation of NF-kappa B and caspase-1-dependent cytokine processing. J Biol Chem 277:29874–29880

Williams KL, Taxman DJ, Linhoff MW, Reed W, Ting JP 2003 Cutting edge: monarch-1: a pyrin/nucleotide-binding domain/leucine-rich repeat protein that controls classical and nonclassical MHC class I genes. J Immunol 170:5354–5358

DISCUSSION

Abbas: In the autoimmunity field in general the focus has been on looking at control molecules and T and B cells, because the tools have been good. There is a whole world out there of control mechanisms and innate immunity. Other than MHC we have looked at nothing in antigen-presenting cells (APCs) that might be influencing autoimmunity. As we go from association studies to genes, I wonder how many will turn out to be genes involved in regulating antigen presentation or regulating innate immunity. It may be a large number.

Bowcock: That is what I wanted to say. The role of dendritic cells (DCs) in autoimmunity is an important question.

Abbas: We don't know anything about what regulates DC survival and function. The only thing we have looked at is MHC. Details are beginning to emerge about the control of DC survival, but not function.

Cookson: You said that they don't bind antigens but they recognize them.

Ting: TLR is in the same boat, in that there is no evidence that TLR molecules bind to their agonists. The way most of these experiments were done with NOD1/NOD2, is that a contaminant of LPS stimulates NOD1/NOD2. The authors fractionated LPS until they found this fraction which activated cells with NOD1 or NOD2. But they never showed that NOD1 or 2 bound to these specific bacterial products.

Cookson: In the plant homologues, the variation in LRRs does seem to induce different responses to different antigens. But you are saying that this has nothing to do with recognition of the antigens. Do you think there is something else on top of this?

Ting: I'm not a plant biologist, in many of the reviews people have looked extensively for a direct interaction. Using the two-hybrid system, once in a while plant biologists can find an R protein that binds to its corresponding product.

These are called *Avr* products. *In vivo*, however, this is rarely seen. In other instances people have found that the R protein may require another protein, which binds to the virulence factor.

Cookson: Doe the LRR of CIITA protein have a ligand?

Ting: When we look at the evolutionary relationship, CIITA seems to be off on a branch. It may be more of a cousin than a sibling. The LRR molecule is important for protein–protein association in those cases. There are over 20 proteins, and if they can undergo heterodimerization (considering that the Apaf1 protein can form a septamer) the combinatorial possibilities are endless. However, you have to look at a time point where these proteins are expressed together to believe that they can undergo heterodimerization. People who are doing protein association experiments are not always concerned about when they are co-expressed. If it is truly a recognition system it would be equivalent to TCR or Ig.

Cookson: It is highly polymorphic then. It is potentially a pattern recognition receptor that has quite a bit more polymorphism.

Ting: The only one I can comment on is the CIAS gene, which has about 35 mutations that are linked to the three diseases I talked about. Most of them are smack in the middle of the nucleotide binding domain yet they cause three different diseases.

Abbas: Have you overexpressed Pexin1 constitutively in the mouse and seen whether it does anything?

Ting: No.

Abbas: Do we have good promoters for overexpression in DCs?

Ting: There are debates about that. There are some data in myeloid DCs but not plasmacytoid DCs.

Abbas: Very little has been done looking at *in vivo* manipulations of these genes so far.

Ting: One thing we are doing is trying to put these RNAi DCs back.

Abbas: You could also try overexpression of the Plexin family to see whether they will give you inflammatory disease.

Ting: One interesting point is that very little if any is found in T cells, B cells or activated macrophages.

Abbas: Is caspase recruitment quite irrelevant to all these CARD proteins?

Ting: No it is very relevant. One of the points we haven't delved into is cell death. This is being looked at now.

Bowcock: Does γ interferon induce caspase 3?

Abbas: Yes, and caspase 8.

Foote: I am interested in the subtelomeric location of these genes. As you said, there are many examples of subtelomeric location. This is a good example where there is an increased amount of exon shuffling to generate novel genes and also a large degree of haplotypic variance. Is there a greater amount of haplotypic variance at these loci than you would otherwise anticipate?

Ting: We are in the process of looking at this. The other group of genes that are subtelomeric in location are the olfactory genes. Why does a system which has to sense so many different things have subtelomeric genes? This system might also be sensing many different things. There are lots of questions.

Wakeland: Olfactory receptors are fairly broadly distributed in the genome, aren't they?

Ting: There is a group that has looked at several olfactory genes. They are preferentially located in the subtelomeric region.

Kere: Gene density is higher in general in the subtelomeric regions. I wonder whether there is a true bias?

Ting: We have 17 out of 22 genes located here.

Rioux: Are any of those duplications?

Ting: On chromosome 19 there may be two or three that are more similar than others. But there are nine on chromosome 19.

Cookson: I wanted to follow-up the apoptosis story. People don't comment on it but it is there. Is it an adaptive sort of response in the same way as it is in a leaf? Do your intestinal epithelial cells die to protect other cells?

Ting: In infection the idea is that cell death is a prominent pathway to control macrophages. This is also a means to kill off the pathogen. Many people are concentrating on the importance of these genes in cell death.

Cookson: Is cell death an alternative to NF-κB?

Ting: NF-κB is a great assay because it is so easy, but I never know quite what to do with it. You can argue that NF-κB is linked to cell death because it is anti-cell death. We did this but we also did cytokine assays which I think are a bit more biological.

Abbas: This genotype–phenotype issue keeps cropping up. You mess up these broadly acting regulatory genes and get a peculiar phenotype.

Ting: Mutations in the CIAS genes map in the same domain but you get three different diseases.

Wakeland: There are multiple members in this family. When you disrupt any one or two, there are several others still firing. This could be why you only see minor shifts in specificity.

Goodnow: Why is it triggered by cold and what is the pathogenesis of this syndrome?

Ting: This is unknown. We put cells in the cold room. CIAS mutants and wild-type proteins do not behave differently.

Index of contributors

Non-participating co-authors are indicated by asterisks. Entries in bold indicate papers; other entries refer to discussion contributions.

A

Abbas, A. K. **1**, 9, 23, 26, 27, 28, 41, 42, 43, 44, 52, 53, 55, 56, 67, 69, 70, 71, 72, 73, 74, 75, 91, 92, 108, 109, 110, 111, 134, 135, 136, 137, 138, 139, 141, 142, 143, 160, 161, 162, 163, 164, 175, 176, 178, 193, 195, 196, 197, 212, 213, 214, 216, 217, 218, 230, 239, 240, 241

B

*Baechler, E. C. **145**
*Bahlo, M. **31**
*Bauer, J. **145**
Behrens, T. W. 12, 72, 93, **145**, 160, 161, 162, 163, 175, 196, 212, 216
Bowcock, A. 11, 12, 21, 22, 27, 55, 70, 71, 72, 73, 74, 110, 136, 142, 143, 178, 217, 239, 240
*Burfoot, R. **31**
*Butzkueven, H. **31**
*Byrne, M. C. **165**

C

*Chamberlain, G. **57**
*Clark, J. **57**
Cookson, W. 9, 10, 12, 22, 24, 26, 29, 45, 53, 54, 70, 72, 73, 91, 107, 108, 111, 135, 137, 138, 140, 141, 143, 164, 177, 194, 212, 216, 217, 239, 240, 241
*Cumiskey, A. M. **57**

D

Daly, M. J. **2**, 11, 12, 19, 25, 29, 40, 41, 43, 44, **94**

*Dickinson, J. L. **31**
*Dustin, M. L. **165**

F

*Farwell, L. **94**
*Feske, S. **165**
Foote, S. J. 12, 22, 28, **31**, 39, 40, 41, 42, 43, 44, 55, 56, 65, 66, 67, 68, 70, 110, 162, 164, 198, 213
*Fraser, H. **57**

G

*Gaffney, P. M. **145**
*García-Cozar, F. **165**
*Garner, V. E. S. **57**
*Gillett, C. **145**
Goldstein, D. B. 8, 9, 10, **14**, 19, 20, 21, 22, 24, 28, 29, 39, 40, 41, 42, 43, 44, 45, 55, 163, 175, 176, 177, 179
*Gonzalez-Munoz, A. **57**
Goodnow, C. C. 9, 23, 27, 29, 41, 42, 45, 53, 55, 69, 70, 72, 74, 75, 89, 90, 92, 135, 136, 137, 138, 139, 140, 141, 142, 161, 174, 177, 179, **180**, 193, 194, 195, 196, 197, 198, 213, 214, 217, 218, 230, 241
*Graham, R. R. **145**
*Gregersen, P K. **145**
*Gregory, S. **57**
*Groom, P. **31**
*Gu, H. **165**

H

Hafler, D. A. 10, 20, 24, 26, 27, 28, 40, 41, 42, 44, 55, 66, 67, 71, 72, 73, 74, 75, 91, 92,

INDEX OF CONTRIBUTORS

137, 139, 143, 161, 163, 174, 175, 176, 178, 192, 193, 195, 197, 214, 217, 218
*Healy, B. **57**
*Heissmeyer, V. **165**
*Hippen, K. L. **145**
*Holmes, T. **219**
*Horton, H. F. **165**
*Howlett, S. **57**
*Howson, J. **57**
*Hunter, K. **57**

I

*Illés, Z. **200**
*Im, S.-H. **165**

J

*Johnson, L. **31**

K

Kere, J. 10, 22, 23, 26, 27, 28, 29, 40, 42, 43, **46**, 52, 53, 54, 55, 56, 68, 69, 72, 74, 111, 136, 137, 139, 140, 141, 143, 164, 176, 212, 241
*Kilpatrick, T. J. **31**
*Kingsnorth, A. **57**
Kuchroo, V. K. 54, 69, 70, 75, 90, 109, 137, 161, 163, 164, 178, 193, 194, 195, 197, **200**, 212, 213, 214, 218
*Kyogoku, C. **145**

L

*Langefeld, C. D. **145**
*Lichtenthaler, S. **219**
Lindgren, C. 137, 178
*Liston, A. **180**
*Liu, Y.-C. **165**
*Lyons, P. A. **57**

M

*Macián, F. **165**
*Moser, K. L. **145**
*Moule, C. L. **57**

N

*Na, S.-Y. **219**

O

*Ortmann, W. A. **145**

P

*Penha-Goncalves, C. **57**
*Peterson, E. **145**
*Peterson, L. B. **57**, **200**

R

*Rabizadeh, S. **219**
*Rainbow, D. **57**, **200**
*Ramos, P. S. **145**
Rao, A. 24, 27, 55, 56, 69, 73, 74, 75, **165**, 174, 176, 177, 178, 197, 198, 212, 213, 217, 229, 230
*Richardson, A. **94**
Rioux, J. D. 9, 12, 19, 20, 21, 24, 30, 44, 45, 67, 73, 74, **94**, 107, 108, 109, 110, 111, 112, 134, 135, 136, 139, 140, 141, 143, 161, 163, 174, 175, 218, 241
*Rogers, J. **57**
*Rubio, J. P. **31**

S

*Sale, M. **31**
Seed, B. 20, 23, 27, 43, 44, 54, 67, 69, 72, 73, 90, 93, 134, 135, 137, 177, 178, 195, 213, **219**, 229, 230
*Sharpe, A. S. **200**
*Slavik, J. M. **200**
*Smink, L. J. **57**
*Speed, T. P. **31**
*Stankovich, J. **31**
*Subramanian, S. **76**

T

*Taylor, B. **31**
*Terhorst, C. **94**
*Tiffen, P. **57**
*Ting, A. **219**
Ting, J. 24, 52, 75, 88, 108, 109, 139, 160, 174, **231**, 239, 240, 241
*Todd, J. A. **57**

U

Umetsu, D. 54, 110, 137, 214, 216, 217, 218

V

*van der Mei, I. A. F. **31**
*Varma, R. **165**
*Venuprasad, K. **165**
*Vijayakrishnan. L. **200**
Vyse, T. J. 25, 69, 70, 92, **94**, 140, 143, 162, 196, 198

W

Wakeland, E. K. 23, 24, 25, 27, 28, 29, 45, 68, **76**, 88, 89, 90, 91, 92, 93, 137, 160, 175, 198, 212, 213, 241
*Walsh, E. **94**
*Wapenaar, M. C. **113**
Wicker, L. S. 29, **57**, 66, 67, 68, 69, 70, 71, 74, 140, 141, 142, 143, 161, 162, 163, 164, 175, 176, 193, 196, **200**, 212, 213, 217
Wijmenga, C. 9, 75, 89, 108, 110, **113**, 134, 135, 136, 137, 138, 139, 140, 198
*Wilkinson, C. **31**
Worthington, J. 12, 112, 162

X

Xavier, R. **219**

Subject index

A

AAA1 48
abacavir 8, 9
ADAM33 47, 48
admixture 20
Affymetrix chips 13, 50, 52–53
African-Americans, multiple sclerosis 20
Africans
 multiple sclerosis 20
 recombination 25
AIRE 183, 184, 190, 194–196
Aire 183–185, 189
anti-epileptics 18, 24
AP-1, NFAT cooperation 167–168, 172
APLP1 228
APOE4 8, 9
apoptosis 157, 241
Arabidopsis genome 232
ASC, NF-κB modulation 235–236
asthma
 AAA1 48
 ADAM33 47, 48
 CELIAC2 116
 chromosome 7p 47–48
 CTLA4 116
 DPP10 48
 GPRA isoform B 48, 54
 hepatitis A virus 215–217
 IL9 111
 IL9R 49
 IL13 111
 infection link 218
 PHF11 48
 positionally cloned genes 26, 47–48
 SNPs 10
 SPINK5 111
 susceptibility genes 47–48, 214–216
 TIM1 215–216
atopy
 GPRA 54
 TIM1 215

autoimmune polyendocrinopathy syndrome
 type 1 (APS1) 183, 184, 190, 195, 196
autoimmune threshold 188–189
autoimmune thyroid disease
 CELIAC2 116
 coeliac disease 115
 PTPN22 R620W 155
autoimmunity
 immune system genes 21
 infection link 217–218
 resistance 190
 suppression 84–86
Avr 232
Avr products 232, 240

B

BAC transgenic 68
BACE1 228
bacterial product sensors 234–235
balancing selection 21–22, 23–24
Bardet-Biedl syndrome 11
Bim 188, 189
Blau syndrome 234

C

C1q, lupus 45, 146
candidate genes, data dredging 65–66
carbamazepine, pharmacogenetics 18
CARD15 (NOD2)
 Blau syndrome 234
 Crohn's disease 9, 19, 96, 97, 110, 234
 DLG5 and 100
 expression 97
 functional aspects 97
 IBD5 and 100, 101
 inflammatory bowel disease 24, 96–97,
  100–101, 122
 irritable bowel disease 234
 muramyl dipeptide receptor 97
 NF-κB 96, 97
 Paneth cells 97

CATERPILLER 232
  CARD domain 233
  CIAS/cryopyrin 236
  diversity generation 236–237
  immune disorders 233–235
  Monarch 1/*PYPAF7* 235–236
  pyrin domain 233
Caucasians
  Crohn's disease 19
  inflammatory bowel disease 24
  multiple sclerosis 20
Cbl 174
Cbl-b, type 1 diabetes 58
CblB 169
CCR5, balancing selection 21
CD4, balancing selection 21
CD25, type 1 diabetes 58
CD28, costimulation with CTLA4 201–202
Cd28 201
CD48 103
Cd48 78
CD84 103
Cd84 78
CD229 103
Cd229 78
CD244 103
Cd244 78
cDNAs, large-scale screens 219–229, 230
CDSN 50
CELIAC2 116, 117
CELIAC3 116, 117
CELIAC4 116–117, 125
central tolerance 58
  monogenic lesions 183–185
  polygenic lesions 185–188
chromatin tolerance 77, 78–80
CIAS 234, 236
CIAS1 236
CIITA 232, 233–234, 240
CINCA 236
CIS gene 240
coalescence 21, 23, 28
coeliac disease 113–134
  autoimmune thyroid disease 115
  CELIAC2 116, 117
  CELIAC3 116, 117
  CELIAC4 116–117, 125
  clinical presentation 115
  'common variant/common disease' model 121–122

  'common variants/multiple disease' model 117
  comorbidity 115, 117
  CTLA4 116, 121
  diagnosis 115, 117, 121
  dosage effect 137
  functional candidate genes 121
  gender bias 113
  gene expression profiling 123–125
  genomewide linkage studies 116–121
  gluten-free diet 115
  gluten response 113, 135, 138
  HLA-DQ2 115–116
  HLA-DW3 115
  intestinal biopsy 115, 117, 121
  locus 6q21 117
  locus 9p21–p13 117
  Marsh classification 113
  microarrays 123–125, 134
  multifactorial disorder 115–116
  prevalence 113
  qRT-PCR 123, 125
  selective advantage 137
  sibling risk 115
  symptoms 115
  twin studies 115
  type 1 diabetes 115
  unrecognized 113
'common variant/common disease' model 83, 121–122
'common variants/multiple disease' model 117
  comorbidity 115, 117, 180
  complement, lupus 146
complex disease 94–95
  haplotype blocks 10, 11
  probabilistic risk factors 3
Crohn's disease
  CARD15 9, 19, 96, 97, 110, 234
  Caucasians 19
  CELIAC4 117
  environmental factors 110
  haplotype maps 4
  IBD1 96, 109
  IBD5 19, 99, 101
  locus5q31 4
  OCTN1 99
  OCTN2 99, 111
  sibling risk 95
  SNPs 97
  Th-1 mediated disease 111
  twin studies 95

SUBJECT INDEX

cryopyrin 236
CS1 103
Cs1 78
Csk 153
CTLA4
  artificial form, therapeutic use 58
  CD28 and 201–202
  cell cycle checkpoints 202
  conservation 201
  full-length 203–205, 208–209
  functions 202, 213
  genetic susceptibility to autoimmune disease 202–203
  IL2 inhibition 202
  ligand independent 60–61, 62, 203–205, 208–209, 210
  molecular mechanisms 202–209
  peripheral tolerance 202
  PP2A 202
  SHP2 202, 205, 208
  soluble 63–64, 66, 201, 203, 210
  T cell costimulation with CD28 201–202
  TCRζ 202, 205, 208
  three bands 203
CTLA4
  asthma 116
  autoimmune disease risk 143
  coeliac disease 116, 121
  Graves' disease 116
  PTPN22 interaction 176
  type 1 diabetes 57–58, 62–64, 116
Ctla4 201
  diabetes 60, 201
  full-length 203, 209
  ligand-independent 203, 209–210
  soluble 203
CYP2D6 21
CYP3A, selection 29
cystic fibrosis, private mutations 10–11

D

dendritic cells (DCs)
  lupus 157, 160
  role in autoimmunity 239
deterministic risk factors 3
diabetes *see* type 1 diabetes
diet
  IBD and CARD15 24
  pharmacogenetics 20–21
DLG5 99–100

DPP10 48
drift 22, 29
drug metabolism 18
  diet 21

E

E3 ligases, T cell anergy 168–170
EAT-2 81, 103
EBP50 136
ectodomain shedding 228
environment
  Crohn's disease 110
  epidemiological studies 24
  lupus 156
epistatic interactions 76–88
Epstein-Barr virus, lupus link 156
experimental autoimmune encephalitis (EAE)
  CLTA4 209
  genomewide scans 109, 163–164
expression cloning 219
extended haplotype homozygosity 28–29

F

factor V Leiden mutation 9
familial cold autoinflammatory syndrome 236
Fc receptors, lupus 146
FcRII 84
fine localization 9–10
FoxP3 195

G

gender bias
  coeliac disease 113
  lupus 101, 145
GENEHUNTER 34
genetic variation 2–8
  expense of testing 3
  HapMap 4–6, 12
  linkage disequilibrium 4
  mosaic in mice 6
  population-based approach 3
genomic mining 231–239
gluten response/tolerance 113, 135, 138
GPRA isoform B 48, 54
graft rejection 26–27
GRAIL 169
Graves' disease
  CTLA4 116
  Ctla4 201

Graves' disease (cont.)
  PTPN22 58
  PTPN22 R620W 155
green fluorescent protein (GFP) 220, 221, 222

H

haplotype
  blocks, complex disease 10, 11
  extended haplotype homozygosity 28–29
  HapMap 4–6, 12
  multiple sclerosis 31–39
  reconstruction 33
  tagging, pharmacogenetics 14–19
HapMap 4–6, 12
Hashimoto's thyroiditis
  Ctla4 201
  PTPN22 R620W 155
HCR 49–50, 52
hepatitis A virus 215–217
HLA
  balancing selection 23–24
  lupus 146–152
HLA-C, psoriasis 49
HLA class II genes, type 1 diabetes 57–58
HLA-DQ2, coeliac disease 115–116
HLA-DW3, coeliac disease 115
HLA genes 104

I

IBD family 96
IBD1 96–97, 109
IBD5
  CARD15 and 100
  Crohn's disease 19, 99, 101
ICOS, type 1 diabetes 62
Icos 201
Idd 59, 185–186, 188
  Idd3 59, 66, 68
  Idd5.1 59, 60–62, 201
  Idd5.2 59
  Idd9.1 59
  Idd9.2 59
  Idd9.3 59
  Idd10 59
  Idd18 59
Iddm1 189
Iddm2 189
IDDM15 117
Il2 66
IL2RA, type 1 diabetes 58
IL4 46, 47
IL9R 49
immune complexes 157
immune system genes, autoimmunity 21
indirect association 4–5
infection
  asthma link 218
  autoimmunity link 217–218
  susceptibility 25–26
inflammatory bowel disease (IBD) 95–101
  CARD15 (*NOD2*) 24, 96–97, 100–101, 122, 234
  CELIAC2 116
  diet 24
  DLG5 99–100
  genetic risk factors 95
  genomewide searches 96
  genotype–genotype interactions 100
  genotype–phenotype interactions 100–101
  IBD1 96–97
  IBD1–*IBD6* 96
  IBD5 99, 100
  OCTN1 99
  OCTN2 99
INS, type 1 diabetes 57–58
insulin, thymic expression 58
insulin-specific T cells 58
interferon (IFN) pathway, lupus 157, 160, 162–163
interleukin 2 (IL2) 58, 66, 67, 69, 202
interleukin 9 (IL9), asthma 111
interleukin 13 (IL13), asthma 111
International Human Haplotype Map Project (HapMap) 4–6, 12
IRAK-M 236
Itch 168–169
ITSM motifs 81

L

lambda sub S (λ_s) 72
Lck 153
linkage disequilibrium
  data set 15
  genetic variation 4
  high-density 5
  proof of concept 8–9
linkage studies, underpowered 71–72, 96, 109, 139
LINKPREP 34

SUBJECT INDEX

lpr 84
Ly9 78
Ly108 78, 81, 103
LYP see PTPN22

M

major histocompatibility complex (MHC) 104
  balancing selection 21
  MHC-II, CIITA 234
malaria susceptibility 12
Mediterranean fever 233
MEKK1 228
Mendelian disorders 2–3, 10
Mendelian-like mutations 3
MERLIN 34
MHC-II, CIITA 234
Monarch 1 235–236
monogenic disorders 2–3, 10
mouse
  genome segments 7
  mosaicism 6
  positional cloning 6
  quantitative trait locus mapping 6–7
Muckle–Wells syndrome 236
multiple sclerosis
  African-Americans 20
  Africans 20
  Caucasians 20
  chromosome 6 38, 117
  chromosome 10 38
  Ctla4 201
  family studies 32
  haplotype association 31–39
  haplotype reconstruction 33
  locus 6q21 117
  simple sequence length polymorphism markers 32
  special populations approach 32
  susceptibility genes 32, 35–38
  twin studies 31
muramyl dipeptide 97, 235
Myelin P0 189
Myo9B 134
MyoH9 134, 136

N

NACHT motif 232
NALP 233
Nedd4 168–169
neglect 181

NFAT
  AP-1 cooperation 167–168, 172
  T cell anergy 166–168, 172, 177–178
NF-κB
  ASC modulation 235–236
  CARD15 96, 97
  cell death 241
  CIAS regulation 236
  measurement 108
  screens 220, 221, 222, 224, 228, 230
NOD family 233
NOD mouse
  CTLA4 208–209
  cure and age 70
  diabetes susceptibility 200–201
  limitations 59
  thymic clonal deletion 185–188, 189, 194
NOD1 232, 234–235
NOD2 11–12, 232, 234, 235
NOD2 see CARD15
NOMID 236

O

OCTN1 111
OCTN1 99
OCTN2 111
OCTN2 99, 111, 112

P

PAN 233
Paneth cells, *CARD15* 97
PD1, lupus 146
PEDCHECK 34
pedigree disequilibrium test 147
pemphigus 55
PEP 152–153
peripheral tolerance, CTLA4 202
pGCIRES vector 203
pharmacogenetics
  diet 20–21
  haplotype tagging 14–19
  simple trait 14–15, 18
phenytoin, pharmacogenetics 18, 24
PHF11 48
Photinus luciferase 224, 228
physical selection 220
PKA 228
PKCθ 168, 169, 170–171, 172
plant disease resistance genes 231–232
'plate to well' dimension 221

PLCγ1 168, 169, 170–171, 172
pool subdivision screens 220
population-based approach 3
positional cloning
    asthma genes 26, 47–48
    complex phenotypes in mice 6
positive selection 181
PP2A 202
PREST 34
pristane-induced lupus, SAP 82
probabilistic risk factors 3
proof of concept, linkage disequilibrium 8–9
proxies 4–5, 10
PSOR1 49–50
psoriasis
    balancing selection 21
    candidate genes 26
    CDSN 50
    HCR 49–50, 52
    HLA-C 49
    identifying at risk individuals 55
    PSOR1 49–50
    reported loci 71
    RUNX1 binding 122
    SLCA3R1 122
    susceptibility locus 21, 26
PTPN22 152, 153–155
PTPN22 58, 152
    CTLA4 interaction 176
purifying selection 23
PYPAF7 235–236
PYRIN 233

Q

quantitative RT-PCR 123, 125
quantitative trait locus mapping 6–7

R

R genes 231–232
R proteins 231, 232, 239–240
    mammalian R-like proteins 232–233
RasGAP 168
recombinational hotspots 5, 10, 24–25
Renilla luciferase 228
rheumatoid arthritis
    CELIAC2 116
    Ctla4 201
    locus 6q21 117
    OCTN2 111, 112
    PTPN22 58
    PTPN22 R620W 154–155
SLC22A4 122
    Zap70 136
rice genome 232
RNA, regulatory function 55–56
roqin mutation 77
RUNX1 122

S

SAP 81, 82, 103
selection 20, 21–23, 29
serum response element screen 224, 228
SH-2 81
SHIP-1 81
SHP2 202, 205, 208
SIBMED 34
sib-selection screens 220
simple sequence length polymorphism markers 32
single nucleotide polymorphisms (SNPs)
    asthma genes 10
    choosing the best 6
    Crohn's disease 97
    HapMap 4, 5
    hidden 5
    HLA genes 104
    proxies 4–5
    redundancy 6
    subset tagging 5
    tagging 15–18, 19
    type 1 diabetes 58, 59–60
SLAM 103
SLAM/CD2 family 78, 80–82, 83, 102–104
SLAM/CD2 haplotype 2 80, 82, 83
SLC22A4 111
SLC22A4 122
SLC22A5 111
SLCA3R1 122
Sle1 77, 84, 89, 102
Sle1a 77
Sle1b 77, 78–80
Sle1d 77, 88
Sle2 77, 102
Sle3 77, 88, 102
Sles1 84, 86, 88, 89, 90
special populations approach 32
SPINK5, asthma 111
sunlight, lupus 156
systemic lupus erythematosus (SLE) 101–104, 145–160
    anti-nuclear autoantibodies (ANAs) 76, 77, 80, 145–146, 156

SUBJECT INDEX

apoptosis 157
B-cell receptor editing 157
C1q locus 45, 146
'common variant/common disease' model 83
complement 146
Ctla4 201
dendritic cells 157, 160
environmental factors 156
Epstein-Barr virus 156
Fc receptors 146
FcRII 84
gender bias 101, 145
genetic complexity 76
gradation of risk 156
HLA 146–152
IFN pathway 157, 160, 162–163
immune complexes 157
incidence 101
lpr 84
lymphocyte apoptosis 157
modelling initiation and progress 155–157
non-European populations 101
NZM2410 murine model 76, 77
PD1 146
PTPN22 58
PTPN22 R620W 154–155
rare variants 83
roqin mutation 77
sibling risk 101
SLAM 78, 80–82, 83, 102–104
Sle1 77, 84, 89, 102
Sle1a 77
Sle1b 77, 78–80
Sle1d 77, 88
Sle2 77, 102
Sle3 77, 88, 102
Sles1 84, 86, 88, 89, 90
sunlight 156
susceptibility genes 77, 102, 146
twin studies 101–102
Yaa 77, 84, 89, 91

T

T cell anergy 166
  CblB 169
  E3 ligases 168–170
  GRAIL 169
  immunological synapse stability 170–171
  Itch 168–169
  multistep model 171

NFAT 166–168, 172, 177–178
PKCθ 168, 169, 170–171, 172
PLCγ1 168, 169, 170–171, 172
programme 171–172
RasGAP 168
Tsg101 170
TCRζ, CTLA4 202, 205, 208
TEAM database 125
therapy, artificial CTLA4 58
thymic T cell clonal deletion 180–192
TIM1 215–216
Tim1 215
Tim3 215
transglutaminase 134, 135–136
Tsg101 170
type 1 diabetes
  Cbl-b 58
  coeliac disease 115
  CTLA4 57–58, 62–64, 116
  Ctla4 60, 201
  genes causing 57–59
  HLA class II genes 57–58
  ICOS 62
  IDDM15 117
  IL2RA/CD25 58
  INS 57–58
  ligand independent CTLA4 60–61, 62
  locus 6q21 117
  mouse models 59
  PTPN22 58
  PTPN22 R620W 154–155
  SNPs 58, 59–60
  soluble CTLA4 63–64

U

ulcerative colitis
  epistasis between *CARD15* and *IBD5* 100
  sibling risk 95
  Th-2 mediated disease 111
  twin studies 95

W

'well to well' dimension 221
'winner's curse' 99

Y

Yaa 77, 84, 89, 91

Z

ZAP70 189
Zap70 27, 136